Health Care Transformation in Contemporary China

Jiong Tu

Health Care Transformation in Contemporary China

Moral Experience in a Socialist Neoliberal Polity

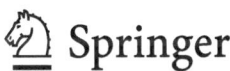 Springer

Jiong Tu
School of Sociology and Anthropology
Sun Yat-sen University
Guangzhou, Guangdong
China

ISBN 978-981-13-0787-4   ISBN 978-981-13-0788-1   (eBook)
https://doi.org/10.1007/978-981-13-0788-1

Library of Congress Control Number: 2018944328

Printed on acid-free paper

This Springer imprint is published by the registered company Springer Nature Singapore Pte Ltd.
part of Springer Nature
The registered company address is: 152 Beach Road, #21-01/04 Gateway East, Singapore 189721,
Singapore

Acknowledgements

First, I would like to thank Dr. Peggy Watson, my Ph.D. supervisor, for her advice, encouragement, and support over the years. Her meticulous guidance accompanies this research from conception to completion.

I owed great gratitude to the people in my field site, who kindly helped me during the fieldwork and sincerely shared their stories, worries and hopes. Without them, the work would be impossible.

I am very grateful to Prof. Jan Sundin, who read my Chap. 6 and offered helpful advice, Prof. Patrick Brown, who read my Chap. 5 and provided useful comments. I would like to thanks my friends and colleagues, C. Y. Ho, Gong Yidong, and Xiao Zhimin, who read different parts of my chapters and gave me very useful suggestions. Professor Therese Hesketh and Darin Weinberg gave me many helpful suggestions on my work, and I really enjoyed the inspirational conversation with them during the viva.

I would like to express my sincere gratitude to the people who stimulated my intellectual growth and accompanied my sociology study: Prof. Yuan Tongkai, Xuan Chaoqing, Peng Huamin, Liu Huaqin, Bai Hongguang, Jan Sundin, Sam Willner, Marja-Liisa Honkasalo, Isabelle Baszanger, C. Y. Ho, Xiao Zhimin, Gong Yidong, Alejandro Miranda, Ana Isabel Aranzazu, Mei Xiao, Wang Wei, and others.

Also, I would like to thank Cambridge University Fieldwork Funds, Department of Sociology, and Homerton College for funding my field research, the Foundation for the Sociology of Health and Illness, the Society of Social Medicine, BSA Medical Sociology Group, Cambridge Philosophical Society for aiding my conference attendance during my Ph.D. study.

Thanks to the Springer team for their work and dedication in making the book published.

Last, but most importantly, I would like to thank my family, for their support and encouragement over these years, especially my husband, Bo, who gave me innumerable support and accompanied me through the ups and downs during the writing up. The book is also dedicated to my daughter Tutu, who came to my life and opens a new window for me.

Contents

Abbreviations

CASS	Chinese Academy of Social Sciences
CCP	Chinese Communist Party
CMS	Cooperative Medical Scheme
CPG	Central People's Government
DXY	Ding Xiang Yuan (a famous Chinese doctor online forum)
EMS	Emergency medical service
GDP	Gross domestic product
MOH	Ministry of Health
MOHRSS	Ministry of Human Resources and Social Security
MOPS	Ministry of Public Security
MOT	Ministry of Transport
NHFPC	National Health and Family Planning Commission (since 2013, the Ministry of Health and the Family Planning Commission were reorganised to form the NHFPC as a ministry-level organisation)
NPC	National People's Congress
OECD	Organisation for Economic Cooperation and Development
PRC	People's Republic of China
TCM	Traditional Chinese Medicine
USA	United States of America
WHO	World Health Organisation

List of Figures

List of Tables

Notes

Chinese names and words in the book are written in pinyin.

Official exchange rate between Chinese Yuan and British Pound is about 10:1 at the time of this research

Chinese Glossaries

danwei	Work units
guanxi	Relationship, network and connections
hongbao	Red packet, envelope containing cash
hukou	Household registration
nao	Speaking or acting violently
renqing	Favour, human affection, or the emotional feeling of obligation and indebtedness
suzhi	Social merit and quality
xiushen	Cultivating the self or life
yangsheng	Nurturing life
yinao	The medical disputes waged by patients' families against medical personnel and medical institutions that involve violent or illegal means. It can also refer to the people who use violence in medical dispute

Abstract

Since the 1980s, when China began to adopt market reforms, its health system experienced a transition from fully state-run and financed system towards more private financing and delivery of health care. These changes led to soaring medical fees, minimal medical insurance coverage, and poor access to affordable medical services. These negative consequences have undermined public perceptions of the Chinese government. In response, since 2009, China has been implementing a new round of healthcare reform that is attempting to reverse the market character of earlier trajectories. The change has been accompanied by the shifts in values, ideologies, and governance. Drawing on Foucault's concept of governmentality and its critical use by other researchers, this research explores the configurations of governmental power, rationality, techniques, and subjectivity in the Chinese health sector.

From 2011 to 2012, I did fieldwork in Riverside (a pseudonym) County of Sichuan province. The research involved semi-structured interviews and conversations with patients, health professionals and administrators about their healthcare (medical practice) experiences. I took participant observation in medical clinics, community health centres, public and private hospitals to see how health care was carried out and talked about in daily practice setting. Local archives, county gazetteers, official regulations, and government reports about health care changes and administrations were searched and collected. This book supplies an ethnographic analysis of people's moral experiences during healthcare transformation over the past decades and outlines the complexity, messiness and contradictions within individual experiences, institutional practices, and government rationales.

Chinese health policy and governance are marked by an extreme form of hybridity with the collision and convergence of market values, neoliberal technologies, authoritarian rule, and a strong, state-led socialism. The combination of these seemly contradictory rationalities and techniques of governance enables the making of governable subjects in the health sector, but also creates increasingly resentful individuals with insufficiently protected rights. Healthcare functions as a biopower, maximising the energy and capacity of individuals and institutions while prohibiting certain acts, ensuring that certain members of the population are nurtured and have entitlement while others are marginalised and neglected. Health care is the site of contestation, rebuilding and legitimation of governance. It makes the government itself subject to the normative discourses of morality and modernity. The Chinese healthcare reform is an ongoing ideological and moral project in the party-state's renewal and reinvention of itself and is tackling unprecedented challenges as it progresses to actually improve people's healthcare experience.

Chapter 1
Introduction: The Politics and Morality of Health Care Transformation in China

1.1 Moral Experience of Health Care Change

In March 2012, a young man in the city of Harbin in northern China stabbed four members of hospital staff; one of the victims, a junior doctor, died shortly afterwards. The attacker complained that he had been refused treatment by the doctors, while the hospital staff explained that the patient had a particular illness which required treatment in another hospital first (Hesketh et al. 2012; ScienceNet 2012). The case was widely discussed on China's social media sites. In an internet survey conducted after the killing, the participants were asked how they felt about the incident by choosing between four responses: 'happy', 'angry', 'sad', and 'sympathetic'. Of the 6161 people who responded to the survey, 4018 indicated that they were 'happy' while only 879 felt 'angry', 410 'sad' and 258 'sympathetic' (Sina 2012). The results beg the obvious question: how could so many people feel 'happy' at hearing that a doctor who had been violently killed?

During the Chinese National People's Congress in March 2013, the message, 'Doctors Sadly Question the Minister of Health about Ten Issues' (*yisheng hanlei shiwen buzhang*), was widely circulated among the deputies and on the internet

© Springer Nature Singapore Pte Ltd. 2019
J. Tu, *Health Care Transformation in Contemporary China*,
https://doi.org/10.1007/978-981-13-0788-1_1

(Xinhua Net 2013a, b, c, d, e).[1] The post, written by a young doctor, raised concern about the ambiguous nature of the Chinese health sector, the chaotic medical market, the low salary of health professionals, the difficult, risky medical work, the tense doctor-patient relationship, the dilemma about rescuing the patient first or demanding money first, and the responsibility of the government and administrative agencies. The post conveyed doctors' general puzzlement and anxiety regarding China's health care transformation over the past decades.

China's health care has undergone a three-stage transformation, from the historically socialist healthcare system, and drastic marketization since the 1980s, to the new socialist-characterised healthcare reform of the 2000s (see Appendix A).

In the collective era, the state built a public health system that provided inexpensive and accessible medical care for virtually all, albeit at a relatively low level. Since the 1980s, when China began to adopt the market reform, its healthcare system underwent a transition, from offering fully state-run, financed care to providing more privately financed and delivered health care. These changes led to soaring medical fees, lower medical insurance coverage, and poor access to affordable medical services. The former universally available (basic) health services were no longer available to all. Individual patients were left to shoulder their own health care expenses. Some even fell into poverty due to illness. Health care became one of the most explosive social problems, being named by the public as one of the new 'three big mountains'[2] that fell on people's shoulders. Various surveys find

---

[1]Issue One: Is our (health) industry a service industry? If yes, why cannot we maximise the profit? Issue Two: Where does your (the health minister's) salary come from? Do you know where we doctors' salary come from? Have you given (sufficient) salary to us? Issue Three: If the tense doctor-patient relationship is caused by our insufficient communication, do you wish all the health professionals to be as talkative as officials and lawyers? We are just doctors. Issue Four: If you have been overworked through the whole year, how can you always have good mood and good attitude? As far as I know, no doctor in the hospital works only five days a week, we work for night shift, work at the weekend if patients come, overwork is just too common to talk about. Issue Five: Have you visited hospitals below the municipal level outside Beijing? Issue Six: What exactly has the Ministry of Health done? Issue Seven: Are doctors protected by the labour law? If yes, why should we frequently work at weekend to check patients? At midnight, we take taxi to treat emergency patients, have you given us overwork fees and taxi fees? Issue Eight: The medical market is chaotic. The rich businessmen opened (private) hospitals everywhere, advertising widely to cheat the people. How could you prove these are not related with the retired personnel from the Ministry of Health? Issue Nine: Should hospital save patient first or charge money first? Do you know how many patients evade the medical bill every year? Who paid these bills (to hospital), you or the Civil Affair Bureau? Issue Ten: The doctor-patient relationship is very tense, should the doctors take the main responsibility? Is it relevant with (the regulations in) the 'Ordinance on the Handling of Medical Malpractice'?

[2]The 'three big mountains', which (according to the official discourses) the Communist Party led the Chinese people overthrew, had been widely used to describe people's sufferings from 'imperialism', 'feudalism' and 'bureaucratic capitalism' in revolutionary time during 1919–1949 prior to the founding of the People's Republic. Now the new 'three big mountains' denotes the difficulties in getting education, buying house, and getting access to health care. As Fewsmith (2008: 273) records, by the early years of the new century, people were widely complaining that 'health care reform had meant that doctors were too expensive to see', 'housing reform meant that homes

that the health care satisfaction rate was one of the lowest aspects of life satisfaction (CASS 2007; Guangzhou Public Opinion Centre 2010).[3] The study of rural people's attitudes towards health care shows that less than 40% felt satisfied with it (Wang 2008). Besides, patients have become increasingly dissatisfied with health professionals, as shown by the rising amount of conflict and dissension. For health professionals, their satisfaction with their job, income (DXY 2013),[4] and the current healthcare system fell very low during the post-reform era (Zhou et al. 2003; Lim et al. 2004). Without sufficient material rewards, many public doctors generate revenue though drug kickback, over-prescription, moonlighting, and bribery. Health professionals experience a conflict between material rewards and their moral position, between the hospital bureaucratic requirements (with regard to work efficiency and financial contribution) and patients' care demands. Facing rising attacks by patients and their relatives, a survey conducted by the Chinese Medical Professional Organisation finds that 74.29% of health professionals felt that their rights and interests were not being protected (Lei and Jiang 2006). During this period, China has changed from being one of the most equal societies to one of the least equal in terms of wealth distribution and social welfare provision.[5] In 2000, it was ranked close to the bottom (188th out of 191 member countries) in terms of the fairness of health care financing and ranked 141st in terms of the health system's overall performance by the World Health Organisation (2010). These negative consequences have undermined the public perception of the Chinese government. In response, since 2009, China has been implementing a new round of healthcare reform that is attempting to reverse the market character of earlier trajectories.

The new healthcare reform agenda (CPG 2009) can be summed up as 'one goal, four beams, and eight columns' (*yige mubiao, siliang bazhu*), symbolising the efforts to build a traditional house. The 'one goal' is to establish a state-sponsored health system that provides universal (basic) health care coverage. The 'eight columns' refer to the eight functional mechanisms that support the healthcare reform operated by various government departments: the healthcare administration, medical institution operation, financing, pricing, governance and surveillance,

---

were too expensive to purchase', and 'educational reform meant that parents could not afford to send their children to school'.

[3]Research carried out by the Institute of Sociology of the Chinese Academy of Social Sciences (2007) shows that 'inaccessible and expensive medical services' has become the social issue which mostly concerns the public. The survey carried out by Guangzhou Public Opinion Centre (2010) finds that in Guangzhou health care satisfaction rate was one of the lowest in life satisfaction, and health care was listed on the top of public wish for change.

[4]The 2012–2013 Chinese doctor income survey conducted by Ding Xiang Yuan (a famous Chinese doctor online forum) shows that 88.4% of the over 20,000 researched doctors felt unsatisfied with their current income, while only 7.8% felt satisfied.

[5]China has changed from one of the most equal society to one of the most unequal society, as shown in its Gini coefficient which has risen from 0.31 in 1985 to 0.42 in 2001 (Wu and Perloff 2004) and 0.53 in 2004 (Han and Whyte 2009:194). The actual number could even be higher due to hidden wealth and illegal incomes of certain groups. The inequality is shown not only in income difference, but also in the rising gap between rural and urban areas, and between different regions.

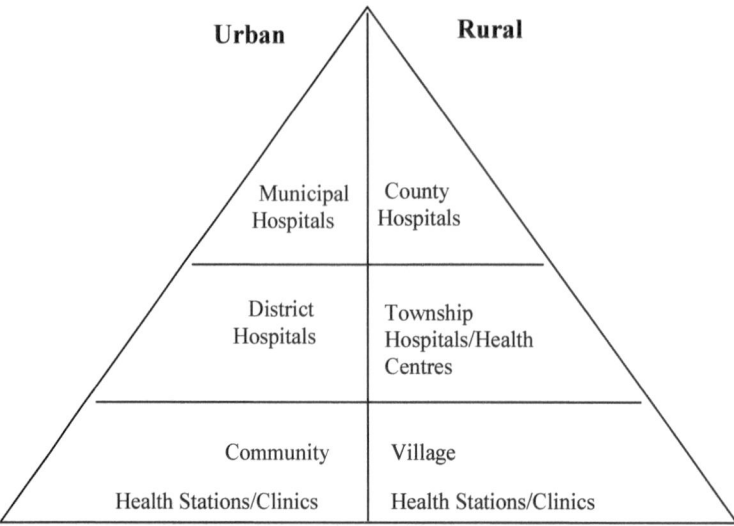

Fig. 1.1 Health care system pyramid—three tiered structure (the figure is drawn by the author)

medical technology innovation and human resources, health information system, and legislation mechanisms. These 'four beams' are the main reform contents, i.e. the four systems that the reform aims to build: a public health system geared towards both rural and urban residents; a healthcare system that makes basic healthcare available to all citizens through a three-tiered structure (see Fig. 1.1); a health insurance system that provides health insurance coverage for all, including health insurance for urban employees and unemployed urban residents, and a new cooperative medical insurance scheme for rural residents; and a medicine provision system for securing safe, affordable medication. The state has started to increase public investment, widen health insurance coverage, expand the public health services, and rebuild the primary and preventive healthcare system.

The new healthcare reform has also encouraged the private sector to play a wider role in providing healthcare services to meet the growing demands of the ageing population. The new reform plan indicates that qualified doctors will be encouraged to start a business and open their own clinic to provide people with convenient access to healthcare services (CPG 2009). It also encourages well-funded enterprises, charities, foundations and commercial insurers, as well as overseas investors and eligible individuals to run the medical institutions (CPG 2012). The parallel process of building public healthcare institutions and the encouragement of private medical practices signify the character of the new reform, which seeks to restore the public welfare nature of health care while using the market forces to satisfy the varied, growing health care needs.[6]

Despite this dramatic transformation of the Chinese health sector, little has been heard directly from the patients and health professionals. Most of the existing discourses arise from the official routes, such as the public media, surveys, public policies, and government reports. The internet seems to provide a new channel for public discussion about health care.[7] Almost every health care change and new policy sparks wide discussion on the internet, where opinions are expressed that differ from the official ones. However, to what extent does the internet reflect the views of the general public? Duckett and Langer (2013: 7) describe the media's reporting on healthcare reform in China as 'elites [who] dominate paternalist populism' where 'elites and the media spoke *for* "the people" and debated their needs and benefits, but gave them little opportunity to voice their own views and preferences'. The media, despite contributing to the diverse debate on the Chinese healthcare reform, are mainly elite voices which rarely mention patients' rights and choices (Kornreich et al. 2012; Duckett and Langer 2013). It is difficult to establish the actual beliefs and conduct of the ordinary citizens. Patients may not understand all of the technical and clinical issues, but they observe and experience the whole process of health care, and are the best witnesses of the health system and its reform. Yet, their voices are frequently ignored in the Chinese health sector. Health professionals also tend to be invisible in the discussion of healthcare reforms. This is partly attributed, for example, to the fact that doctors are strictly controlled under the *danwei* (work unit) system, are powerless before the state (Henderson and Cohen 1984; Yang 2008), and they are beneficiaries of the existing system and the target of criticism (Sina 2007). However, health professionals are a diverse, differentiated group, with varied social and economic characteristics. Many health professionals (such as village doctors, as described in Chap. 7) have suffered due to recent reforms and show rising resentment in their medical work, but little information is available about what the health professionals actually think and experience, and how they view and handle the conflicts and dilemmas associated with their daily work.

---

[6]In early 2012, the central government released several new, vital reform targets for the 12th Five-year Plan (2011–2015) period, including the reform of public hospitals, the expansion of basic health insurance coverage, the perfection of the country's essential medicine system, and the improvement of community-level clinics and hospitals (CPG 2012).

[7]For instance, the new healthcare reform agenda was put online, opening to public to comment at the end of 2008 before its formal release. Within one month, the National Development and Reform Commission got 35,260 responses (CPG 2008). Balla (2014) has done research about political participation on the Chinese Internet based on these online responses. He finds that the health system reform commenting process offered citizens the opportunity to gain exposure to democratic principles and the process of articulating interests but, currently and in the immediate future, online consultation is likely to remain as an instrument for communications between government decision-makers and a limited set of socially advantaged, politically sophisticated Chinese citizens.

The Chinese healthcare reform has attracted increasing academic attention in recent years (see Duckett 2008, 2011; Eggleston et al. 2008; Gu 2008; Hu et al. 2008a, b; Liu et al. 2008; Milcent 2016, 2018; Yip and Hsiao 2008; Wang and Fan 2013; Zhou et al. 2014), but the literature about the health care transformation in China is often statistical in nature or policy analysis within the disciplines of public health, social policy and health economy. There is relatively limited long-term, fieldwork-based research to provide a rich, nuanced understanding of people's experience of the healthcare reform or facilitate the exploration of the complexity, messiness and contradictions associated with the changing health sector. The book fills this lacuna by undertaking an ethnographic analysis of people's moral experiences during the healthcare reform over the past decades. This book situates health care change among the overall changes in Chinese society, analysing the links between experience, subjectivity and governance. The following section develops a theoretical framework to explore the transformation of values, subjectivities, practices, and governance in the changing health sector.

1.2   Moral Experience in the View of Governmentality

'Moral experience' in this book refers to Kleinman's definition, which is about what is most at stake for the actors in a local social world and is 'practical engagements in a particular local world, a social space that carries cultural, political, and economic specificity' (Kleinman 1998: 365). Actual moral experience, for Kleinman, is contextual and specific in a given local world. Kleinman (1998, 2004, 2007) has promoted a new ethnography of moral experience, requiring researchers to enter the local world to see the social interactions, social practices and social discourses, to observe the daily lives of ordinary people as they make decisions, face challenges, and pass judgements, which underlie people's worldview, their way of seeing the world and transition, and the way in which they frame their understanding of human and state-society relations. My research adopts the concept of 'moral experience' in order to explore what is most at stake for Chinese patients and health professionals in a period of health care transformation.

For Kleinman, 'experience' is defined as the felt flow of interpersonal communication, negotiation, contestation, and other sorts of engagement. 'What characterises experience is an orientation of overwhelming practicality' (2004: 270). Experience for him is inherently moral inasmuch as it involves practices, negotiations, and contestations with others (1998: 358–359). Kleinman puts 'experience' as evidence and empirical foundation in which analysis is based, but did not question experience itself, the process of its construction through which power is exercised, or how it constitutes subject and identity. To complement this, the book employs the Foucauldian concept of governmentality.

For Foucault, experiences and subjects are not factual givens. It is discourse that produces human experience (rather than vice versa). Foucault explores the 'discursive formation' (Foucault 1972) of experience, the power and ideology involved in the construction of experience, and the subjectivity and the identity formed in the process of experience. The moral core of experience is about how the configuration of political, economic, and medical institutions shapes the modes of subjectivity. Experience here is understood not as incontestable evidence: 'it is not individuals who have experience, but subjects who are constituted through experience' (Scott 1991: 779). Joan Scott proposes historicising experience as well as the identities it produces, exploring the ways in which subjectivity is produced, the constitutive forces and ideology involved, and the discursive processes by which identities are ascribed, resisted, or embraced. People's experience then becomes not the origin of explanation, but what we need to explain (1991: 797). The book focuses on the constructive nature and discursive character of experience, exploring how different experiences are established, operated, and contested, and how and in what ways they constitute subjects. 'Governmentality' provides a useful conceptual tool to explore the ways through which experience and subjects are constructed.

Governmentality refers to all endeavours involving 'how to govern oneself, how to be governed, how to govern others, by whom the people will accept being governed, how to become the best possible governor' (Foucault 1991: 87). It captures the subtle and complex ways in which the lives of individuals or collectives are guided and directed socio-historically. It is about the 'conduct of conduct'—'a form of activity aiming to shape, guide or affect the conduct of some person or persons' (Gordon 1991: 2)—through shaping their hopes, desires, and environment, in contrast to sovereign power that governs through cruder and coercive measures. Governmentality includes self-government where certain values and knowledge are implanted in individual's social behaviour, enabling one 'to bridle one's own passions, to control one's own instincts, to govern oneself' (Rose 1999: 3). The operation of government to govern individuals, population, society, political and economic life, thus is not just through official bureaucracy, but through institutions and individuals beyond the state.

Governmentality is fundamentally moral activity, 'if morality is understood as the attempt to make oneself accountable for one's own actions, or as a practice in which human beings take their own conduct to be subject to self-regulation' (Dean 2010: 19). The morality of the government encompasses the policies and practices of government which involves value and knowledge of what constitutes good, moral, proper behaviour, and the ways through which the government seeks to engage in people's self-government (Dean 2010: 20). Foucault links people's moral experience with power and dominance. He writes: 'In order to protect capitalist wealth it was necessary to constitute the populace as a moral subject' (Foucault 1980: 41), while elsewhere he states that the moralisation of the working class is 'the strategy which allows the bourgeois class to be the bourgeois class and to exercise its domination' (Foucault 1980: 203). Besides, he (1987: 20) makes a distinction between 'morality' (as sets of rules that impose requirements and restrictions on the individual) and 'ethics' (as the ways in which individuals conduct themselves and negotiate in relation to such sets of rules, or what he refers to as the moral practices of the self). Moral governance thus concerns how particular values and ideologies are harnessed by the state to meet the economic, social and political ends; the aspects of morality and ethics that involve disciplining and governing people, institutions and social relations; and the ethical discourses and practices embedded in people's everyday life that require the self-discipline, self-cultivation, and self-control of individuals to constitute themselves as a moral agent. The moral practice by individuals may deviate from the subscript moral codes, encompassing individual subjects' challenge to the moral governance.

The book differentiates the levels at which governmentality operates: governance on individuals and the population (ordinary patients and health professionals, in this research); the self-government of individuals; and the governance of the state itself (including the public institutions, bureaucrats, officials, and policy-makers that constitute the state). It explores the ideologies, rationalities, techniques and processes of the state to direct and shape people's behaviour in the health sector. It also encompasses the practice of the government in projecting itself as a moral agent, in the process subject itself to the forces of governmentality. In other words, it is about not only moral economy in the domain of health care, but also the moral economy of the state. With this differentiation, it would be possible to see the discrepancies and contestations within and between the different levels: how government rationales and ideas are converted into concrete techniques and practices; how these government activities were conceived, constituted, negotiated and resisted by the people; and the configuration of the political rationalities, discourses and ideologies in the changing government itself. The concept of governmentality well links the power, experience, and subjectivity of individuals by exploring the ideologies and constitutive forces involved in the contested construction of experience. It also enriches the research on experiences and subject formation by looking at multiple factors within and beyond the state. Researching people's health care experience in the view of governmentality thus allows us to see the political and economic circumstances within which people's subjectivity takes shape and contests, as well as the relationship of the individual to the powerful epistemological and political realities.

1.3 Moral Experience of Health Care in the Transitional Chinese Governance

To use governmentality in a non-western, non-liberal context, different from the one from which it originates, the book needs critically to explore its applicability in relation to the history and political economy of the specific locale.

1.3.1 Chinese Governance in Transformation: A Socialist Neoliberal Governmentality?

Scholars have questioned the use of governmentality in non-Western contexts (see Kipnis 2008; Ferguson 2009; Yang 2011; Joseph 2009, 2012). Generally, they make several points: the imposition of techniques of (neoliberal) governmentality in countries outside those where they initially developed is lifting governmentality out of its social context; governmentality in a liberal West is based upon its structural and legal constraints on sovereign power, but governance in other parts of the world may not have clear constraints on sovereign power, or may have to rely on cruder disciplinary practices and coercive forms of power; in international relations, the rudely thrust-upon neoliberal governmentality in developing countries may subject them to the strategies and techniques of the advanced liberal countries while being locked into the social conditions of their own uneven development. Despite these concerns, the book regards that 'governmentality' could be a useful conceptual tool if it concerns 'how we govern and are governed within different regimes, and the conditions under which such regimes emerge, continue to operate, and are transformed' (Dean 2010: 33) with multiple knowledge, techniques, practices, and identities.

There is a growing body of research that employs the concept of governmentality in the Chinese context (Anagnost 2004; Farquhar 2002; Farquhar and Zhang 2005; Festa 2006; Greenhalgh 2003, 2009, 2011; Jeffreys 2009; Keane 1999, 2001a, b; Kohrman 2004, 2005; Lee 2006; Powell and Cook 2000; Sigley 1996, 2006; Yan 2003; Yang 1989, 2011). Many of these researches find that there is a gradual *transition* from sovereign power to governmentality, and that a *shift* from the concept of 'government' to one of 'governance' accompanied China's post-1978 entry into the global market. However, most researches also admit that it would be a mistake to regard China as now experiencing a process whereby the form of governance is *replacing* the sovereign power of government. Transformation in contemporary China embodies highly contradictory strategies and policies. It sees the simultaneous retreat of the state in certain areas and the strict control in other areas, the adoption of new modes of governance as well as the continuity of coercive forms of power. Many regard the changing governance in China as not the state 'retreat' from governing, but the modes of governance 'regrouping' (Sigley 2006) into different mixes. Pieke (2009) writes about a combination of centralisation, strengthening and selective retreat of the state, and a mixture of Leninist organisational discipline, modern governmental bureaucracy, and neoliberal marketization in China. Zhang (2011) records the coexistence of different modes of power—sovereignty, governmentality, and the power of communist revolution (which sometimes serve to enhance sovereignty and sometimes reinforces governmentality) in China. Sigley (2006: 489) notes the shift from a concept of 'government' as a task of 'planning' and 'administration' to one of 'governance' and 'management' with a hybrid socialist-neoliberal form of political rationality 'that is at once authoritarian in a familiar political and technocratic sense yet, at the same time, seeks to govern certain subjects, but not all, through their own autonomy'. Research on environmental city-building notes, the mechanisms of governing (market logics, quantification, and decentralisation/localisation) consti-tute part of the wider shift from detailed state planning (*jihua*) to more macro-level supervision (*guihua*) (Hoffman 2009). In population control, there is also a shift from a Leninist approach in the 1980s dominated by the state to an increasingly neoliberal approach in the early 2000s (Greenhalgh and Winckler 2005), and recently the shift from one of economic governance aimed at a rapid fertility decline and GDP growth to one of social and even human governance aimed at population optimisation—the development of population quality and human capital (Greenhalgh 2009), yet the new configuration remains a kind of 'Leninist neolib-eralism in which the state monitors and tries hard to manage the politics of life' (Greenhalgh 2011: 157). These mixes of governance technologies and rationales in post-reform China are named by scholars 'neoliberal sovereignty' (Ren 2010: xiii), 'neo-socialism' (Pieke 2009), 'socialism with Chinese characteristics' (Hann and Hart 2009; Vickers 2009),[8] 'neoliberalism with Chinese characteristics' (Harvey 2005), and 'socialism with neoliberal characteristics' (Ren 2010: 162).

The hybridity of governance in China is not particular. As Foucault (1991: 102) writes, 'we need to see things not in terms of the replacement of a society of sovereignty by a disciplinary society and the subsequent replacement of a disci-plinary society by a society of government; in reality one has a triangle, sovereignty-discipline-government'. The coexistence of multiple modes of power, technologies and rationales could also be found in other countries, such as post-Soviet Russia (Collier 2005a) and Africa (Ferguson 2009). As Ferguson (2009: 183) writes:

> "[I]f there is a really socialist governmentality, then it is not hidden within socialism and its texts. It cannot be deduced from them. It must be invented". [Quote from Foucault (2008: 94)] But invention in the domain of governmental technique is rarely something worked up out of whole cloth. More often, it involves a kind of bricolage (Lévi-Strauss 1966), a piecing together of something new out of scavenged parts originally intended for some other purpose. As we pursue such a process of improvisatory invention, we might begin by making an inventory of the parts available for such tinkering, keeping all the while an open mind about how different mechanisms might be put to work, and what kinds of purposes they might serve.

Tracing the purposes, this book will show that the coexistence of multiple modes of power, techniques and rationales in Chinese governance is the result of the continuous and creative efforts of the party-state to reinvent it and to find new legitimacy and effective governance. Pieke (2009: 13) notes that governance in China is an ongoing effort to build new institutions, mould the agents of the state and realise a particular vision of China's modernity; in the process, the Chinese reforms borrow many ideas and techniques of government from neoliberal thought and practice in the West, which are blended with indigenous socialist ideas and

---

[8]It is also the word used in the party's official discourse, indicating the special characteristics of China's socialist modernity as it has been guided by the market.

practices. Hai Ren (2010: 6) also shows that China has developed its own neoliberal path since the late 1970s in the Chinese communist party (CCP)'s exploration of legitimacy, imposing 'neoliberalism as a fundamental legitimizing principle in developing, shaping, and reconstructing nation states'. The Chinese state in the past few decades has ceaselessly reinvented and regenerated itself and its governance. In the continuously changing and adjusting process, the party-state actively adopts various technologies to serve political projects. Health care transformation is a case in point here.

The adoption of specific technologies may not mean accepting the relevant ideology. Collier (2005a, b) makes a distinction between specific techniques and political-economic projects, the relation of which is 'polymorphous and unstable', and the former are frequently 'deployed in relation to diverse political projects and social norms' (2005a: 2). He suggests that, to review the neoliberal reforms in a non-Western context, what is required is a 'shift from questions of value to questions of technique' (2005b: 389). In their 'Introduction' to *Privatizing China*, Ong and Zhang (2008: 9–10) similarly advocate analysing neoliberalism as 'a mobile set of calculative practices' that could be adopted by any political regime in a contingent manner 'without changing its entire state apparatus or character', and the adoption of neoliberal practices in China is such a case. Andrew Kipnis (2008) in particular notes Nikolas Rose's conceptualisation that 'neoliberal governmentality'—governing from a distance, calculability, and the promotion of self-activating, disciplined, individuated subjects—can actually be found in a variety of governing cultures that are historically distant from western neoliberalism, such as China, whose culturally specific traditions of governmentality often involve ways of disciplining and cultivating the self, governing from a distance, and calculating value; but the use of neoliberal technologies in a local Chinese context may serve certain purpose in the management of social relations and lead to non-liberal results, rather than accepting the neoliberal ideology.

Following the above distinction between government technologies and government ideologies/political projects, this book will explore the dynamic practice of particular technologies in the Chinese health sector and their effects on the overall governance. As Kipnis rightly notes, neoliberal technologies may be implemented incompletely and in modified ways in the face of 'resistance, transformation, and subversion by those who are its objects' (Dunn 2004: 23, cited in Kipnis 2008: 285). The changing governance (with neoliberal characteristics) in China does not mean a reduction in the involvement of the party-state, but instead the party-state continues to occupy a central position in the reforms over the past few decades. This may not be well captured by Foucault's concept of 'governmentality' that shifts attention away from a direct state role towards an understanding of the mentalities, rationalities, and techniques of government (Kohrman 2004a, b, 2005a, b).[9] Using multiple techniques

---

[9]Kohrman (2004a, b, 2005a, b) points out that the problem inherent to early governmentality theory when using it in the Chinese context is Foucault's reluctance to grant the state a greater role in socio-political formation. He suggests, in the context of China where the state remains so pivotal to social organization, it is important to see how state and non-state entities are complicit in the

to serve the polity, China thereby sees the coexistence of neoliberal practices and illiberal forms of state controls. Besides the role of the party-state that is still crucial and frequently occupies a central position in initiating reforms, this research also identifies elite or interest groups (including government officials, all levels of health administrators, public hospitals, and doctors on the frontline who gain from the market mode of health care) within the health sector. Post-reform China sees that many reforms, policies, and discourses are the result of deliberate strategies of the elite or interest groups, who actively promote or resist certain reform measures, influence the policy making, and use new reform agendas to reap more profits. The political and economic elites form a powerful alliance, making the market reforms and socialist governance support each other. Under the new healthcare reform, although policy is still mainly decided by the state, the reform process itself shows varied local implementation, resistance from market forces and commercialised hospitals, increasingly diversified voices from vibrant intellectual and public debates, and the involvement of several budding interest groups.[10] The relations between the party-state, interest groups, and the market are reconfiguring the healthcare reforms as well as impacting on the implementation of government technologies and the direction in which healthcare reform is moving.

China's governance is filled with contradictions, and is far more complicated than a socialist or neoliberal turn. Health care is one of the key programmes of the state concerning the welfare of the population, occupying the central aspect of 'governmentality'. It is an area where state morality and legitimacy can be built, has been the center for political debate in many countries. This research sees health care as a specific government project, and China's health sector, with its dramatic transformations in recent decades, is especially useful for exploring the configurations of governmental power, rationality, techniques, and subjectivity.

1.3.2 Moral Economy of the State: Health Care as a Modern Project and Political Task

The book is about the Chinese government's self-exploration of how to regenerate itself as a moral agent, its impact on the health sector, and the way in which power is exercised and contested in the health sector. Thornton (2007: 2) notes that the projection of the state and its leaders as moral actors has played a central role in the Chinese state-making process, 'not because they served to cloak more fundamental material or political interests behind a mask of legitimation, but because

---

creation of forms of truth and practices, how governmental regulatory agencies discursively problematize people's lives, their forms of conduct, and their selves (2004a, b: 229).

[10]Wang and Fan (2013) even name the Chinese new healthcare reform as a 'consensus decision-making process' that all parties, interest groups, and the people have a say in the reform agenda, which displays a picture different from the western depiction of the Chinese governance mode as authoritarianism.

state-making and moral regulation are in fact co-constituting historical processes'. Ong (1999: 64) uses 'the moral economy of the State' to describe the social contract whereby the government guarantees economic and social well-being in return for economic discipline and social conformity on the part of the population. Health care is such an arena through which the government builds its moral economy. The transformation of the Chinese health sector is debated and decided mainly by the central leadership, with distinct political and economic concerns (Duckett 2011; Huang 2014).[11] Through healthcare reform, the state negotiates a variety of values and techniques from different historical periods to form a new moral narrative and reinforce its moral governance. The Chinese healthcare reforms over the past few decades are also a consistent state effort of modernisation. Placed in the grand trajectory of recent Chinese history, health care pertains to state-building, political legitimacy, and the broad workings of modernity.

In the early 20th century, facing the Western encroachment and the humiliating discourses of the 'sick man of East Asia' (*dongya bingfu*), the elites became increasingly concerned about medicine, hygiene, and the health of the population, which were correlated with the prosperity and strength of the nation-state, with China's place in the world, and with the race and ethnicity of what it means to be 'Chinese' (Rogaski 2004; Sigley 1996). The association of *weisheng* (health, hygiene) with questions of China's place in the modern world compelled the state to chase 'hygienic modernity'—creating a hygienically modern nation in order to counter the spectre of national deficiency from the late 19th century to the mid-20th century (Rogaski 2004). In this period, science and democracy were widely accepted as the most effective Western formulae for transforming China into a modern nation (Tu 2001). Traditional Chinese medicine (TCM hereafter) was attacked as unscientific, backward, and was a hindrance to the development of the nation, while 'scientific' modern biomedicine began to be promoted in China. The Republican government (1919–1949) had made efforts to set up a modern health system, but these efforts largely went in vain in the turbulent social and political environment.

Since the socialist revolution started in the 1920s, the CCP has pursued the project of modernity and committed to medical modernisation in the wider context of state-building. In the early period of the PRC (People's Republic of China), the party-state adopted the Soviet model of health care, placing emphasis on health care in the urban areas. Health care was embedded in socialist revolution practices and used for political rhetoric by the party-state to counter imperialism and capitalism. The 'Patriotic Health Campaigns' that started in the 1950s framed mass public health and sanitation programmes as 'patriotic' actions to restore the Chinese nation

---

[11]Duckett (2011) shows that the result of the Chinese state's retreat from health care in the 1980s and 1990s reflected the priorities of decision-makers in the context of China's evolving political system, bureaucratic interests, the role of ideology and ideas, and the inability of the people to defend their interests. Huang (2014) also notes that the changing scope and generosity of healthcare benefits have reflected the strategies adopted by the Chinese central leadership of different generations, with distinct political and economic priorities in mind.

to good health in order to combat American imperialism (Perry 2013: 10–11). The early socialist public health programmes also promoted health subjects as the wealth of the nation (Chen 2001: 166). Later, in the 1960s, with the deterioration of the Sino-Soviet relationship and Mao's efforts to find a distinctive Chinese road, the indigenous barefoot doctor and cooperative medical scheme (CMS hereafter) were introduced to shift health care attention to the rural areas. The barefoot doctor movement was part of the state-driven project of medical modernisation which effectively expanded the state medical system to the rural areas (see Fang 2012), and TCM was promoted to provide cheap health care in times of economic and resource restraints. Health care provision in this period was 'dedicated to the people's health (*yiqie weile renmin jiankang*)' and centred on 'healing the wounded and rescuing the dying (*jiusifushang*)'.

Since the 1980s, the health care arrangements of the collective era have been viewed by the government as lagging behind the global development. The rural CMS and barefoot doctor system were regarded as 'backward' and unable to meet the social needs and modern development (Wang 2013). They were abandoned subsequently. The party sought to set its legitimacy after the Cultural Revolution through a modernisation road by adopting western knowledge and technology, the capitalist modes of production, and market economy. To prioritise economic efficiency, health care sector also learnt from western countries (especially the US) in choosing a neoliberal road with the state retreat from service provision. The market reform of health care was to remove development barriers, to help China's health sector to achieve technological development, and to improve health care quality and efficiency. The previous prevention-focused mode of health care was replaced by a curative mode. The humanitarian value dominated health care provision in the previous period was replaced by the value of market exchange, under which medical institutions and health professionals work to maximise profits and patients had to pay for most care they received.

However, as time went by, the market-oriented healthcare reform led to many problems. The retreat of the state from health care provision left the legitimacy issue wide open to be questioned. The state implemented several remedial measures in the 1990s and early 2000s: rebuilding the rural CMS and attempting to 'institutionalize, routinize, and normalize' public health after the 1989 Tiananmen crisis to improve the relationship between the Party and the masses (Huang 2013);[12] and the build-up of the health insurance system for urban employees in the late 1990s due to increasing concern over social stability when the state-sector was restructuring (Huang 2014). Partly owing to these remedial measures, China did not witness a

---

[12]Huang (2013: 85) records the words used by Li Tieying (the State Councillor in the early 1990s): there is 'direct relevance of the health work to the blood-and-flesh links between the party-state and the masses'.

measurable decline in people's overall health status, as witnessed in Eastern Europe and the former Soviet Union (Huang 2013: 85–86), although these tentative healthcare reforms were considered 'basically a failure'.[13]

In the post-reform era, the health and health care of the Chinese population are being increasingly linked to social stability, economic development, the strength of the nation state, and China's place in the world. Public health challenges such as SARS in 2003 triggered the state's response largely because they were deemed a threat to economic prosperity, socio-political stability, and/or national security (Huang 2013). The anti-SARS campaign was presented as a 'patriotic health campaign', concerned not only people's life and health, but also China's image and responsibility in the international community. In the post-SARS era, the state has promoted the image of more open, transparent government in dealing with pandemic outbreaks and infectious disease in the international stage. It also began to increase health insurance coverage to the peasants (since 2003) and urban non-employed residents (since 2007). At the 17th Party Congress in 2007, a general consensus was reached within the government—'health care is correlated with political stability and with the integrity of the state'.[14] The 2008 global financial crisis further increased people's sense of uncertainty and possible instability (Bo and Chen 2009; Duckett 2010). Thus, a new round healthcare reform was officially initiated in 2009. The government aims to increase the availability of the health service as a social palliative to reduce public resentment and resolve the conflicts surrounding the market reform. It is central to the establishment of a 'harmonious Society'—the political agenda promoted by Hu-Wen leadership since 2004 (Gao 2005; Wong 2010). From 2016, under the leadership of Xi Jinping, a 'Healthy China' action plan is launched, aiming to promote healthy lifestyles, improve health services and the health industry, and build a sustainable health system to provide essential health services to every citizen (Fu et al. 2018). The plan is based on four core principles—health as a priority, reform and innovation, scientific development, and equity and justice, which concerns China's social, economic stability and its global image overall.[15] Thereafter, in almost every state meeting, health care issues are regularly mentioned and frequently dominate the headline. All these demonstrate the government's dedication to investing in health and there is a return to the state responsibility in health care provision. The new healthcare reform constitutes part of the government's efforts to improve its moral and political legitimacy by meeting people's needs and shifting from economic priority policies towards more 'responsible', 'human-centred' governance.

Currently, the Chinese health system is complicated by the coexistence of a market and a planned system: the adoption of a market mechanism in health care

---

[13]In 2005, Ge Yanfeng from the Development Research Centre of the State Council expressed in an interview that the previous healthcare reforms had basically failed (People's Net 2005).

[14]From my interview of an official in the Riverside County Health Bureau (Interview D8).

[15]World Health Organization, 'Healthy China 2030', retrieved 28 March, 2018 (http://www.who.int/healthpromotion/conferences/9gchp/healthy-china/en/).

management and provision on the one hand, and the tight state control on medical pricing, personnel, and administration, and increasing state investments in health care on the other. Chinese scholars and officials have widely debated the hybrid 'socialist market' system of healthcare. Some (such as Professor Li Ling of Beijing University and officials in the Ministry of Health) blame the health care issue mainly on the market and advocate a return to the state's responsibility for health care. Others (pro-market experts represented by Professor Gu Xin of Beijing University, officials from the Ministry of Finance and the Ministry of Human Resources and Social Security) attribute health care problems not to the market but to improper state intervention in the market. They advocate further a free medical market to stimulate competition or rebalance between the market mechanism and state intervention instead of diminishing the market force (see Duckett 2011; Kornreich et al. 2012: 183–184). The two sides of the health sector represent the new left and neoliberal thoughts that have emerged in China since the 1990s. The relation between the state and the market is the central debate across the economic and social arenas by the new-left and liberal scholars.[16] It is also the struggle between the left- and right-wings of the party. The radical articulation of neoliberalism in the 1990s and the left-turn in the 2000s in China are manifested in the health sector, within which there has been a shift from 'state retreat' in the 1990s to 'state re-intervention' recently (Gu 2010). The actual social and political situation, however, does not constitute a clear-cut division between neoliberalism and new-leftism. The Chinese health sector is a combination of centralisation, regulation, marketization and the selective retreat of the state in various degrees over time. The state continuously reinvents and modernises itself by adopting all kinds of governmental technologies and ideologies. In the current system, it adopts liberalism and a market mechanism while continuing many socialist principles, indicating the mutual support between the market and state power. It balances between increasing state investment and emphasizing individual responsibility in health care. After decades' reform and years since the new round of healthcare reforms,

---

[16]The liberal intellectuals dominated China's academia and significantly influenced the government's social and economic policies in the 1990s and early 2000s. The market reform and the state's withdrawal from social welfare provision in this period paralleled the neoliberal development in Western countries and the new waves of globalisation. The new left criticised neoliberalism, defended the interests of the poor, and emphasised more government involvement in social and economic arenas. The new left school influenced the policies of the Hu-Wen leadership when they took power in 2003. This leadership regarded the new left as a viable force to outset the unfavourable market outcome and steer China's transition. A series of social policies and welfare programmes were initiated in this period to reduce the disparities between regions, tackle rural-urban disparities, build a more equitable people-centred society, and improve social justice (Wang 2008; Li 2010). The global financial crisis further provides avenues for the new left to voice their concerns. They prefer the gentler capitalism of European model than the US model (which was taken as an example to follow in the 1990s), and urge the policy-makers to learn from the European development model and its socialist welfare tradition (Bo and Chen 2009). While the neo-liberals still heavily influence the official policies (on economic reforms and the pro-market approach of governance), there has been a left turn of social policies since the Hu-Wen leadership.

it is good time to review how does this influence people's life with regard to health care, and how does it impact on the way people are governed and the formation of individual subjectivity?

1.3.3 Moral Experience of Health Care in Chinese Governance

Many scholars note the emergence of neoliberal governance and neoliberal citizenship in post-reform China (Anagnost 2004, 2008; Keane 2001a, b; Yan 2003; Ren 2010). In the market, medical practices are reoriented according to economic rationales. Hospitals are public service institutions, but function like private enterprises to maximise profit. Hospital administrators are required to become entrepreneurs, managing hospitals based on careful calculations of costs, profits, and efficiency. Health professionals are required to be responsible for generating money and promoting their own development. They are evaluated in terms of their market competitiveness and economic productivity, and increasingly make medical decisions based on patients' ability to pay. Patients are required to be responsible for their own health care, to be 'deserving' or 'worthy' individuals for social benefits, and to be capable consumers to make the right decision in the market. Individuals are increasingly viewed as autonomous, rational providers or consumers. This proposes the profound ethical implication that moral, worthy people are those who earn their own livelihood, work hard and succeed in the market.

While admitting the powerful influence of neoliberal values among Chinese patients and health professionals, this research also questions the neoliberal turn, as people in my fieldwork display ambivalent, complex values in terms of health care and daily life. Many people, especially those who have experienced the transition from the collective era to the market era, do not exhibit the ideal neoliberal subjectivity. Patients use different discourses, including traditional values, collective ideals and market rationales, in their commentaries on health care and health professionals. They negotiate health care in the reconfiguration of hybrid notions about obligation, entitlement, right, and need (Chap. 3). The body is used by the state and hospitals to produce economic value, but is also used by patients to argue for existential needs and proper health care. Health care is continually seen by many patients as a humane service which cannot be commercially calculated. Besides, individual responsibility is continually being emphasized, oriented towards a common good and serves a collective end, which reinforces authoritarian power rather than neoliberal governance. Doctors, too, constantly negotiate with themselves and their institutions, making medical decisions in relation to the codes and rules set out by the government bodies in complex and sometimes conflicting ways. Many health professionals still value medical practice as humanitarian work rather than the exchange of commercial products, but they have to work in an institutionally environment that increasingly put economic consideration at priority.

Moreover, the recent reform direction also demonstrates the authorities' ambiguous attitude toward neoliberal governance. Since the new health reform in 2009, the state has continuously increased its investments in health sector, and many measures are taken to alleviate individual's burden in health care, yet people's average out-of-pocket expenditures in health care are continually rising.[17] How to achieve good governances in China's health care is a challenge faced by the party-state.

In the Chinese health sector, there is an assemblage of techniques, rationales, powers, and knowledge that shapes the conduct of individuals, extracts economic utility from human body and controls the population, while rendering individuals and the population politically docile. Later chapters will demonstrate that the governance within the health sector takes multiple forms: 'visible' supervision and prohibition, the use of policy and institution to coordinate people's activities, the more subtle and intangible guiding and shaping of people's values, desires, and dispositions, and letting them govern themselves. Health policy is one in which power is exercised. Health policies promote tactical interventions, form systems of discipline and knowledge, and constitute new subjects. Health insurance schemes serve to discipline individual conduct and control the population—its health, quantity, mobility and stability (Chap. 4). Moreover, the official discourses frequently individualise and moralise systemic issue: a failure to rescue patients is attributed to the moral problem of individual doctors (Chap. 2); *nao* (speaking or acting violently) is an illegal, backward practice by patients (Chap. 5); gift-taking is a corrupt, immoral behaviour of doctors (Chap. 6). These further justify the state's control of individuals. The authority issues a series of rules and laws to regulate people's conduct, sometimes with coercive elements. The hybrid forms of socialist neoliberal governmentality do not universally govern the population. The social rights of certain groups (for instance, the disadvantaged and poor patients, as shown in Chap. 3, the migrant workers recorded in Chap. 4, and the village doctors described in Chap. 7) have not been sufficiently protected during recent transformation.

The book also considers how certain government activities were negotiated, resisted, and modified by individuals. Foucault has often been criticised for his insufficient recognition of the extent to which disciplinary power is routinely contested, but some scholars identify that Foucault, later in life, did affirm that power addresses 'individuals who are free to act in one way or another' (Gordon 1991: 5), and that the 'conduct of conduct' necessarily entails a capacity for resistance whereby individuals can think and act in various ways, that are sometimes not foreseen by the authorities (Dean 2010: 21). Foucault discusses the 'strategic reversibility' of power relations that the conduct of conduct or the practices and techniques of the self might sometimes develop into dissenting 'counter-conduct' or resistance (Cordon 1991: 5; Dean 2010: 21). Governance involves the reflections, practices, and manoeuvres of the subjects, who may desubjectify themselves and challenge certain normative rules and power.

---

[17]See Zhu (2018).

This book thus also explores how people negotiate with the state's 'discursive regimes' in daily practice and to what extent people may transgress or challenge the state-regulated moral category to defend their own interests. There are overlaps, conflicts, and contestations between the official regulations of 'things should be' (the rules that should be followed), the individual ethical reasoning of 'I should be' (the practice of the self), and the public discourse about how the authority should be (the moral sense of the rightness of power). In the health sector, these are revealed by the conflicts between the official discourses of obligations and rights and people's concrete experiences of articulating their rights and needs, between the moral codes put forward by the administrative agencies and the actual requirements of the daily medical environment for health professionals. Doctors in medical practices are frequently discouraged from, and even punished for, lifesaving behaviour that fails to generate profits or causes an economic loss for the hospital. Yet, the state regulates on health professionals' compulsory obligation to save lives. For health professionals, there is a lack of consistent moral guidelines related to their daily medical practice. The competing and sometimes contradictory ideas, claims, and moral judgements involved in medical practice in a changing social context require individual doctor constantly to readjust themselves in searching for meaningful practice, to act upon themselves, to monitor, question, improve and transform themselves. For patients, the official discourses regulate health care as both needs and rights that should be secured by the state. Yet, patients face structural obstacles to accessing health care, such as the household registration system and the categories and qualifications regulated by health insurance. People experience disappointment, feel contradictions, navigate the system, and act to confirm, contest, and transform the existing power structure and state discursive regime in order to defend their interests. Patients (and their relatives) and doctors (and hospitals) also compete with each other in a struggle over the control of their interests and safety, as well as their moral definitions of justice and rights. This book reveals a nuanced picture of interwoven compliance and resistance as people asserted their interests and rights in the health sector during the historically unprecedented merging of the socialist system with the neoliberal market reform.

The book situates individual moral experience and changing subjectivity in the wider social transformations, and moves between government policies and people's lived experience. It explores the power configuration among patients (who seek qualified care and engage in struggles for their well-being), health professionals (who are in search of meaning medical practice while preserving their interests), medical institutions (that try to maximise profits while maintaining their public service nature), local state agents (that promote economic development, conceal local problems and preserve stability), and the central state (that attempts to improve health care, preserve moral and political legitimacy, and promote social harmony) in the healthcare reforms in China. The following chapters will provide detailed accounts of the social and value shifts produced by the market reforms and by the recent reverse in the market trajectory, the changing forms of governance, and the formation of new identities and subjectivities in the health sector.

1.4 Field Site and Research Methods

1.4.1 The Field Site

From 2011 to 2012, I conducted fieldwork in Riverside (a pseudonym) County of Sichuan Province, a historically less-developed[18] and less-researched region of southwest China (see Fig. 2.2). China has over 2000 counties. Sichuan Province embraces 181 counties. The county lies in the middle of the administrative hierarchy,[19] connecting the rural and urban areas. Health care delivery at the county level is vital for both rural and urban residents. Besides, the county is the lowest level of the state health administration, managing health professionals, medical institutions, and health care funding. While much media and academic attention has focused on health care in the larger, central cities, it is these thousands of small but rapidly developing counties around the country host the most Chinese people, who have experienced the diversity, inequality, and turbulence of the health care changes that have taken place over the past few decades. It is also these thousands of middle-sized and smaller cities at the county level, that have gone unnoticed, that have hosted the majority of urbanised population in recent years.

Riverside County has a population of 1.04 million, of whom about 300,000 live in the county capital (Riverside City hereafter). Riverside County has undergone a profound transformation in recent years. The urban population of Riverside has increased rapidly, as many village residents have moved to the towns and the city, holding an urban *hukou* (household registration) status.[20] Riverside has several local industries that employ many urban citizens, but large numbers of rural population (mainly the young and middle-aged) migrate to work in the coastal areas and big cities. The government records show that Riverside has sent out around 250,000 migrant workers annually in the past few several years, constituting about a quarter of its population.[21] The county in recent years has seen growing differences among people, as shown in the increasing numbers of gated communities in the city, big villas as well as poor huts in the villages, private schools for the rich, and so on. The city and its nearby areas have expanded at a rapid pace through the impressive construction of high buildings, new roads, parks, and shopping centres, but some of the county's remote rural areas have lagged behind in terms of development. In 2010, the local urban per capita disposable income was 13,226

---

[18]In 2011, Sichuan province was ranked 25th for GDP per capita among the 31 provinces in China (see http://news.xinhuanet.com/local/2012-02/07/c_122667889.htm, retrieved 15 January, 2014).

[19]There are five practical levels of local government in China's administrative hierarchy (from the higher to the lower): the province, the prefecture, the county, the township, and the village. The county normally has a medium-sized city as its centre, and is the intermediate zone between the rural and urban areas.

[20]When I carried out my master's study in Riverside County in 2009, the local records of urban population was 250,000 (see Tu 2010: 14). When I did the Ph.D. fieldwork in 2011 and 2012, the number already surpassed 300,000 and is continually increasing.

[21]The data come from local government website.

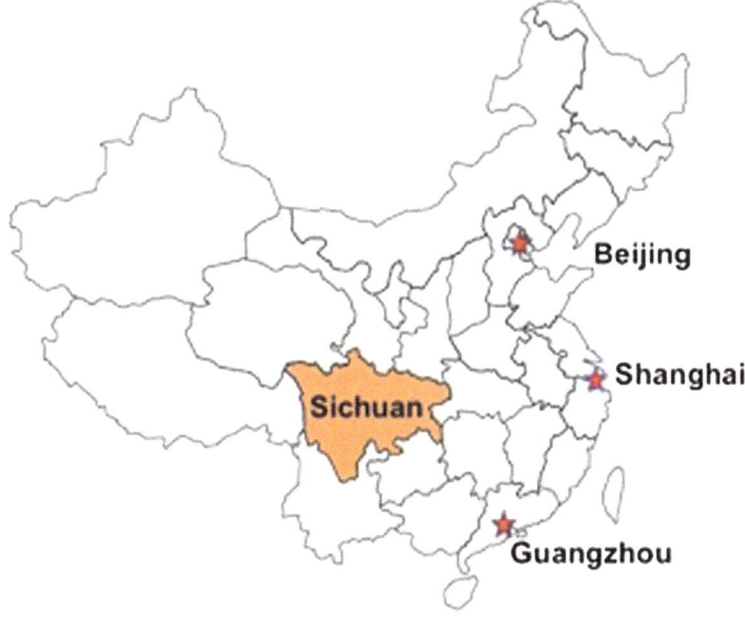

Fig. 1.2 Field province Sichuan in China

Yuan, whereas the rural per capita net income was a mere 5,920 Yuan.[22] The national average for that year was 19,109 Yuan in the urban areas and 5919 Yuan in the rural areas (People's Net 2011). The local average income was lower than the national level. Riverside is considered by the locals to be comparatively 'backward' and less developed. Yet, the county was once listed in the 'top 100 counties' in China, which is considered by local people as a source of both pride and pity. The locals complained that the former governors gained 'facade achievement' by putting the county's name in the top list, but that this good name also stopped the county from obtaining substantial subsidies for poor areas from the central government.

In Riverside County, there were 3109 (registered) health professionals (including 1468 traditional Chinese medical professionals) by 2007 (see Table 1.1).[23] A secondary medical school is located in the city, which has trained large numbers of primary medical professionals to serve the local areas, but there exists a shortage of

---

[22]The data come from local government website.

[23]Health professionals include both physician and other health workers. The number of physicians in the county is not available. The local number of health professionals is increasing. The recorded number varies in different government reports. In another local document I collected, it states that the county had 3268 health professionals by the end of 2007 (see Riverside County Health Department. 2008. 'The Work Summary of Building Advanced Traditional Chinese Medicine County in Rural Areas, Riverside, Sichuan').

high level medical professionals. There were 1087 medical institutions by 2007: two county hospitals (the People's Hospital and the Hospital of Traditional Chinese Medicine, hereafter TCM Hospital); one County Centre for Disease Control and Prevention; one Maternal and Child Health Centre; one Health Care Supervision Institute; 30 township health centres (one in each of the 30 towns) and two township Traditional Chinese Medicine hospitals; 810 village clinics; four private hospitals and 236 private clinics.[24] Apart from the township medical institutions, village health stations and certain private clinics situated in the countryside, all of the other medical institutions are located in the city—the capital and administrative centre of the county. Since the new healthcare reform, the medical facilities in Riverside have improved quickly. By 2012, four new community health centres had been set up in the four districts of the city.[25] Each covers several residential neighbourhoods and keeps health records for over 50,000 residents. In the rural area, township health centres and village clinics that were privatised or were bankrupt during the previous market reform are being rebuilt. Private hospitals are encouraged to develop to complement the public healthcare system. By 2012, there were eight private hospitals and the number is increasing.

In addition, there are many chemist shops, massage and acupuncture clinics, and medical equipment shops that offer various products and therapies in the city and towns (see Fig. 1.3). In the squares, streets and markets of the city and towns, stalls are set up by merchants dressed as medical professionals or wearing Tibetan, Qiang, or Uyghur ethnic dress, selling special drugs and therapies (see Figs. 1.4, 1.5, and 1.6).[26] Non-medically qualified acupuncturists and folk healers work in these places with ambiguous identities. Religious healing practices have also revived since the market reform. Street peddlers seek marketing niches, selling medicine for rare and minor illnesses around the city. Folk doctors and peddlers also travel around the towns and villages in search of household consumers to buy their products and services. These activities are often outside the purview of government regulation.

The healthcare reform policies are frequently implemented with local variations. Governance is also multiple and uneven, considering the unevenness of the social economic development within China. The experience in this inland county may differ from that in other parts of China. However, research on a specific locale remains empirically and theoretically significant in that it constitutes an important 'case' (Gerring 2007; Yin 2003) that can illustrate the dynamics, limits and potential in a period of structural transformation. It is hoped to reveal the various forces as they intersect in health care, and to reveal the logic, conflict and characters that generally exist in the Chinese health sector. Besides, research in a specific

---

[24]Riverside County Health Department. 2008. 'The Work Summary of Building Advanced Traditional Chinese Medicine County in Rural Areas, Riverside, Sichuan'.

[25]Riverside County Health Department. 2008. 'The Arrangement Planning of Community Health Institution in the Riverside County'.

[26]Sichuan province is famous for its production of traditional pharmaceutical products and various therapies and formulae from diverse ethnic groups.

Table 1.1 Health professionals in riverside county

	Western medical professionals	Traditional medical professionals	Total
County level	590 (73%)	194 (27%)	719
Town level	631 (59%)	437 (41%)	1068
Village level	485 (37%)	837 (63%)	1322
Total	1641 (53%)	1468 (47%)	3109

Data Source Riverside County Health Department 2007 (Riverside County Health Department. 2007. 'Statistical Overview of Western and Traditional Health Professionals in the County')

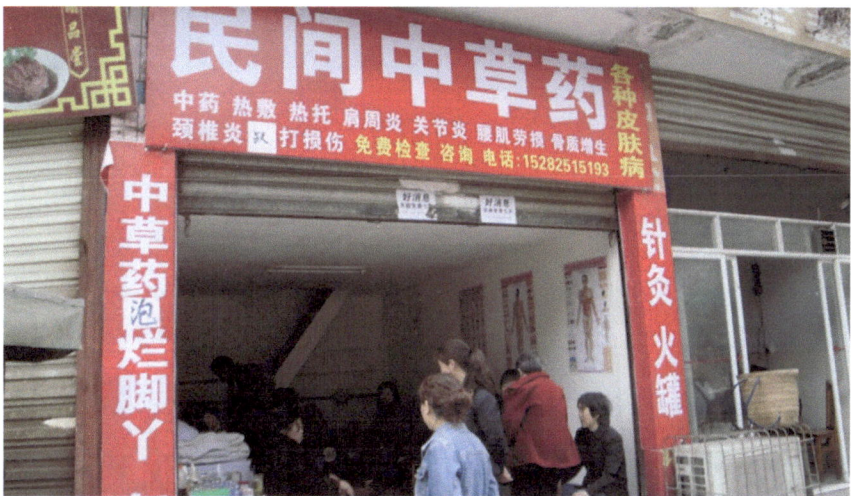

Fig. 1.3 Popular local Chinese medicine and herb therapy shop

location for a relatively longer period of time would yield the depth and richness of materials necessary to understand the practices and perceptions of the healthcare reform, as well as facilitate the creation of a narrative of change over time. This research puts the local into the national and global—the local experience in an increasingly national and global context of change. It is also a 'localisation of national', as the national policies and reforms are adjusted to suit the local context.[27]

---

[27]I got inspiration from Oxfeld's (2010: 167) use of 'localisation of the global' in her research on moral discourse in a Chinese village, by which she means that the global discourses are pulled into the local world of gossip, moral judgement, and status revaluation.

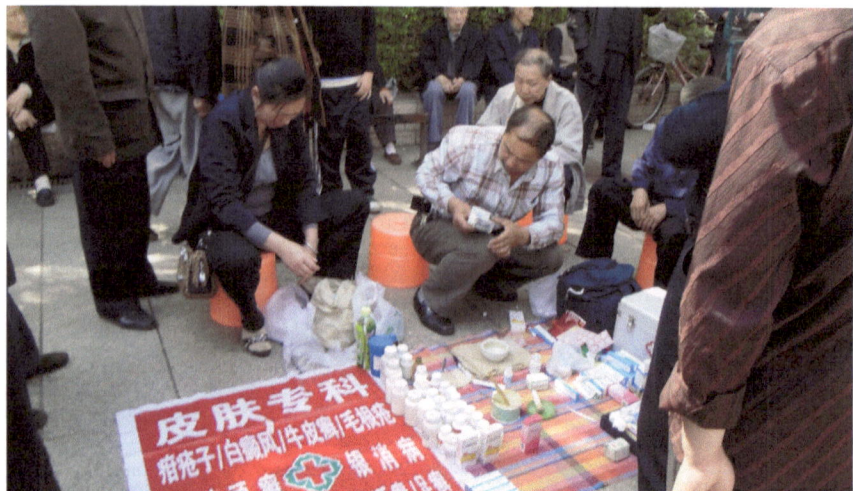

Fig. 1.4 Medicine sale in a square—medicine for various skin diseases

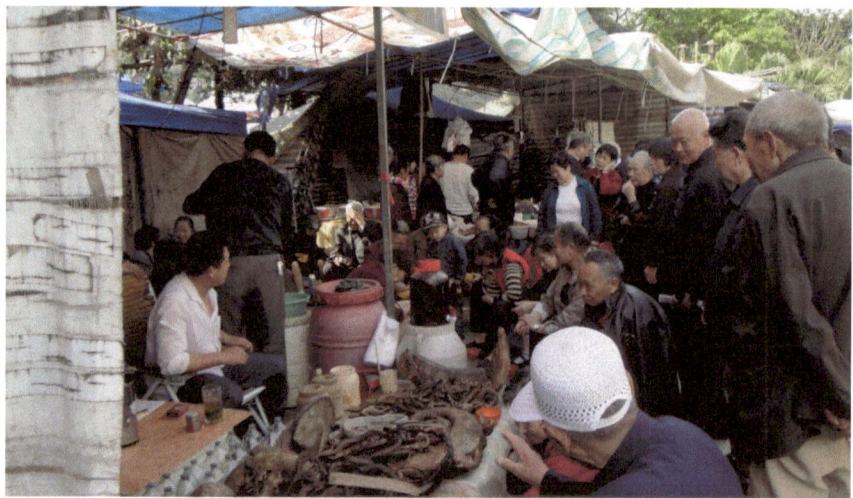

Fig. 1.5 Medicine sale in a square—medicated liquor and secret family formulae

1.4.2   Research Methods

The fieldwork took place over two periods mainly: October 2011–April 2012 (six months) and September 2012–October 2012 (two months), involving semi-structured interviews and conversations with patients, health professionals, health administrators and officials, participant observation in medical institutions,

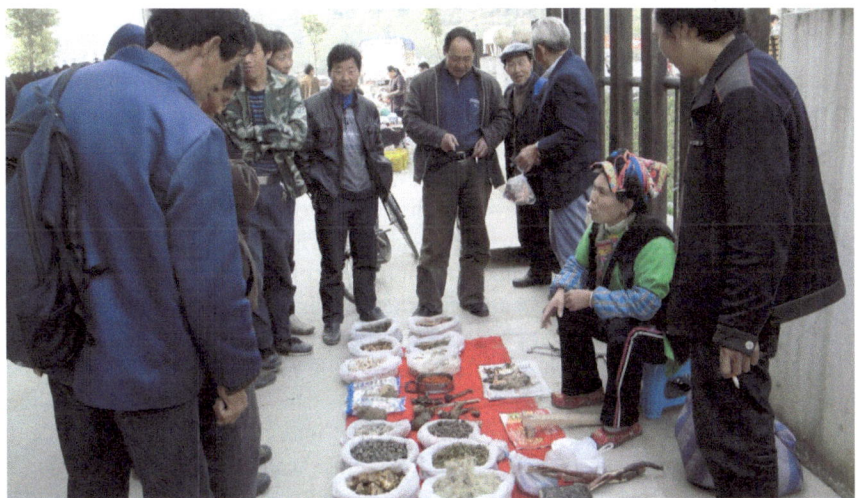

Fig. 1.6 Woman in ethnic clothing selling herbal medicine in a market

and document research. Before these researches, I conducted my master's research on private medical practice at the same site for three months, from June to August 2009, and my preparations had involved informal conversations, interviews and observations in Riverside County in summer 2010 and 2011. Following the fieldwork, I maintained contact with several of the informants and remained informed about the recent changes within the local health sector. Afterwards, I had periodic visits back to the field. The longitudinal fieldwork has enabled me to trace the ongoing healthcare reform continuously over the past few years.

From 2015, I began to work in Guangzhou city, a metropolitan in the developed costal area where many policies and reform measures were first experimented (see Fig. 1.2). I continued following China's healthcare reforms and its implementations and impacts on local patients and health professionals in Guangzhou. The familiarisation with health policy makers in Guangzhou offers me further insight on how the authority rationalise and implement its reform policies, and how a policy change or reform experiment in a capital city radiate to the whole province including many counties like Riverside. It provides me a top-down perspective to supplement the bottom-up perspective of my research in Riverside County. The social, economic and political environment of the costal capital Guangzhou differs much from the interior rural county of Riverside, yet the situation in Guangzhou provides me an opportunity for comparison and enables a better understanding of the particularity and generality of Riverside within China. The two very different, yet strategic locations, offer me insight into the complex health care experiences in China. I update some recent reform changes based on my follow up studies in Riverside and Guangzhou, but this book is still mainly based on the fieldwork in Riverside.

The fieldwork in Riverside involves in-depth, semi-structured interviews and conversations with various actors in the health sector. I conducted 80 interviews with health professionals, administrators, and officials, mostly individually apart from four focus group interviews with health professionals (see Appendix B). An informant who worked in the local health sector was the key person who introduced me to the health officials and hospital administrators. The interviews with health professionals were arranged through introductions by my acquaintances in the city, towns and villages. I carried out 50 interviews with patients and local residents, 14 of which were individual interview and the rest involved groups of two or more individuals (see Appendix C). Local residents were visited and interviewed in their daily life settings: their home, local community, water bar, coffee shop, teahouse, or park, where locals gather to play cards and chat. The interviews focused on people's health care experience (medical practice experience for health professionals) in the past and currently. The majority of interviewees were middle-aged (late 30s to 50s) and elderly (over 60), with experience of health care before the major market reforms of the 1980s and early 1990s. Only five interviews with local residents involved young people in their 20s, and 21 young health professionals under 35 were interviewed. These interviews were semi-structured, with many open-ended questions. Interviews are centred on three themes: perception toward health care change and reform, health professional-patient relationships, health care responsibility, entitlement and rights. I had some key topics in mind (health care costs, health care experience, the doctor-patient relationship, attitudes towards health professionals and hospitals, health care responsibility and rights, the fairness of the health system, insurance arrangements, problems in health care, and so on), and opened the interview to the locals' accounts. The ethnographic, open-ended interviews allowed the locals to address what was most at stake for them. These interviews were supplemented with many casual conversations during my observations of the medical institutions and the local residents' daily life.

I made visits and undertook observations in a variety of medical institutions: private clinics, village clinics, community health centres, public and private hospitals, and the local medical school, which covered 13 of the 30 towns in Riverside County. Local hospitals and outpatient clinics are like public spaces, where people walk in and out freely, especially the county hospitals, which many people visit daily. This enabled me to spend time in these institutions and observe, after receiving authorisation from the hospital administrators. In addition, after getting to know some of the interviewees, I accompanied them when they sought health care from various medical institutions. Whenever any of my acquaintances went into hospital, I visited them and stayed with them there for as long as I could. I also visited the health professionals I met over time and shadowed them at work for a while, when the situation allowed but, without expert knowledge, I could do little to help with these processes. Generally, the health professionals from the public hospitals were so busy that I felt guilty when they found a moment to talk to me when so many tasks and patients were awaiting them. The overburdened, overcrowded hospital setting did not allow me to enter the inpatient department to make a long-term observation and I could not obtain permission to observe the medical dispute resolution process which took place behind closed doors between the hospital and the patients' relatives. Later in April 2012, I visited a township hospital in northern Sichuan, where one of my relatives worked as a doctor. There, I shadowed health professionals' daily life for a week, attending their meetings, working with them to distribute preventive medicine to local residents, aiding in their health checks for children, and helping with their paper work. The visit allowed me to enter a hospital and gain first-hand experience of being a health professional, which I could not achieve in Riverside County.

County gazetteers, local documents, and government reports about health care were searched and collected (see lists of these materials in Appendix D). Media reports and internet discussions were also collected and studied. I followed blogs, micro-blogs, health professionals' websites, and medical forums over time, which were filled with lively discussions about health care (see Appendix D). The online information, albeit fragmented, supplied the important background information to deepen my understanding of the local context. These multiple sources of data were compared with each other and also with empirical materials that I gathered locally. Official documents, together with interviews with local health officials, provide a view from within the structure of the authority with respect to the policy agenda. These official discourses and policies are powerful tools for analysing the process and agencies of government (Shore and Wright 1997), enabling me to see how the government is responding to the changing situation and enacting governance.

These ethnographic interviews, conversations, participant observations, and archive research enable a rich, nuanced understanding of people's experience of the healthcare reform. These methods offer unique insights into the analysis of the contradictions and inconsistencies between people's discourses and actions, between the official regulations and the actual practices, which may remain invisible to researches based on the quantitative survey or a single method.

My own background, as a native who grew up in Riverside County, gave me ready access to the local society. I returned 'home' to carry out my fieldwork, mainly because I had already accumulated some fieldwork materials from this site previously, which would help me to trace the long-term changes as the new healthcare reform progresses. Also, some of the existing networks would help me to access the research targets. Even so, I still encountered difficulties when meeting local officials, some of whom treated me with caution, avoidance or rejection.[28] Many local healthcare data thus proved unobtainable from the government offices. In the field, on the one hand, I spoke the local dialect and understood the local culture, which helped me to hear the natives' voice and to see things from the locals' point of view. On the other hand, I left Riverside to study elsewhere in China and abroad in 2004, and have only returned for annual visits. Influenced by my cultural and social experiences elsewhere, I needed to 'refamiliarise' (Yan 2004: 204) myself with my native county. Besides, to the health professionals who I studied, I was an outsider to their medical practices. My academic knowledge,

---

[28]I have written about my experience of encountering officials in my field in a short article —'Encountering Chinese Officials: Bureaucratism, Politics and Power Struggle' (see http://blogs. lse.ac.uk/fieldresearch/2014/10/21/encountering-chinese-officials/).

based on institutional training, was also strange to the locals. The research thus placed me as both an insider and an outsider, and also required me carefully to balance the emic (insider's) and etic (outsider's) perspectives.

In the field, a researcher frequently constitutes the local society he or she tries to figure out. The researcher could become a tool of politics, constitute part of local propaganda, or become the target of avoidance or surveillance. Local health officials sometimes avoided me or openly rejected my interview. Even for the ones who accepted my interviews, some might speak certain words in specific context and time, and provided particular information but not others to influence the perspective of the researcher (for instance, the Head of the County Health Bureau introduced me to the Northern City Community Health Centre for research because it was the best established among the four in the city). Ordinary people also become increasingly conscious to use the influence of media and researchers to express their opinions when there are few formal channels to make their voices be heard. In my field, patients told me endlessly about their unhappy experiences with health care and their individual stories of being defrauded by hospitals and doctors, in the hope that my research could warn other patients from falling into a similar trap or get somebody from higher up to correct the local wrongdoing. Doctors practically express their views in the hope that my research could help them solve their issues or deliver their appeals to a higher level authority. The group of elderly village doctors is such a typical case (Chap. 7). They heard my fieldwork and contacted me, complained to me their dissatisfactions with current health reform policies and their pension issue. Many saw me as a prospective advocate for them. Yet I frequently found myself not doing much more to patients and doctors than lending a sympathetic ear or giving a few simple policy advices. When some interviewees found I could not make any immediate change, they left in the middle of an interview (in one interview—Interview 79, the number of village doctors reduced from about 15 at the beginning to around five doctors in the end). There was a gap between researcher and locals in terms of expectations and understandings of research. The awkward positions of both the local people and the researcher were defined by the current modes of governance, of policy making, and of politics. These governance, policy making and politics are exactly what constitute the 'field' and what this research tries to explore. In the field, researchers have to learn to interact with local people and consider the interests and motivations of people involved. The encounter itself shows a profile of how local society works, constitutes a significant part of the research of local society. Yet the process itself poses challenge to the researcher who needs to cultivate relationship with locals while reflecting on this relationship, to familiarise oneself with a local society while keeping certain distance to uphold a neutral position, and to get insider's knowledge while avoiding being solely guided by a group's voice. The process needs a researcher to constantly reflect on his or her position in the field, and uphold fluid identities (as researcher, acquaintance, or friend) in relation to the local people. This is exactly what I tried very hard in the field.

The interviews recorded digitally in the field were transcribed verbatim. The interviews recorded by hand were transcribed on the day to ensure accuracy. All the interviews and transcriptions were carried out in person. The process makes me familiar with the data collected. The over 700 pages of field notes include observations, conversations, my personal experiences, and interview transcripts.[29] I went through these materials several times, identifying the thematic topics, phrases and issues that came up repeatedly. The analysis was informed by thematic analysis outlined by Braun and Clarke (2006). I carefully read and re-read data transcriptions and field notes, highlighted important passages in different colours according to topics, making notes in the margins that represent particular concepts, issues, or comments. After this initial coding, I went through my codes and notes again, refine and differentiate the categories.[30] I wrote down repeated ideas and questions, identified a large array of recurring concepts, phrases, and topics, which are further sorted into potential themes. There were more themes and topics identified than that could not be incorporated into this book. In reviewing and refining writing themes, I chose to address the most significant aspects and themes that there were sufficient data to support. The book is thus organised in thematic order that each chapter focuses on an emerging or prominent issue in current Chinese health sector (what people talked about most): the conflicts and dilemmas associated with medical practice (Chap. 2); the reconfiguration of health care obligations, rights, and needs over time (Chap. 3); discrepancies between the state's regulations and people's lived experience, between policy design and local implementation (Chap. 4); informal exchanges in daily health care access and medical practice (Chap. 5); the increasing medical disputes between patients and health professionals (Chap. 6); and the sense of a changing morality and profound loss associated with the transformation from the Maoist era to the market era (Chap. 7). Underneath these different topics in each chapter, there are similar structure and theoretical framework. Beside the above general coding, I also employed selective coding to generate thematic domains and categories for a single case or theme (for instance, in Chap. 5, I tried to categorise people's perception of gift practice in the health sector, the pattern in their accounts of gift change; in Chap. 6, I focused on analysing people's accounts of *yinao*, the shared views expressed in patients' and local residents' accounts, the doctors' views in contrast with the local residents', the changing trend of government policies on *yinao* governance). As I wrote the book, I constantly compared phenomena, cases and concepts, and frequently went back to the original materials to interpret meaning in the context. The writing weaves together individual narratives, institutional change, policy analysis, and historical

---

[29]Except some interviews that were transcribed on the day of interview, other interviews recorded digitally were transcribed after leaving the field, which are put in a separate sheet outside the field note. The transcription per se has taken me several months. Among all the interviews, 27 important interviews have been further translated partly or wholly from Chinese into English, covering over 200 pages.

[30]The analysis process tries to identify key themes around people's experience of the health reforms. I did coding, but did not strictly follow the coding process as in methods such as grounded theory. I did not code line by line, sentence by sentence, but more generally paragraph by paragraph, case by case.

and social investigation. Sometimes I use people's account as fact in order to present original materials—such as people's recounts of historical incidents, cases, and data. Most times I use people's accounts as subjective interpretive accounts which are analysed with the Foucauldian constructionist perspective.

To protect the participants' privacy, I use pseudonyms for all place names under the provincial level. The interviewees' names are either pseudonyms or based on how I addressed them in the field. Quotes are translated from the local dialect into English, containing an interview number at the end. The interviews are numbered Dx and Px: D1 means the first interview with doctors, widely referring to all health professionals and administrators; P1 indicates the first interview with patients and local residents. In discussing health care now and in the past, people frequently refer to three periods: 'before the Liberation' (*jiefang qian*) suggests the time before the communist victory (in liberating China) and the founding of the PRC in 1949; the 'collective era' or 'Maoist era' is the time between the founding of the PRC and the 'reform and opening up' in 1978; the 'post-reform era' is the time since the market reform in 1978. Following the locals' usage, this book employs the 'post-reform' or 'market' era (emphasising the period since the market reform of the late 1970s) and the 'post-collective' or 'post-Mao' era (emphasising the period since the end of the collective era) interchangeably according to the context to refer to the third period—the main focus of this research. I also use the new healthcare reform as a point of time division. Broadly speaking, the new healthcare reform started in 2003 with the outbreak of SARS, the subsequent rebuilding of the public health facilities and the implementation of the new rural cooperative medical scheme. It has been narrowly implemented since 2009, when the new healthcare reform plan was officially released. Albeit adopting these time divisions, the book will show that the past and the present are not ruptured in people's moral experiences and in terms of governance, but involve both continuities and changes.

References

Anagnost, Ann. 2004. The corporeal politics of quality (suzhi). *Public Culture* 16 (2): 189–208.
Anagnost, Ann. 2008. From "class" to "social strata": Grasping the social totality in reform-era China. *Third World Quarterly* 29 (3): 497–519.
Balla, Steven J. 2014. Health System Reform and Political Participation on the Chinese Internet. *China Information* 28 (2): 214–236.
Bo, Zhiyue and Gang Chen. 2009. Global Financial Crisis and the Voice of the New Left in China. East Asian Institute, National University of Singapore. Retrieved September 22, 2013. http://www.eai.nus.edu.sg/BB443.pdf.
Braun, Virginia, and Victoria Clarke. 2006. Using thematic analysis in psychology. *Qualitative Research in Psychology* 3 (2): 77–101.
Central People's Government, PRC. 2008. The Development and Reform Commission: The New Healthcare Reform Draft Received 35,000 Feedbacks. Retrieved February 7, 2011. http://www.gov.cn/jrzg/2008-11/15/content_1150149.html.

Central People's Government, PRC. 2009. *Opinions of the CPC Central Committee and the State Council on Deepening the Health Care System Reform* (Zhonggong zhongyang guowuyuan guanyu shenhua yiyao weisheng tizhi gaige de yijian). Retrieved January 27, 2011. http://www.gov.cn/jrzg/2009-04/06/content_1278721.html.

Central People's Government, PRC. 2012. *Chinese Government to Raise Health Insurance Subsidies*. Retrieved March 3, 2012. http://english.gov.cn/2012-02/22/content_2074190.htm.

Chen, Nancy N. 2001. *Health Wealth and the Good Life*. In *China Urban: Ethnographies of Contemporary Culture*, edited by N. N. Chen. 165–182. Durham: Duke University Press.

Chinese Academy of Social Sciences. 2007. *The Analysis and Prediction of the Situation of Chinese Society in 2007* (2007 nian: zhongguo shehui xingshi fenxi yu yuce). Beijing: Chinese Academy of Social Science Press.

Collier, Stephen. 2005a. *The Spatial Forms and Social Norms of "Actually Existing Neoliberalism": Toward a Substantive Analytics*. International Affairs Working Paper. New York: New School University.

Collier, Stephen. 2005b. Budgets and biopolitics. In *Global Assemblages: Technology, Politics, and Ethics as Anthropological Problems*, edited by A. Ong and S. J. Collier. 373–390. Malden, MA: Blackwell.

Dean, Mitchell. 2010. *Governmentality: Power and Rule in Modern Society*, 2nd ed. London: Sage Publications.

Ding Xiang Yuan. 2013. *2012–2013 Chinese Doctor Income Survey Report* (2012–2013 niandu zhongguo yisheng xinchou qingkuang diaocha baogao). Retrieved December 5, 2013. http://vote.dxy.cn/report/dxy/id/64391.

Duckett, Jane. 2008. Health NGOs: A second generation of policy advocates? *China Review* 42 (6): 16.

Duckett, Jane, 2010. Economic Crisis and China's 2009 Health Reform Plan: Rebuilding Social Protections for Stability and Growth? *China Analysis: Studies in China's Political Economy* 80: 1–14. Retrieved September 12, 2012. http://eprints.gla.ac.uk/47463/2/id47463.pdf.

Duckett, Jane, 2011. *The Chinese State's Retreat from Health: Policy and the Politics of Retrenchment*. London: Routledge.

Duckett, Jane and Ana Inés Langer. 2013. Populism versus Neo-liberalism: Diversity and Ideology in the Chinese Media's Reporting of Health System Reform. *Modern China* 39 (6): 653–680.

Dunn, Elizabeth C. 2004. *Privatizing Poland: Baby food, big business, and the remaking of labor*. Ithaca, NY: Cornell University Press.

Eggleston, Karen, Li Ling, Meng Qingyue, Magnus Lindelow, and Adam Wagstaff. 2008. Health service delivery in China: A literature review. *Health Economics* 17 (2): 149–165.

Fang, Xiaoping. 2012. *Barefoot Doctors and Western Medicine in China*. Rochester, NY: University of Rochester Press.

Farquhar, Judith. 2002. *Appetites: Food and sex in post-socialist China*. Durham: Duke University Press.

Farquhar, Judith, and Qicheng Zhang. 2005. Biopolitical Beijing: Pleasure, sovereignty, and self-cultivation in China's capital. *Cultural Anthropology* 20 (3): 303–327.

Ferguson, James. 2009. The Uses of Neoliberalism. *Antipode* 41 (S1): 166–184.

Festa, Paul E. 2006. Mahjong politics in contemporary China: Civility, Chineseness, and mass culture. *Positions: East Asia Cultures Critique* 14 (1): 7–35.

Fewsmith, Joseph. 2008. 'Staying in Power: What does the Chinese Communist Party Have to do?' In *China's Changing Political Landscape: Prospects for Democracy*, edited by C. Li. 212–226. Washington, DC: Brookings Institution Press.

Foucault, Michel. 1972. *The Archaeology of Knowledge*. New York: Pantheon Books.

Foucault, Michel. 1980. *The History of Sexuality*. New York: Vintage.

Foucault, Michel. 1987. The Ethic of Care for the Self as a Practice of Freedom: An Interview with Michel Foucault on January 20, 1984 in The Final Foucault: Studies on Michel Foucault's Last Works. *Philosophy & Social Criticism* 12 (2–3): 112–131.

Foucault, Michel. 1991. 'Governmentality'. In *The Foucault Effect: Studies in Governmentality*, edited G. Burchell, C. Gordon, and P. Miller. Chicago: University of Chicago Press.

Fu, Wei, Shuli Zhao, Yuhui Zhang, Peipei Chai, and John Goss. 2018. Research in health policy making in China: Out-of-pocket payments in healthy China 2030. *BMJ* 360: k234.

Gao, Qiang (the Minister of the Ministry of Health). 2005. Developing medical and health work, making contribution to build a socialist harmonious society (Fazhan yiliao weisheng shiye, wei goujian shehuizhuyi hexieshehui zuo gongxian). *People's Net*. Retrieved April 13, 2011. http://politics.people.com.cn/GB/1027/3590082.html.

Gerring, John. 2007. *Case Study Research: Principles and Practices*. Cambridge, UK: Cambridge University Press.

Gordon, Colin. 1991. Governmental Rationality: An Introduction. In *The Foucault Effect: Studies in Governmentality*, edited G. Burchell, C. Gordon, and P. Miller. 1–52. Chicago: University of Chicago Press.

Greenhalgh, Susan. 2003. Planned births, unplanned persons: "Population" in the making of Chinese modernity. *American Ethnologist* 30 (2): 196–215.

Greenhalgh, Susan. 2009. The Chinese biopolitical facing the twenty-first century. *New Genetics and Society* 28 (3): 205–222.

Greenhalgh, Susan. 2011. Governing Chinese life: From sovereignty to biopolitical governance. In *Governance of Life in Chinese Moral Experience*, edited by E. Zhang, A. Kleinman, and W. Tu. 146–162. New York: Routledge.

Greenhalgh, Susan, and Edwin A. Winckler. 2005. *Governing China's Population: From Leninist to Neoliberal Biopolitics*. Stanford, CA: Stanford University Press.

Guangzhou Public Opinion Centre. 2010. *Guangzhou Annual Survey Report of the Public Evaluation on Personal Life Experience (2010)* (Guangzhou geren ganshou gongzhong pingjia niandu diaocha baogao 2010 nian). Retrieved February 7, 2011. http://www.gzporc.com/newsview.asp?cid=2andid=142.

Gu, Xin. 2008. *Towards Universal Coverage of Healthcare Insurance: The Strategic Choices and Institutional Frameworks of China's New Healthcare Reform* (Zouxiang quanmin yibao: zhongguo xin yigai de zhanlue yu zhanshu). Beijing: China Labour and Social Security Publishing House.

Gu, Xin. 2010. Public finance transformation and the retaking of government health funding responsibility (Gonggong caizheng zhuanxing yu zhengfu weisheng chouzi zeren de huigui). *Social Sciences in China (Zhongguo shehui kexue)* 2: 103–120.

Han, Chunping and Martin King Whyte. 2009. The Social Contours of Distributive Injustice Feelings in Contemporary China. In *Creating Wealth and Poverty in Postsocialist China*, edited by D. Davis and F. Wang, 193–212. Stanford, CA: Stanford University Press.

Hann, Chris and Keith Hart, eds. 2009. *Market and society: The Great Transformation Today*. Cambridge: Cambridge University Press.

Harvey, David. 2005. *A Brief History of Neoliberalism*. Oxford: Oxford University Press.

Henderson, Gail, and Myron Cohen. 1984. *The Chinese Hospital: A Socialist Work Unit*. New Haven, CT: Yale University Press.

Hesketh, Therese, Dan Wu, Linan Mao, and Nan Ma. 2012. Violence against doctors in China. *BMJ: British Medical Journal* 345. Retrieved August 10, 2013 (http://www.bmj.com/content/345/bmj.e5730).

Hoffman, Lisa. 2009. Governmental rationalities of environmental city-building in contemporary China. In *China's Governmentalities: Governing Change, Changing Government*, edited by E. Jeffreys. 120–137. London: Routledge.

Hu, Shanlian, Shenglan Tang, Yuanli Liu, Yuxin Zhao, Maria-Luisa Escobar, and David de Ferranti. 2008. Reform of how health care is paid for in China: Challenges and opportunities. *The Lancet* 372 (9652): 1846–1853.

Hu, Xiaojiang, Sarah Cook, and Miguel A. Salazar. 2008. Internal Migration and Health in China. *The Lancet* 372 (9651): 1717–1719.

Huang, Yanzhong. 2013. *Governing Health in Contemporary China*. New York: Routledge.

Huang, Xian. 2014. Expansion of Chinese social health insurance: Who gets what, when and how? *Journal of Contemporary China* 23 (89): 923–951.

Jeffreys, Elaine (ed.). 2009. *China's Governmentalities: Governing Change, Changing Government*. London: Routledge.

Joseph, Jonathan. 2009. Governmentality of what? Populations, states and international organisations. *Global Society* 23 (4): 413–427.

Joseph, Jonathan. 2012. *The Social in the Global: Social Theory, Governmentality and Global Politics*. Cambridge, UK: Cambridge University Press.

Keane, Michael. 1999. Television and civilization: The unity of opposites? *International Journal of Cultural Studies* 2 (2): 246–259.

Keane, Michael. 2001. Redefining Chinese citizenship. *Economy and Society* 30 (1): 1–17.

Kipnis, Andrew. 2008. Audit Cultures: Neoliberal Governmentality, Socialist Legacy, or Technologies of Governing? *American Ethnologist* 35 (2): 275–289.

Kleinman, Arthur. 1998. Experience and its moral modes: Culture, human conditions and disorder. In *The Tanner Lectures on Human Values*, edited by G. B. Peterson. 357–420. Salt Lake City: University of Utah Press.

Kleinman, Arthur. 2004. Ethics and experience: An anthropological approach to health equity. In *Public Health, Ethics, and Equity*, edited by S. Anand, F. Peter, and A. K. Sen. Oxford: Oxford University Press.

Kleinman, Arthur, 2007. *What really matters: Living a moral life amidst uncertainty and danger*. Oxford: Oxford University Press.

Kohrman, Matthew. 2004. Should I quit? Tobacco, fraught identity, and the risks of governmentality in Urban China. *Urban Anthropology and Studies of Cultural Systems and World Economic Development* 33 (2–4): 211–245.

Kohrman, Matthew. 2005. *Bodies of Difference: Experiences of Disability and Institutional Advocacy in the Making of Modern China*. Berkeley: University of California Press.

Kornreich, Yoel, Ilan Vertinsky, and Pitman B. Potter. 2012. Consultation and deliberation in China: The making of China's health-care reform. *China Journal* 68: 176–203.

Lee, Haiyan. 2006. Governmentality and the Aesthetic State: A Chinese Fantasia. *Positions* 14 (1): 100–129.

Lei, Zhichun and Jilu Jiang. 2006. How to build harmonious hospital and patient relation (Qiantan ruhe goujian hexie yihuan guanxi). *Chinese Hospitals (Zhongguo Yiyuan)* 10 (11): 74–75.

Li, He. 2010. Debating China's economic reform: New leftists versus liberals. *Journal of Chinese Political Science* 15 (1): 1–23.

Lim, Meng-Kin, Hui Yang, Tuohong Zhang, Zijun Zhou, Wen Feng, and Yude Chen. 2004. China's evolving health care market: How doctors feel and what they think. *Health Policy* 69 (3): 329–337.

Liu, Yuanli, Keqin Rao, Jing Wu, and Emmanuela Gakidou. 2008. China's health system performance. *The Lancet* 372 (9653): 1914–1923.

Milcent, Carine. 2016. Evolution of the health system: Inefficiency, violence, and digital healthcare. *China Perspectives* (2016/4): 39–50.

Milcent, Carine. 2018. *Healthcare reform in China: From violence to digital healthcare*. Springer.

Ong, Aihwa. 1999. Clash of civilizations or Asia liberalism? An Anthropology of the State and Citizenship. In *Anthropological Theory Today*, edited by H. L. Moore. 48–72. Cambridge: Polity Press.

Ong, Aihwa and Li Zhang. 2008. Introduction: Privatizing China: Powers of the self, socialism from Afar. In *Privatizing China: Socialism from Afar*. 1–20. Ithaca, NY: Cornell University Press.

Oxfeld, Ellen. 2010. *Drink Water, but Remember the Source: Moral Discourse in a Chinese Village*. Berkeley: University of California Press.

People's Net. 2005. *China's Healthcare Reforms Violate the Basic Rules of Healthcare Development* (Zhongguo yigai weibei le weisheng shiye fazhan jiben guilv). Retrieved September 12, 2012. http://www.people.com.cn/GB/news/37454/37462/3445267.html.

People's Net. 2011. *National Bureau of Statistics: The National per Capita Disposable Income of Urban Residents Increased by 7.8% in 2010* (Guojia tongjiju: 2010 nian quanguo chengzhen jumin renjun kezhipei shouru zeng 7.8%). Retrieved January 10, 2013. http://politics.people. com.cn/GB/1026/14026625.html.

Perry, Elizabeth. 2013. *Cultural Governance in Contemporary China: "Re-Orienting" Party Propaganda.* Harvard-Yenching Institute Working Paper Series. Retrieved January 11, 2014. http://www.harvard-yenching.org/sites/harvard-yenching.org/files/featurefiles/Elizabeth% 20Perry_Cultural%20Governance%20in%20Contemporary%20China_0.pdf.

Pieke, Fank. 2009. *The good communist: Elite training and state building in today's China.* Cambridge, UK: Cambridge University Press.

Powell, Jason, and Ian Cook. 2000. "A Tiger Behind, and Coming Up Fast": Governmentality and the Politics of Population Control in China. *Journal of Aging and Identity* 5 (2): 79–89.

Ren, Hai. 2010. *Neoliberalism and Culture in China and Hong Kong: The Countdown of Time.* London: Routledge.

Rogaski, Ruth. 2004. *Hygienic Modernity: Meanings of Health and Disease in Treaty-Port China.* Berkeley: University of California Press.

Rose, Nikolas. 1999. *Powers of Freedom: Reframing Political Thought.* Cambridge, UK: Cambridge University Press.

ScienceNet. 2012. *Murder in Harbin Medical University Hospital, an Intern was Killed* (Hayida yiyuan fasheng xuean, yi shuoshi shixiyihseng bei kansi). Retrieved March 27, 2012. http:// news.sciencenet.cn/htmlnews/2012/3/261751.shtm.

Scott, Joan W. 1991. The Evidence of Experience. *Critical Inquiry* 17 (4): 773–797.

Shore, Cris and Susan Wright. 1997. Policy: A new field of anthropology. In *Anthropology of Policy: Critical Perspectives on Governance and Power,* edited by C. Shore and S. Wright. 3– 42. New York: Routledge Press.

Sigley, Gary. 1996. Governing Chinese bodies: The significance of studies in the concept of govermentality for the analysis of government in China. *Economy and Society* 25 (4): 457–482.

Sigley, Gary. 2006. Chinese governmentalities: Government, governance and the socialist market economy. *Economy and Society* 35 (4): 487–508.

Sina. 2007. *China's Healthcare Reform: Why Doctors Keep Silent?* (Zhogguo yigai: yisheng weihe chenmo). Retrieved 14 January, 2011 http://news.sina.com.cn/c/2007-12-05/ 135914455943.shtml.

Sina. 2012. *Survey Shows 60% People Feel "Happy" for the Killing Incident in Harbin Medical University Hospital* (Diaocha cheng 6 cheng minzhong dui hayida shayian 'gaoxing'). Retrieved March 27, 2012. http://finance.chinanews.com/jk/2012/03-27/3775529.shtml.

Thornton, Patricia M. 2007. *Disciplining the State: Virtue, Violence, and State-Making in Modern China.* Cambridge, MA: Harvard University Press.

Tu, Weiming. 2001. The ecological turn in new confucian humanism: Implications for China and the world. *Daedalus* 130 (4): 243–264.

Tu, Jiong. 2010. Privatisation of Health Care in Transitional China: A Study of Private Clinics at the County Level. Master thesis, Tema Health and Society, Linköping University. Retrieved April 7, 2013.

Vickers, Edward. 2009. Selling "socialism with Chinese characteristics" "thought and politics" and the Legitimisation of China's developmental strategy. *International Journal of Educational Development* 29 (5): 523–531.

Wang, Chaojun. 2008. Less than 40% peasants satisfied with health care (Nongmin kanbing manyidu buzu sicheng). *Chinese Health (Zhongguo Weisheng)* 1: 65.

Wang, Shaoguang. 2013. Making clear about the advantage of the Chinese system to avoid being fooled (Zhongguo tizhi de youshi yao jiangtou, yimian bei huyou). *Huanqiu.* Retrieved December 28, 2013. http://opinion.huanqiu.com/opinion_china/2013-08/4303248.html.

Wang, Shaoguang and Peng Fan. 2013. *The Chinese model of consensus decision-making: A case study of health reform* (Zhongguo shi gongshi xin juece). Beijing: China Renmin University Press.

Wong, Linda. 2010. *Mending the Chinese Welfare Net: Tool for Social Harmony or Regime Stability?* Paper presented on 7th EASP Conference: Searching for New Policy Paradigms in East Asia: Initiatives, Ideas and Debates. Retrieved 13 April, 2011 (http://7th.welfareasia.org/2010/08/mending-the-chinese-welfare-net-tool-for-social-harmony-or-regime-stability.html).

World Health Organisation. 2010. *World Health Report 2000*. Retrieved December 20, 2010. http://www.who.int/whr/2000/en/.

Wu, Ximing and Jeffrey M. Perloff. 2004. *China's Income Distribution over Time: Reasons for Rising Inequality*. Publication for Department of Agricultural & Resource Economics, UCB. Retrieved December 12, 2013. https://escholarship.org/uc/item/166747gz#page-1.

Xinhua Net. 2013a. *Huang Jiefu, Vice Minister of the Ministry of Health, Answer the "Ten Questions to Minister"* (Weishengbu fubuzhang Huang Jiefu weiyuan huida 'Shiwen buzhang'). Retrieved March 7, 2013. http://news.xinhuanet.com/2013lh/2013-03/07/c_114937378.htm.

Xinhua Net. 2013b. *11 Departments will jointly Carry out a Special Task to Fight Medically-related Illegal and Criminal Actions* (Woguo 11 ge bumen jiang lianhe kaizhan daji sheyi weifa fanzui zhuanxiang xingdong). Retrieved March 25, 2014. http://news.xinhuanet.com/2013-12/20/c_125893851.htm.

Xinhua Net. 2013c. *Man unable to Pay Medical Fee, Cut Off His own Right Leg* (Nanzi youbing wuqian zhi zi ju huanbing youtui). Retrieved May 22, 2014. http://news.xinhuanet.com/health/2013-10/11/c_125511492.htm.

Xinhua Net. 2013d. *"Only 10% Patients Trusted in Doctors" is a Serious Warning* (Jin 10% huanzhe xinren yisheng shi ji chenzhong jingzhong). Retrieved August 26, 2013. http://news.xinhuanet.com/health/2013-03/11/c_124442435.htm.

Xinhua Net. 2013e. *Xi Jinping Explain "China Dream"* (Xi Jinping zongshuji chanshi 'zhongguomeng'). Retrieved December 12, 2013. http://news.youth.cn/gn/201303/t20130317_2988865.htm.

Yan, Hairong. 2003. Neoliberal governmentality and neohumanism: Organizing Suzhi/value flow through labor recruitment networks. *Cultural Anthropology* 18 (4): 493–523.

Yan, Yunxiang. 2004. Native anthropologist, longitudinal fieldwork, and experience-near ethnography. In *New Reflections on Anthropological Studies of (Greater) China*, edited by X. Liu. 204–213. Berkeley: Institute of East Asian Studies, University of California Press.

Yang, Mayfair Mei-hui. 1989. The gift economy and state power in China. *Comparative Studies in Society and History* 31 (1): 25–54.

Yang, Jingqing. 2008. *The Power Relationships between Doctors, Patients and the Party-state under the Impact of Red Packets in the Chinese Health-care System*. PhD dissertation, Department of Social Science and International Studies, University of New South Wales. Retrieved April 9, 2010. http://handle.unsw.edu.au/1959.4/43116.

Yang, Mayfair Mei-hui. 2011. Postcoloniality and Religiosity in Modern China: The Disenchantments of Sovereignty. *Theory, Culture & Society* 28 (2): 3–44.

Yin, Robert K. 2003. *Case Study Research: Design and Methods*. London: Sage.

Yip, Winnie Chi-Man and William C. Hsiao. 2008. The Chinese Health System at a Crossroads. *Health Affairs* 27 (2): 460–68.

Zhang, Everett Yuehong. 2011. Governmentality in China. In *Governance of Life in Chinese Moral Experience: The Quest for an Adequate Life*, edited by E. Zhang, A. Kleinman, and W. Tu. 1–30. London: Routledge.

Zhou, Xu Dong, Lu Li, and Therese Hesketh. 2014. Health system reform in rural China: voices of healthworkers and service-users. *Social Science & Medicine* 117: 134-141.

Zhou, Zijun, Mingjian Lin, Hui Yang, Tuohong Zhang, Wen Feng, and Yude Chen. 2003. Investigation on satisfactory degree of doctors in parts of cities (Bufen shengshi yisheng manyidu diaocha). *Chinese Hospital Management (Zhongguo Yiyuan Guanli)* 23 (5): 3–6.

Zhu, Hengpeng. 2018. After eight years health reform, do you have a "sense of gain"? (*yigai banian, ni you huodegan ma?*). *Caixin Net*. Retrieved March 12, 2018. http://m.opinion.caixin.com/m/2018-02-09/101209601.html.

Chapter 2
Rescue First or Money First? Commercialised Institutions, Calculating Professionals, and Neoliberal Governance

One afternoon, in Dayu Town, I was chatting to a few local residents in the main street. Suddenly, people began to gather in front of a teashop run by an old couple. The news quickly spread that the old lady had collapsed at home and was unconscious, so the neighbours had dialled 120 (the emergency service). I joined the many neighbours waiting on the street outside the teashop. Shortly afterwards, an ambulance arrived, and the doctor and nurse went inside. Around 20 min later, the doctor and nurse emerged, and informed the old man that his wife had died. He appeared shocked by her sudden death. Sitting at the reception desk, he began to ring his adult children. His neighbours began to organise the immediate death rituals: someone was sent to buy spirit money,[1] candles and incense; some went to fetch hot water to wash the body; and others went to prepare clothes in which to dress the body. The doctor fetched a form from the ambulance, and came to the neighbours standing outside the teashop to ask information about the deceased, but the neighbours focused on the imperative death rituals, responding to her only occasionally. For a few minutes, the doctor and nurse, waiting beside the ambulance outside the teashop, seemed to be forgotten. The doctor then took the form into the teashop to look for someone to fill it in and pay the fee, but returned with an empty form. Walking back to the ambulance, she shouted very angrily at the neighbours outside the teashop: 'We're leaving now. You wouldn't respond to us. If, later, you can't get a death certificate, it's your fault, not ours'. With these words, she got into the ambulance and slammed the door. Two neighbours quickly approached the ambulance and pleaded with the doctor: 'Please understand [the situation]. The couple's children are elsewhere. Only the old man's here. He's on the phone now. We're just neighbours trying to help out'. The doctor then informed them that there was a 98 Yuan (about £10) fee to be paid, and asked whether it would be paid then or later. The neighbours glanced towards the old man who was

---

[1]Spirit money, also called ghost money (*zhiqian*, *mingqian*), is the paper representation of real money, used as burnt offering to the dead soul to use in another world of the afterlife.

J. Tu, *Health Care Transformation in Contemporary China*,
https://doi.org/10.1007/978-981-13-0788-1_2

still on the phone and then told the doctor that the deceased's family would pay it later. Thereupon, the ambulance departed immediately (From field notes on 1 February, 2012).

In China, patients must pay for emergency services. The emergency medical service (EMS) system comprises three sectors: the pre-hospital emergency service, the in-hospital emergency department and the intensive care unit (Hung et al. 2009). Theoretically, the emergency service is a non-profit undertaking, established and funded by the government (the provincial and city bureau of public health) (Dai et al. 2003; Hung et al. 2009), but, in practice, private payments are becoming an increasingly important source of funding for the daily operations of the EMS due to a lack of finance from the government. The daily operational fees (covering ambulances, emergency treatment, and labour) are collected from the patients. Sometimes, the decisions regarding the dispatch of an ambulance or acceptance of emergency patients are based on the patients' ability to pay. The locals told me various stories about ambulances leaving patients unattended after hearing that they were unable to pay, and patients without money being left to die in hospital. The media regularly reports that emergency doctors are being attacked by angry patients because of medical charges (see, for instance, People's Net 2013). Patients and their families who face sudden illness or death are often in shock and agony. Hearing a demand for a fee, they can feel that the doctors are ruthless and some family members even become outraged. People frequently compare the high charge for 120 (the first aid service) with the free 110 (police) and 119 (fire) services, and feel increasingly dissatisfied with the first aid service, but the first aid charge for doctors is also a troubling issue. In Riverside, the emergency services are provided and managed by the nearby public hospitals in terms of both pre- and in-hospital emergency care.[2] The ambulances are staffed by medical workers from the hospital. In the market era, public hospitals are being asked to become self-sufficient with reduced state investment. Hospital services have inevitably become the target for cost-benefit calculations. The first-aid service involves the use of ambulances, petrol, and equipment, together with the costs associated with health professionals and drivers. If an ambulance is called out in the evening, this will also incur overtime payments. All of these costs are transferred to the patients. In the above case, the emergency doctor, after the rescue effort, needed to find the family to pay the fee, who however were in shock and agony, and were busy attending to the immediate death rituals. The doctor was angry not only that people were ignoring her, but also about the procedure whereby she was compelled to request payment. This endangers the integrity of doctors, who must change from being a life saver one minute to being a money demander the next.

---

[2]Generally there are five different models of emergency services in China: independent emergency service centre, pre-hospital emergency services without in-patient beds, pre-hospital emergency service supported by a general hospital, unified communication command centre with pre-hospital emergency care to be handled by different hospitals, and three-level emergency service network in small cities (Dai et al. 2003). Different places have their own model. In Riverside County, emergency services are provided by general hospitals.

This chapter explores the 'rescue first or money first' dilemma of Chinese doctors and the frequent occurrence of 'letting die' incidents in the Chinese health sector. It traces these problems to the market transformation of the Chinese health sector and the neoliberal transition of governance. It explores how these transformations shape the operations of the medical institutions and the conduct of health professionals in accordance with market logic, how hospitals and doctors confront moral dilemma and navigate through the differing or even opposing requirements of the recent healthcare reforms, and the power configuration of the state, the local authorities, hospitals, health administrators and professionals in the neoliberal change.

2.1 Rescue First or Money First?

2.1.1 Troubling Emergency Treatment

One afternoon, in the emergency department of TCM Hospital, I was chatting with Xiao Luo, an old friend and an emergency doctor, when an ambulance arriving with a male patient and his wife. The patient, lying on a stretcher, was brought out of the ambulance and left in the corridor outside the consulting room. The doctor from the ambulance invited the patient's wife to follow him into the consulting room. Several minutes later, the middle-aged woman came out the consulting room. She was on her mobile, asking the person she had rung to bring several thousand Yuan to the hospital immediately. She then rang someone else, asking to borrow 1000 Yuan. All this time, the patient was left in the corridor, unattended. In recent years, there have been many sensational media reports about patients being left in hospital without treatment until they have paid a fee (See reports like Xinhua Net 2003a; People's Net 2012). Yet, when I witnessed it myself, I was still shocked. I asked Xiao Luo why the 'emergency' patient was left there, and he explained calmly that, if the patient's condition was stable, they would ask the family to register for hospitalisation (by paying a deposit) first to avoid fee evasion (*taofei*). Xiao Luo further explained that, although charging money was not a doctor's business, the doctor in charge would be fined if the patient evaded the medical bill. Emphasising the pressure that doctors are under, Xiao Luo added that they would still provide basic treatment for seriously-ill patients even if they were unable to pay for it at that time. He told me that, in the Intensive Care Unit, a patient who had been badly injured in a fight had been treated for several days although the hospital had not received a penny from him (From field notes on 6 February 2012).

Facing high medical charges, patients sometimes evade their medical bills after treatment. Before the 1980s, the government took on most of the financial burden of the public hospitals, and would cover their annual deficit at the end of each year. Following the market reform, the public hospitals were asked to become self-sufficient. When patients evaded medical bills, the hospitals would suffer the loss, without receiving compensation from any party. In this situation, the cost of the services became the focus of intense scrutiny and hospitals transferred the pressure of securing up-front payments to the health professionals. If patients evaded medical bills, the doctors who treated them could be punished. In response, doctors demand that patients pay a sum of money in order to be admitted to hospital. Patients and their family are even threatened that the treatment will only start or continue once cash has been paid up-front. Even for people with insurance, reimbursement follows the treatment, so they too are required to pay a large sum of money in advance first. This easily leads to people feeling that hospitals and health professionals are unrelenting.

During interviews, the locals frequently question why the emergency departments are open 24 h a day, 364 days a year, but fail to help patients in an emergency, why 120 ambulances fly around the county but refuse to take certain patients. They feel that they are being betrayed by the 'helping' professionals and hospitals. Complaining about health care today, the locals frequently brought up the Maoist past when doctors were kind and gentle and hospitals were not profit-centred. The locals generally recounted that, during Mao's era, one could be treated in hospital for a small fee or be treated first and pay later, but now patients must pay a large sum in advance of their treatment. The contrast between 'rescue first' and 'money first' has become one of the key differences between health care in the collective era and that today, according to people's accounts. Health care in the collective era, although of low quality, was remembered as being provided by dedicated doctors. Doctors tried to save patients and frequently acted heroically, according to people's memories. In the post-reform era, patients have become increasingly disillusioned and sceptical about medical professionals who are regarded as putting profit above the patients' interests. The hospitals are also regarded as being profit-motivated rather than patient-centred. The frequent occurrence of 'letting patient die' incidents encroach on people's moral economy, and violate universal medical ethics and the socialist ideology of 'serving the people'. The taken-for-granted concepts of 'help' and 'rescue' are increasingly being questioned, which increases people's senses of uncertainty, insecurity and dread.

2.1.2   Unpaid Debts in the Post-reform Era: The Bankruptcy of the Credit System

However, the contrast between the 'rescue first' of the past and the 'money first' of today in people's accounts has been a gradual transition rather than a radical change. It involves intense negotiations between patients, health professionals, and medical institutions in a changing institutional environment over the past decades.

In the 70s, 80s, and even early 90s, the local public hospitals continually allowed poor patients to be treated first and pay the hospital later. The hospitals regularly sent staff to reclaim the debts from the patients. Doctor He, a retired doctor, in her late 60s, recalled collecting debts in the late 1970s:

> When I was studying at the People's Hospital for a few years, every year, when the peasants harvested the cotton, we were sent to reclaim the debts. I visited many towns and villages; how difficult life was in those villages! For the very poorest families, if they couldn't repay the money, we asked them to give us proof, a note from their production team, brigade, or commune [all signed], and we took this note back to the hospital to redeem our mission, and then this family's debt was cleared. (Interview P45)

Normally, after several efforts to reclaim the debt, if people were still unable to repay the money, the hospital would wipe off the debt. In the collective era, the work unit, production team, brigade or commune acted as guarantors for patients, and would pressurise them to repay the money. Through the intermediate role of these collectives, the creditor hospitals had some means of recovering the money from the debtor patients, but these 'insurer' institutions were either dissolved or ceased functioning during the market era. Besides, in the post-reform era, the rural insurance scheme was basically dismantled. In the urban area, many workers were laid off from their work unit and were increasingly excluded from the insurance system (see Chap. 4). Without insurance as a guarantee, the mutual obligation and trust between the creditor hospital and the debtor patients were further endangered.

Since the 1990s, when the public hospitals were asked to become self-sufficient or manage with greatly-reduced state investment (in terms of total hospital expenditure), the debt became a heavy burden for public hospitals. In Riverside, hospitals put pressure on their staff to collect the debts. Unless they reclaimed the money, some hospital staff were punished, such as the former accountant of the People's Hospital, who had been in charge of approving debts and was responsible for recovering the money afterwards. When many debts failed to be claimed in the early 1990s, he was sacked. Mrs Zhao, a 78-year-old local resident, vividly recalled the accountant's efforts to collect debts from patients, which however were mostly in vain:

> That year, the accountant went here and there, chasing people, asking them to pay. I met him on the way and asked him: 'What's the point going to these places to claim money? If the peasants don't have any money, they can't pay you back. If they do, they still might not pay you, but continue to live in debt'. That was many years ago, in the 90s… Now, the hospital won't treat you unless you pay…No matter how loud you [the patient] cry [in the hospital], you still need to pay the fee first and then get the medication. (Interview P41)

The hospital accountant encountered great difficulties in collecting the payments and was punished for causing bad debts. Under the market pressure, hospitals changed their strategy. They no longer allowed patients to be indebted to them, but demanded that they pay for all treatment in advance. While the patients attributed this change to the erosion of the socialist spirit, the hospitals justified it as a result of the market reform. People like Mrs. Zhao, who witnessed the difficulty associated with debt collection, displayed a more sympathetic attitude towards the changes in hospitals. Demanding a deposit before treatment has become the best measure to avoid financial loss and has been widely-adopted by almost every hospital in Riverside County since the 1990s.

2.1.3 To Save or Let Die? The Doctor's Dilemma

To save or let die is a problem that is constantly confronted by Chinese doctors. In Riverside, the unspoken rule about medical intervention has been based on informed consent. The 'Medical Institution Administration Ordinance' (CPG 2005a) regulates that medical institutions should rescue emergency patients instantly, but it also notes that 'medical institutions have to obtain the patient's consent before surgery, special tests or other specific treatment; if the patient's opinion cannot be obtained, the consent and signature of the patient's family or other relevant person should be obtained; if the patient, their family and other relevant persons' opinions cannot be obtained, or in other special circumstances, treatment should be provided following approval by the person in charge of the medical institution' (Article 33). The Tort Law of the PRC came into force in 2010 specifies the 'Liability of Medical Malpractice'. Article 56 denotes that 'where the opinion of a patient or his close relative cannot be obtained in the case of emergency, corresponding medical measures may be carried out immediately after the approval from the person in charge of the medical institution or another authorised personnel' (CPG 2009). Under these regulations, if a patient is alone without clear consciousness and is in danger, emergency care should be provided immediately with the approval of the hospital administrators; however, if a patient's family decides to abandon the treatment or the patient is conscious and decides to stop the treatment, the health professionals might not intervene. The latter situation normally involves patients with hopeless conditions who have already spent a large amount of money.

In actual hospital practice, however, if an emergency patient arrives at hospital alone, the first thing the hospital staff do is to contact the family; if the patient's family cannot be contacted, the question of whether treatment will be offered or not will be decided after taking instruction from the hospital management, whose primary focus might be to avoid losing money. Patients, who arrive at hospital alone and do not have cash up front, possess little 'negotiation power' in the face of the hospital's strict rules that require patients to pay money first. They are at the mercy of individual health professionals, who at best might supply basic emergency treatment (such as stopping bleeding, stitching a wound) without further instruction from the hospital administrators. In this process, the treatment of patients in critical conditions is easily delayed.

A well-known incident occurred in 2012 when a migrant worker was left to die under a bridge, a spot where many migrant workers camped at night in Henan

Province (China News 2012). The migrant worker had been ill for more than 20 days. A few days before his death, people called an ambulance. The emergency doctor came and examined him, found that his symptoms were normal, but asked him to go to the hospital for further checks. The patient refused. The doctor discovered that the patient had not eaten for two days. The doctor took some money out of her own pocket and asked another migrant worker to buy some food and drink for the patient. The ambulance then left, leaving the patient untreated. The worker died a few days later. In this case, the treatment decision was based on informed consent. The migrant worker was conscious and had refused to go to hospital, so the ambulance left him. The doctor did not do anything wrong according to the hospital regulations, and even showed kindness in taking money out of her own pocket, but her altruistic action was constrained by the hospital rules. The rescue decision that was once under the jurisdiction of health professionals is now increasingly under the scrutiny of hospital administrators whose primary focus is to avoid losing money. Individual doctors face the painful dilemma of choosing between rescue and self-protection. If they save a patient, if that patient fails to pay the fees, they could be held responsible for the hospital's loss but, if they do not rescue the patient, they violate their professional integrity and face criticism from the patient's family.

Many of the Chinese doctors I encountered demonstrated sincere sympathy for patients. However, they felt powerless to change anything: 'What else can we do? … We also sympathise with patients, but the expenditure of the hospital is enormous, and the investment in these new building and new equipment needs to be earned back' (Interview D5), a local doctor reasoned. The doctors were criticised by the patients for focusing more on making money than caring about the patients' needs. The doctors defended themselves, saying they had no choice. They are hired to serve the interests of the hospital. Their work is judged within the paradigm of market logic, which frequently conflicts with the patients' interests. Their daily medical practices involve ambivalence and contradictions that constantly trouble Chinese doctors. Doctors have to make 'fateful' decisions in stressful, uncertain environments, and the economic considerations at critical moments make this situation even more difficult. The principles of patient autonomy and informed consent, newly-promoted in the market era, thus become the arbiters of the dilemmas encountered by the doctors. In the process, the principles which are designed to protect patients' rights and autonomy become the rationales employed by the medical institutions and practitioners to avoid treatment that may lead to possible economic loss (Fig. 2.1).[3]

---

[3]Cooper (2011b) also shows that the informed consent contract in medical trial effectively serves as a means of limiting the patients' right to litigation in the event of a medical accident, because patients are regarded as a fully informed, responsible bearer of risk, who give up further rights to litigation.

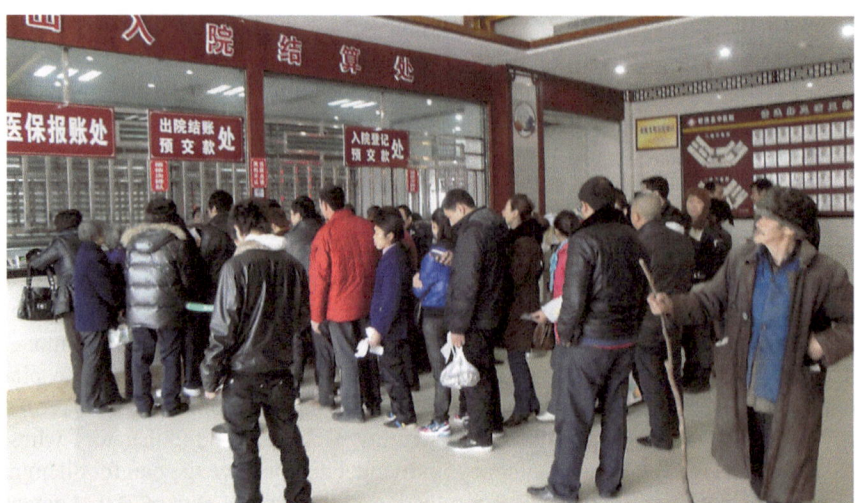

Fig. 2.1 A hospital's cashier window

2.2   Commercialised Institution, Calculative Subjects, and Neoliberal Governance

2.2.1   *Ambiguous Characteristics of Public Hospitals*

The health professionals' dilemmas originated from the ambiguous characteristics of Chinese hospitals. Institutions in China are broadly divided into public-service organisations (*shiye danwei*), enterprises (*qiye*), government administrative institutions (*zhengfu jiguan*) and social groups (*shehui tuanti*). The majority of public hospitals are public-service organisations, which are defined as 'for social welfare purpose, governments or other organisations use state-owned assets to set up social service organisations to take education, science, culture and health activities' (MOT 2008). The public-service organisation originated from the planned system that the government employed for the founding, function and personnel of public-service organisations, and directly administered their activities. According to this arrangement, public hospitals should be state-funded, whereby the state pays the salary of their employees, is responsible for their staff's insurance and welfare, and funds their daily operations.

However, the market reform changed the situation so that the funding of many public-service organisations was greatly reduced. Later, the public-service organisations were divided into three categories: fully state-funded, partly state-funded, and self-funded. Most public hospitals were categorised as partly-funded organisations that the state contributed only a small proportion of their funding; some public hospitals were almost entirely self-funded. In 1978, the central government paid 32% of the national medical costs, the number reduced to 25% by 1990 and

15% in 2002 (Duckett 2007; Hui 2010). The fiscal decentralisation caused the financial subsidies for public medical institutions to be transferred from the central to local levels of government, while the local government also reduced its contribution. In the local People's Hospital, the administrators informed me that they had received a meagre funding of 700,000 Yuan per year from the local government in the past few years. This amount had decreased to about 300,000 Yuan by 2012. Compared with the hospital's actual expenditure and income, this left the hospital almost entirely self-financed. In the municipal hospital, a higher level hospital above Riverside County, the administrator stated:

> We've over 1600 current staff, over 300 retirees, the salaries, subsidies, bonuses and insurance our hospital pays annually [to its staff members] are over a hundred million Yuan. But the state allocates us just over two million Yuan a year. We are called a 'partly-funded' work unit, not fully funded…But this two million is not even enough to cover our [annual] basic expenditure on water, gas, electricity… (Interview 40)

This situation is similar for many other public hospitals in China. In 2006, 93.6% of the income of the general hospitals under the Ministry of Health was obtained via patients rather than government subsidies (Transition Institute 2011).

The management of these hospitals, nevertheless, continues to follow the mode in the planned system that the governments control the public hospitals' service prices, personnel, assets and functions. To maintain the availability of health services to the general public, the state keeps the prices of these services below the actual costs. Instead, public hospitals are given operational autonomy to self-finance. They are allowed to charge a 15% premium for services that employ new diagnostic technologies, and a 15–25% premium for imported drugs and Chinese medication (Hsiao 1995: 1051–1052). Hospitals and health professionals are motivated to increase profits by over-prescribing drugs and tests, and increasing the profit margin by prescribing expensive medicines and high-technology services. Data from 2001 to 2007 show that the income from drugs has become the main source of finance for Chinese hospitals, constituting between 50 and 60% of out-patient medical expenses and 40 to 50% of inpatient expenses (Urio 2010: 148). This leads to the so-called 'selling medicine to sustain healthcare/hospital/health professionals' (*yiyao yangyi*). These revenue-generating activities caused the health care expenditure to grow by 16% annually over the past two decades, which is 7% faster than the average GDP growth (Yip et al. 2010: 1121). The general health care costs have increased at a rate far exceeding the increase in people's average income (Gu 2008: 47). A local hospital director justified their profit-generating activities as follows:

> Our medical devices and products are bought at the market price, while our medical charges are regulated under the planned system. The planned system means that our health service prices are far below the actual costs. The CPI [consumer price index] increased very fast while our service price was at about the same level over the years. The hospital is actually in deficit, and we have to make up the deficit from other channels. (Interview 47)

The hospital director pointed out the key issue in current health system: the provision of pharmaceutical products has been completely marketised, while the provision of health services is still under administrative control following the time of planned economy. When the pharmaceutical products are priced according to the market principle, health services are fixed at extremely low price by the government as public welfare products. The 'policy deficit' therefore forces hospitals to adopt 'other channels' to make money, such as the over-prescription of expensive medicines and profitable tests. Hospitals need to find a balance between preserving their public service nature and chasing profit. Local hospital administrators admitted that their profit-making practices led to a rising burden for patients, but they asked: 'Where can we get the money to sustain this [hospital] expenditure? If not from the patients, where can we get the money?' (Interview 40) Many of my respondents admitted that, in this context, refusing patients who were unable to pay become an unspoken rule in public hospitals that are trying to avoid any possible losses.

2.2.2   Corporatisation of Hospitals

In the market, public hospitals increasingly operate on a commercial basis. A hospital is like a company, the patients are the customers, the doctors are the employees (and even salespersons promoting medical products to patients), the hospital head is the CEO of the company, and the medical services are the commercial products. The hospital directors whom I interviewed in Riverside County gave me similar metaphors. They regarded their role as similar to that of the president of a company, as they needed to manage their hospital in an increasingly entrepreneurial manner by carefully calculating the income, expenditure, investment and returns. The hospital administrators recited in detail their patient increase rate, income growth rate, annual surgery figure, etc., which for them could best demonstrate the improvements that had taken place in their hospital. It is not uncommon to find huge posters in Chinese hospitals celebrating their achievements: 'congratulate our hospital becoming x level hospital', 'the inpatient number in our hospital reached xx (number)', 'celebrate the completion of the new hospital building', 'celebrate the installation of an MRI machine in our hospital', etc. These posters, displayed outside the hospital building, at the hospital entrance, and on the hospital walls, reflect the reigning development ideology. Development means the expansion of the hospital infrastructure, the upgrade of the hospital's level, an increase in patient numbers, and a rise in the hospital's gross income. The scientific management of a hospital includes increasing the investment in the infrastructure, buying new equipment, adopting high-tech treatments, and improving the hospital's efficiency and economic performance. Since the 2009 new healthcare reform, there have been rising health care demands. The willingness of local hospitals to expand and upgrade has become more imperative. During my fieldwork, the People's Hospital had been constructing a new 12-storey building which was completed and has been in use since 2013. The TCM Hospital moved into a new 11-storey building in 2010 and was planning to build another. Both hospitals began to build sub-hospitals on the outskirts of the city, invested heavily in new equipment and recruited highly-skilled professionals. Both devoted great efforts to apply to become a 3-B (Grade 3 Class B) hospital on top of their current 2-A level.[4] The upgrade in the hospital's level means more state investment, higher charges for medical services, and correspondingly greater profits. Fancying a vision of efficiency, economic effectiveness, and high technology, the entrepreneurial hospital leaders were determined to help their hospitals to develop to a higher level.

As hospital directors in the market era, whose institutions gain limited funding from the state and whose performance is evaluated in terms of hard economic figures, they are forced to become entrepreneurs to operate their hospital like a company. Without profit, the hospital cannot buy new equipment, retain top class professionals, or attract patients. Yet, hospital directors also actively become 'entrepreneurs' in the market, where success in making their hospital profitable represents their personal ability, achievement, and 'worthiness' in the market era.

Although official slogans, such as 'serving the people' and 'safeguarding people's health', are still displayed on hospital walls and around the city (see Fig. 2.2), the hospital management has already been replaced by a new set of market rules. Hospitals charge for every possible item, including those beyond medical services: (inpatient) bedding fees, (the use of) a chair, a washbasin, a towel, bike and car parking services, etc. The business has expanded beyond the hospital walls. A well-developed business circle surrounds a hospital, including gift shops, chemists, funeral services, restaurants, retail stores, hotels (for patients' relatives), etc., many of which include the involvement of the hospital administration. The good businesses surrounding public hospitals make the housing costs around the two biggest county hospitals in Riverside several times higher than those in other parts of the city.[5]

When asked about the conflict between the high medical charges by hospitals and the target of reducing medical costs under the new healthcare reform, a local hospital head simply stated that the medical costs are not that high in the light of

---

[4]Chinese hospitals are classified into three grades (Grade 1, 2 and 3), with three classes—A, B and C—in each grade. The Grade 1 Class C (1-C) is the lowest level, while the Grade 3 Class A (3-A) is the highest. The level determines the recourses and subsidies a hospital can get from the state, the medical prices of a hospital's services, etc. The hospital classification has recently caused many controversies. Many hospitals are criticised of competitively chasing higher classification without considering the actual needs of local society. In 2012, the Ministry of Health stopped to grant top level classification to hospitals and claimed back the licences it had already granted to some hospitals that year.

[5]I accidentally got information about the high rent of shops around the county hospitals when interviewing hospital administrators about medical disputes. In one medical dispute, the case was complicated by the financial dispute between the patient's family and the hospital for renting a grocery store outside this hospital. Many properties around the hospital belonged to the hospital, the hospital administration rented out these shops to generate profits for the hospital. The patient's family had rented a store outside the hospital for years, but when the contract expired, the hospital administration would not continue the contract with them, in order to rent the store at higher price to someone else. This financial dispute further complicated the medical dispute which already existed. Later I further checked the housing costs around the two county hospitals with other informants.

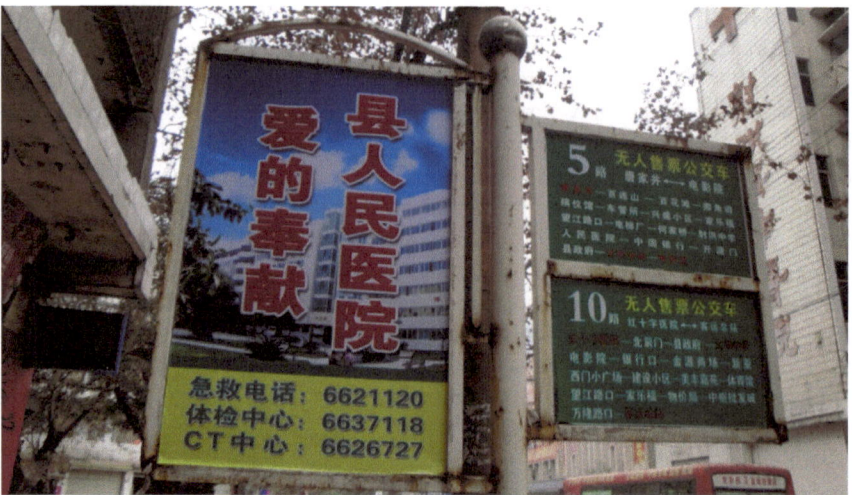

Fig. 2.2 'The people's hospital: love and dedication'—hospital advert at a bus stop

China's high economic growth. He indicated that expensive medical fees were people's psychological perception, influenced by media reports. 'The media influence [the public]. The government and [non-medical] intellectuals talk on TV about "getting high quality care for the cheapest price"; that's rubbish!' (Interview D52) The hospital head then recounted in a nostalgic tone: 'In the 90s the simple measure of marketization enabled our hospital to develop quickly'. His 'ideal free market' is where the hospitals can follow the market rule to maximise profit without intervention by the state. He believed that this would better serve the market needs, and so correspondingly, the needs of patients-consumers. In the last 30 years of the market reform, public hospitals above the county level have accumulated a large amount of wealth, albeit they have lost most of their state investment. In reference to health insurance and other welfare programmes that have been initiated by the state in recent new reforms, this hospital leader expressed his disagreement:

> If we continue the reform like this, the state may even go bankrupt. What will we do if all the money is used up? [JT: but many people at the bottom feel satisfied with these welfare programmes.] Yes, peasants are satisfied, they do not need to pay [the agricultural] tax anymore…But the state forgets one thing. People feel satisfied, but can this counter wars, riots, or invasions by other countries? What really makes a country develop is its economy…What really enables a country to counter invasion is technology…

The emphasis on economic and technologic development is consistent with the party-state's definition of modernity. The director's words also indicate his focus in managing his hospital, that is economic efficiency and high medical technology, which for him means 'development'. This view is shared by many hospaital administeators who reform their hospital by expanding the departments that can make the most profits while putting less attention on, even cutting down the departments that may lose money, investing heavily in 'profitable' high technology equipments while ignoring the 'soft' humanitarian aspect. Yet, the new round of healthcare reform since 2009 seems to interfere with his hospital's existing profit-making behaviour. The new healthcare reform that tries to restore the public welfare nature of health care prevents public hospitals from making money easily by promoting the 'separation of drug sale and health care' (*yiyao fenkai*) and further controlling medical charges. The hospital head expressed his disagreement with the recent reforms, and indicated his determination to make his hospital benefit most from the ongoing healthcare reform rather than lose out (see Chap. 4 about how hospitals are generating profits from the new healthcare reform policies).

2.2.3   Doctors as the Calculative Subject

When a hospital faces pressure to become financially self-sufficient, it transfers this pressure on its health professionals to be productive and competitive. Health professionals are evaluated according to criteria that are in accord with the market economy. Their medical decisions are based on a cost-benefit calculation. Their work is measured in terms of the profits they generate. A technician in the electrocardiogram diagnosis division of a local hospital told me:

> Our work is about a cost-benefit calculation, which means that, what we get from patients, deduct the cost of the machine, the daily expenditure on electricity, water, stationary, etc., count everything in, then it is the amount [profits] left, the hospital gives us a certain percentage of that amount, that becomes our [bonus] income… (Interview D45)

The bonus allocated by the hospital was the overall bonus for the department, which is then distributed to the staff members within the department according to individuals' performance and contribution.

In the market era, a public doctor's income is normally composed of three parts: the regular salary, bonus, and other 'grey' incomes.[6] In the public service sector, the salary includes a fixed low salary supplemented by subsidies according to one's rank, title, years of services, etc. In Riverside County, the public doctors' regular salaries vary from 2000 to over 3000 Yuan (about £200–300) a month. The bonuses that the doctors receive in addition to their regular salaries are a performance-based allocation tied to their workload and the revenue they generate for their hospital. This part is the bonus income that the technician mentioned above. A formal doctor can get over 3000 Yuan as a bonus per month. A senior doctor may earn more income in the form of bonus and rewards than the regular salary. Additionally, doctors have 'grey' incomes: direct kickbacks from the pharmaceutical companies,

---

[6]This analysis of a doctor's income only attempts to show the general situation based on materials collected in Riverside County, rather than a particular doctor's income which varies from one doctor to another. Doctors in different regions also have varied incomes.

Table 2.1 The composition
of a senior doctor's income in
riverside county

Overall monthly income	
Category	Percentage (%)
Regular salary	20–30
Bonus	20–30
Grey incomes	40 to over 50

private payments and *hongbao* (red envelopes containing gifts of money) from patients, income from moonlighting, etc. Some senior doctors acquire over half of their total income from these grey sources. Thus, in the composition of a doctor's overall income, the regular salary only occupies a small proportion (around 20–30%) (see Table 2.1). The other income is positively related to the number of patients treated, the workload, the drugs and tests prescribed, etc.

Performance figures are the evaluation of a doctor's work and the criterion for deciding the bonus distribution. Doctors constantly have numeric figures in their head when making medical decisions about which medicines to prescribe, which patients to enrol, which treatment agenda to choose, etc.[7] They are urged to reflect on their daily medical practice with a profit consideration, contribute more to their department's overall profits, and compete with their colleagues. They face tremendous pressure to satisfy the performance standard laid down by the hospital. If they fail to meet the hospital's target, their bonuses will be deducted; they face demotion, transferral, and blame or ostracism from their colleagues (Hui 2010). The system places doctors in a difficult situation, in that they feel they have no choice but to submit to the hospital's requirements. Doctors are easily objectified by a variety of management and efficiency requirements. Correspondingly, they will 'objectify' patients in order to achieve the hospital's targets and secure their own interests. The system places the health professionals and patients' respective interests in conflict. Saving the poor who cannot pay may lead to the doctor's own salary being reduced. Doctors do not feel secure about making their best efforts to save patients, and increasingly tailor their actions according to their own safety and interests. The 'socialist man' ethos was abandoned in favour of notions of the 'economic man' (Chan 1997: 100). Red and expert are replaced by the ability to make profits, by practices aligned with the market rationales, and by a capacity to exploit the opportunities provided by the market. For many doctors, the change is also about what the health service symbolised to them personally. 'Serving the people' and an 'altruistic contribution' cannot help them to maintain their social status, nor do these bring them any professional recognition. The new standard for evaluating one's worth and status is the ability to generate profits and make money. Struggling in an environment that is increasingly obsessed with economic figures, doctors sometimes feel tired and 'would rather be a simple doctor, focusing on

---

[7]Many quantitative researches have shown the positive correlation between bonus system and the increase in hospital service revenue, and the potential risks of linking remuneration with revenue generation in Chinese hospitals (see researches such as Liu and Mills 2003, 2005).

treatment only'. The inherent conflicts in the medical profession between saving lives on the one hand, and economic motivation and self-protection on the other, remain unresolved.

2.2.4 Hospital, Government and Neoliberal Governance

If a hospital director is the CEO of a hospital corporation, under the government, he or she is merely playing a sub-role and needs to obey the rule of an even bigger corporation—the city or county. Above the local state, there is a 'super firm'—the state itself becomes an enterprise organised by the market rationality (Ren 2010: 12–13). The local governments are part of the 'super firm' of the state. According to the CCP's slogan that 'development is the undisputable truth' (*fazhan caishi ying daoli*), development and modernity are guided by progressive economic rationalisation. Development is easily simplified as economic progress, shown by GDP growth. The party-state relies on economic progress for its legitimacy. Economic performance is also fundamental to the promotion of party secretaries and governors (Choi 2012). Officials, hospitals, administrators and professionals are all subject to the 'audit culture' (Strathern 2000) that evaluates their work mainly according to a set of market rules.[8] Hospitals are evaluated according to their economic efficiency, competitiveness, and the numeric figures relating to their total patient numbers and gross incomes. Hospital administrators and professionals are subjected to monthly and annual appraisals with regard to their economic performance. The 'hegemony of economist language' (Dirlik 1989)—the language of management, efficiency, and productivity—are thus adopted from high to low levels of government, officials, health administrators and ordinary health professionals.

In the 'analytics of government' proposed by Foucault, 'government is accomplished through multiple actors and agencies rather than a centralised set of state apparatuses' (Dean 2010: 37). In the health sector, public hospitals are the institutions and networks through which individual professionals are governed and through which individuals govern themselves. Economic imperatives are institutionalised by hospitals through various indicators, criteria, and calculating metrics, and are internalised by the people within through the entrepreneurial ethic of self-striving and self-responsibility. Public hospitals facilitate the exercise of 'government at a distance', enabling the state power to extend beyond the actual state bureaucracy. The state policies and governance are carried out through these local public institutions, although the process involves not only the 'conduct of conduct', but also the coercive element (such as the punishment of doctors who perform 'unprofitable' rescues).

---

[8]Kipnis (2008) has well documented the audit content and process of Chinese officials and teachers.

The Chinese health sector in the market era displays many characteristics of neoliberalism, if neoliberalism is linked to specific mechanisms of the government and recognisable modes of creating subjects (Ferguson 2009: 171), involving the deployment of new, market-based techniques of government within the terrain of the state itself that leads to the state being run like a business, and the construction of 'active' and 'responsible' rational economic actors and institutions. Yet, the emerging neoliberal characteristics do not mean the retreat of the state. The Chinese health sector remains intensely controlled by the state, and the management of institutions and professionals within involve not only the use of neoliberal techniques but also coercive measures and political administration. Market evaluation and auditing bestow new forms of managerial power on the higher level authorities to control the people below and benefit from the local institutions. Scholars have described this business relationship between local society and government as 'local state corporatism' (Oi 1999) and the 'commodification of state power' (Wank 2001). The local government focusing on GDP performance not only reduces investment in public services, but also uses its administrative power to profit directly from these sectors.[9] The local hospitals are like enterprises that generate prosperity for the local economy and income for the local governments, since public hospitals (especially those at or above the county level) are becoming increasingly profitable in the market. Hospital administrators, besides improving the economic performance of their hospital, need to collaborate with the local state and contribute to local economic performance and government revenue (this is discussed in detail in Chap. 5). This 'commodification of state power' thus reinforces the sovereign power, rather than making a change to neoliberal governance.

2.3   Individualising System Problem

The commercialisation of the health system ignores the basic values of health care and threatens the life-saving impulse of health professionals. It encourages 'rational' profit-driving activities and frequently acts to discourage altruistic behaviour that fails to generate profits. Health professionals are forced to become rational economic subjects and productive labour in the market regime to optimise and regenerate resources and profits, but they risk losing sight of patients as suffering human beings. The commercialisation of the health sector has made the value of (a patient's) life the target of calculation so that a differentiation is made between the lives to be enhanced (making live) and lives not worth preserving (letting die). The economic rationales that dominate hospitals and professionals easily reduce the

---

[9]In Riverside County, since the 1990s, many state-or collective-owned enterprises have been sold to private, and basic social provisions such as health care, water, electricity, and education have been increasingly commercialised.

poor to a 'bare life' (without entitlement or security) (Agamben 1998), leading to the death of a body without 'economic' value (for hospitals to reap the profit).

While the health sector is dominated by the neoliberal logic of governance, the party-state continues emphasizing its moral responsibility toward its people, in terms life, health and security. The 'letting die' incidents obviously breached its promise to secure people's life and health. When such events were reported by the media, the government always reemphasize the public nature of health care provision, and heavily criticise the hospital and health professionals involved. The frequent occurrences of 'letting patients die' are perceived by the public as being an external manifestation of the moral degeneration of health professionals and hospitals. The government and public media also tend to link the 'letting die' phenomenon to the moral failure of individual health professionals. Correspondingly, the authority issues a series of rules, regulations and policies to control health professionals' behaviour.

Over the past few decades, the state has released a series of normative regulations on hospitals and doctors' rescue obligations. In 1988, the Ministry of Health issued a code of conduct for health professionals. The first guide was about 'healing the wounded and rescuing the dying (*jiusifushang*), implement socialist humanitarianism, always thinking for patients, and taking best effort to solve patients' pains'.[10] In 1994, the State Council released the 'Medical Institution Administration Ordinance' which regulates that a 'medical institution should rescue emergency patients instantly' (Article 31) (CPG 2005a). The 'Medical Practitioner Act' released in 1998 notes that 'medical practitioners should take emergent measures to treat patient with critical condition, are not allowed to reject emergency patient' (Article 24) (CPG 2005b).[11] The 2012 new 'Code of Conduct for Medical Institution Professionals' released by the Ministry of Health further emphasises patients' right to be saved (MOH 2012). Although these regulations clearly denote the medical institutions and practitioners' saving responsibility and the patients' right to be saved, they ignore the thorny issue of payment that troubles medical institutions and practitioners.

These ethic regulations are in conflict with the actual hospital operations and requirements placed on the health professionals' daily work. They deflect attention from the system that discourages altruistic behaviour and the government's retreat from responsibility. While the government 'retreat' from investment, subsidies, and funding with regard to health care, which led to many medical facilities being privatised in the 1980s and 1990s, it continues to exert strict control over the

---

[10]The code *Health Professionals' Medical Ethic Criteria and Implemental Measures (Yiwurenyuan yide guifan ji shishi banfa)* has become invalid since 2010 and was replaced by a new one, thus it could not be found from any central government website. But it is still available at some local government websites, such as the Ningbo Health Bureau website at http://www.nbws. gov.cn/wsdj/News_view.aspx?CategoryId=225andContentId=6426, retrieved 21 May, 2013.

[11]Article 37 of the 'Medical Practitioner Act' further lists a set of misconducts of medical practitioners that will be punished, including 'delaying rescue and treatment of emergency patients, which leads to serious consequence'.

medical sector, where the hospital functions, medical pricing, and health profes-sional mobility are all under the scrutiny of the local authorities. Local levels of government even strategically manoeuvre to 'profit' from the health sector. The hybrid market and planned system place dual and frequent conflicting requirements on the public hospitals—both to uphold their public service nature and be self-sufficient. Hospitals have been forced to seek other sources (particularly selling drugs) of income and run like an enterprise. Public doctors have extremely low formal salary and have to reply on grey sources for extra income. In my field, many doctors have not lost their desire to serve the people. They too are questioning the commercialised health system, where the medical practices are reoriented according to economic calculations of cost, profit, and efficiency. Yet, many express a sense of powerlessness to redress the alienation brought about by the market calculation and instrumentalism. In the hospitals, the incentive structures do not reward profes-sionals' rescue behaviour, but punish rescues that lead to economic loss. The ambiguous character of public hospitals under the complex of both a market and planned system continues to cause a dilemma for doctors and forces them to sus-pend their altruistic impulses. The authority tries to control professional behaviour through various professional codes and compulsory rules, while subtly promoting market motivation for professionals to improve economic efficiency. The discrep-ancies between what the policy and professional guidelines require and what is required in concrete medical practice remain a source of conflict for the doctors. The new guidelines on doctors' behaviour, such as compulsory rescue obligation, sometimes ironically deepen the sense of moral alienation and disaffection already being experienced by these doctors.

Recently, China has been gradually changing from an economy-first society to include security, political, economic, ethical, and social factors within its evaluation of national power (Greenhalgn 2009: 217). The new healthcare reform tries to reverse the neoliberal change in health care by rebuilding a state-sponsored health system and providing basic health insurance for all. Recent research shows that 95% of the Chinese population had health insurance by the end of 2011 (Gao et al. 2014). Health insurance is changing the way people pay for medical care. Hospitals have become 'bolder' in treating patients, whose medical bills are partly covered by insurance. Patients can now go into hospital on payment of a small deposit, and are allowed to pay the remaining fees after their treatment has been completed. The newly-promoted health insurance schemes have become the third party between patients and hospitals, serving to share the patients' burden. With this wide insurance coverage, the Ministry of Health has issued guidance to public hospitals to adopt a 'treatment first payment later' approach since 2010 (China Net 2013). After the migrant worker incident mentioned above, the state initiated an emer-gency medical aid system to help emergency patients to access health care (CPG 2013). In 2013, the National Health and Family Planning Commission (the former Ministry of Health and the Family Planning Commission, hereafter NHFPC) issued a new decree on hospitals' and doctors' obligation to save lives, which specified standards and procedures for hospitals to supply basic treatment for emergency patients (NHFPC 2013). Besides, in recent healthcare reforms, the state initiated public hospital reforms,[12] including many measures to prevent public hospitals from allocating numeric tasks to relevant departments and health professionals, and disconnect individual health professionals' income from the amount of drugs and checks they prescribe.

Even so, the patients' families still feel the burden of major illnesses. The new health insurance schemes have not significantly reduced patients' medical expenditure (Gao et al. 2014; Liu et al. 2014).[13] Many treatments, tests and drugs remain uncovered by insurance, and the actual reimbursement rates are not very high. Although government spending on healthcare has increased rapidly under the new healthcare reform, most of the money goes on health insurance, public health, and community and township medical institutions, rather than directly to the public hospitals at or above the county level. Public hospitals must still work under the business model, focusing on maximising profit. Public hospitals can even make money through the newly-promoted insurance schemes: patients are encouraged to go into hospital even for minor illnesses; doctors are encouraged to prescribe heavily to insured patients; and hospitals make claims for services that were medically unnecessary or never provided (this is discussed further in Chap. 4). Hospitals also have new measures for bonus allocation to guide doctors' medical practices. In a system where doctors cannot mobilise freely, they still have to work in the public hospital and make the best efforts to increase their own income. Furthermore, facing rising health care needs of an ageing population and a shortage of health professionals and good medical resources, medical institutions and health professionals in China frequently have to make critical decisions on resource distributions, in terms of who to save and what treatment to provide.

Fundamentally, the rescue issue concerns the current business model of health care. The state that releases the above reform measures itself constitutes the omnipresent economic forces in China. Its recent adjustments of the market trajectory show the competing guiding ideologies of market competitiveness, social justice, efficiency, socialist welfare, and development. The local administrative authorities, health officials and hospital administrators who execute the new reform policies continue to be subject to the measurements of the market criteria within the state's efforts to develop the economy. The state institutions, hospitals, and ordinary health professionals need to navigate through differing or even opposing values and requirements. In a context where the local government, hospitals, administrators, and doctors form a chain to profit from the existing business model of health care, the recent reform measures to change the market trajectory will be contested and resisted. The alliance between the market factor and government power—local administrative agencies and commercialised hospitals in the health sector—has already resisted the state's previous reform efforts from as early as the late 1990s. Under the new healthcare reform, the powerful interest alliance again began to resist the reform measures, such as the essential medicine system, the separation of

---

[12]Central People's Government, PRC (2015).

[13]Also see Zhu (2018).

medicine sale and health care,[14] and the new containment measures on medical charges (this is discussed further in Chap. 4). The reform efforts have yet to change the commercial mode of the medical institutions and tackle the system that discourages doctors' rescue behaviour.

References

Agamben, Giorgio. 1998. *Homo Sacer: Sovereign Power and Bare Life*. Stanford, CA: Stanford University Press.

Central People's Government, PRC. 2005a. *Medical Institution Administration Ordinance* (Yiliao jigou guanli tiaoli). Retrieved 19 February, 2013. (http://www.gov.cn/banshi/2005-08/01/content_19113_2.htm).

Central People's Government, PRC. 2005b. *The People's Republic of China Medical Practitioner Act* (Zhonghua renmin gongheguo zhiye yishi fa). Retrieved 13 May, 2010. (http://www.gov.cn/banshi/2005-08/01/content_18970.htm).

Central People's Government, PRC. 2009. *The Tort Law of the PRC* (Zhonghua renmin gongheguo qinquan zeren fa). Retrieved 21 June, 2013. (http://www.gov.cn/flfg/2009-12/26/content_1497435.htm).

Central People's Government, PRC. 2013. *Guidance on Setting Up Emergency Medical Aid System from General Office of the State Council of the People's Republic of China* (Guowuyuan bangongting guanyu jianli jibing yingji jiuzhu zhidu de zhidao yijian). Retrieved 2 March, 2013. (http://www.gov.cn/zwgk/2013-03/01/content_2342656.htm).

Central People's Government, PRC. 2015. *Guidance on Urban Public Hospital Reform Experiment from General Office of the State Council of the People's Republic of China* (Guowuyuan bangongting guanyu chengshi gongli yiyuan zonghe gaige shidian de zhidao yijian). Retrieved 12 March, 2017. (http://www.gov.cn/zhengce/content/2015-05/17/content_9776.htm).

Chan, Anita. 1997. Chinese danwei reforms: Convergence with the Japanese model? In *Danwei: The Changing Chinese Workplace in Historical and Comparative Perspective*, ed. X Lü and E. J. Perry, 91–113. Armonk, NY: ME Sharpe.

China Net. 2013. *"Treatment First Payment Later" Targeting the Hospitals' Rejection of Patients and High Medical Fees* ("Xian kanbing hou fufei" jianzhi jiansibujiu he kanbinggui). Retrieved 19 February, 2013. (http://news.china.com.cn/live/2013-02/19/content_18706134.htm).

China News. 2012. *Ambulance Failed to Save Dying Migrant, Zhengzhou Government Responded: Patient Refused to Go to Hospital* (Zhengzhou huiying mingong jietou binsi 120 jianerweijiu: huanzhe jujue jiuyi). Retrieved 19 February, 2013. (http://www.chinanews.com/sh/2012/12-02/4374931.shtml).

Choi, Eun Kyong. 2012. Patronage and performance: Factors in the political mobility of provincial leaders in post-Deng China. *The China Quarterly* 212: 965–981.

Cooper, Melinda. 2011. Trial by accident: Tort law, industrial risks and the history of medical experiment. *Journal of Cultural Economy* 4 (1): 81–96.

---

[14]As shown in this chapter, the majority of a doctor's grey income comes from the prescription of medical products. Doctors receive 'commissions' for prescribing drugs, tests, and other medical products from pharmaceutical companies and medical suppliers. Prescriptions also contribute to the profit of the hospital, thus the bonus that doctors can receive from the hospital. Therefore, the separation of medicine sale and health care, which tries to stop doctors and hospitals from making profits directly from drugs, encounters strong resistance.

Dai, Kerong, Xu Zhaochun, and Liulong Zhu. 2003. Trauma care systems in China. *Injury* 34 (9): 664–668.

Dean, Mitchell. 2010. *Governmentality: Power and Rule in Modern Society*, 2nd ed. London: Sage Publications.

Dirlik, Arif. 1989. Revolutionary hegemony and the language of revolution: Chinese socialism between present and future. In *Marxism and the Chinese Experience*, ed. A. Dirlik and M. Meisner, 27–42. Armonk, NY: ME Sharpe.

Duckett, Jane. 2007. Local governance, health finance, and changing patterns of inequality in access to health services. In *Paying for Progress in China: Public Finance, Human Welfare, and Changing Patterns of Inequality*, ed. V. Shue and C. P. Wong, 46–68. London: Routledge.

Ferguson, James. 2009. The uses of neoliberalism. *Antipode* 41 (S1): 166–184.

Gao, Chen, Xu Fei, and Gordon G. Liu. 2014. Payment reform and changes in health care in China. *Social Science and Medicine* 111: 10–16.

Greenhalgh, Susan. 2009. The Chinese biopolitical facing the twenty-first century. *New Genetics and Society* 28 (3): 205–222.

Gu, Xin. 2008. *Towards Universal Coverage of Healthcare Insurance: The Strategic Choices and Institutional Frameworks of China's New Healthcare Reform* (Zouxiang quanmin yibao: zhongguo xin yigai de zhanlue yu zhanshu). Beijing: China Labour and Social Security Publishing House.

Hsiao, William C. 1995. The Chinese health care system: Lessons for other nations. *Social Science and Medicine* 41 (8): 1047–1055.

Hui, Edwin C. 2010. The contemporary healthcare crisis in china and the role of medical professionalism. *Journal of Medicine and Philosophy* 35 (4): 477–492.

Hung, Kevin K.C., C.S.K. Cheung, T.H. Rainer, and C.A. Graham. 2009. EMS systems in China. *Resuscitation* 80 (7): 732–735.

Kipnis, Andrew. 2008. Audit cultures: Neoliberal governmentality, socialist legacy, or technologies of governing? *American Ethnologist* 35 (2): 275–289.

Liu, Xingzhu, and Anne Mills. 2003. The influence of bonus payments to doctors on hospital revenue: Results of a quasi-experimental study. *Applied Health Economics and Health Policy* 2 (2): 91–98.

Liu, Xingzhu, and Anne Mills. 2005. The effect of performance-related pay of hospital doctors on hospital behavior: A case study from Shandong. *Human Resource for Health* 3 (11): 1–12.

Liu, Kai, Wu Qiaobing, and Junqiang Liu. 2014. Examining the association between social health insurance participation and patients' out-of-pocket payments in China: The role of institutional arrangement. *Social Science and Medicine* 113: 95–103.

Ministry of Health, PRC. 2012. *The Code of Conduct for Medical Institution Professionals* (Yiliao jigou congye renyuan xingwei guifan). Retrieved 10 March, 2013. (http://www.moh. gov.cn/mohjcg/s3577/201207/55445.shtml).

Ministry of Transport, PRC. 2008. *Interim Regulation on the Registration and Administration of Public Institutions* (Shiye danwei dengji guanli zanxing tiaoli). Retrieved 22 May, 2013. (http:// www.moc.gov.cn/zhuzhan/renshixinxi/shetuanguanli/200802/t20080225_468807.html).

National Health and Family Planning Commission, PRC. 2013. *Regulation on Treatment to Those Serious or Dangerous Emergency Patients* (Xuyao jinji jiuzhi de ji weizhong shangbing biaozhun ji zhenliao guifan de tongzhi). Retrieved 28 November, 2013. (http://www.nhfpc. gov.cn/yzygj/s3593g/201311/fd8cd0386bd740fa87e2f7714901989f.shtml).

Oi, Jean C. 1999. *Rural China Takes Off: Institutional Foundations of Economic Reform*. Berkeley: University of California Press.

People's Net. 2012. *A Hospital in Sheyang was Suspected of Rejecting Patient, Family Pleased to the Hospital but Nobody Responded* (Sheyang yi yiyuan yi jiansibujiu, jiashu gui qiu ren wurenguowen). Retrieved 19 February, 2013. (http://js.people.com.cn/html/2012/12/18/ 194058.html).

People's Net. 2013. *Emergency Doctor was Assaulted, Drunk man Attacked Doctor due to Medical Charge, Family Made Apology* (Jizhen yisheng zai zao ouda, zuihan yin shoufei wenti daren, jiashu mang daoqian). Retrieved 26 October, 2013. (http://health.people.com.cn/n/2013/1026/c14739-23333797.html).

Ren, Hai. 2010. *Neoliberalism and Culture in China and Hong Kong: The Countdown of Time.* London: Routledge.

Strathern, Marilyn. 2000. Introduction: New accountabilities. In *Audit Cultures: Anthropological Studies in Accountability, Ethics, and the Academy*, ed. M. Strathern, 1–18. London: Routledge.

Transition Institute. 2011. *New Cooperative Medical Scheme: Problems and Outlook* (Xinxing hezuo yiliao: wenti yu zhanwang). Retrieved 22 May, 2014. (http://www.zhuanxing.cn/uploadfile/2011/0606/20110606121329313.pdf).

Urio, Paolo. 2010. *Reconciling State, Market and Society in China: The Long March toward Prosperity.* New York: Routledge.

Wank, David. 2001. *Commodifying Communism: Business, Trust, and Politics in a Chinese City.* Cambridge, UK: Cambridge University Press.

Xinhua Net. 2003a. *Hospital Again Failed to Treat Patient's illness and Save Patient in Danger* (Youjian yiyuan jianbingbuzhi, jiansibujiu), Retrieved 19 February, 2013. (http://news.xinhuanet.com/comments/2003-04/22/content_842674.htm).

Yip, Winnie Chi-Man, William C. Hsiao, Qingyue Meng, Wen Chen, and Xiaoming Sun. 2010. Realignment of incentives for health-care providers in China. *The Lancet* 375 (9720): 1120–1130.

Zhu, Hengpeng. 2018. '*After Eight Years' Health Reform, Do You Have a "Sense of Gain"?*' (*yigai banian, ni you huodegan ma?*). *Caixin Net.* Retrieved 12 March, 2018. (http://m.opinion.caixin.com/m/2018-02-09/101209601.html).

Chapter 3
From 'Care of the Self' to 'Entrepreneur of the Self': Reconfiguration of Health Care Responsibilities, Needs, and Rights

This chapter explores the reconfiguration of health care responsibilities, needs and rights in contemporary China. Health care in the Chinese official discourses is expressed as both rights and needs. At the First National Health Work Conference in 1950, soon after the founding of the PRC, health care was declared as a right. It laid down healthcare guidelines oriented towards 'workers, peasants and soldiers' (Wang 2010). The constitution (CPG 2004), first promulgated in 1954 and later revised many times, denoted that the state should develop various medical and health care facilities to protect people's health (Article 21), that Chinese citizens should have the right to get material help from the state and society when they are old, sick, or lose their working ability, and that the state will develop social insurance, social aid, and medical and health care work to meet these rights of citizens (Article 45). The General Principles of the Civil Law states that citizens have the rights of life and health (Article 98) (NPC 2000). In the collective era, China had provided basic health care to most of its population. Its barefoot doctor system and cooperative medical scheme in the rural areas had been proclaimed by the WHO for securing people's basic health care rights. However, things began to change with the advent of market reforms in the 1980s. Health care rights anchored in the legal system were frequently compromised and differentiated in the post-reform era, and China was listed by the WHO as one of the most unequal countries in term of health care. Not until 2009 did the new healthcare reform re-emphasise citizens' entitlement to (primary) health care as a basic right. It denotes that the government should do its utmost to fulfil its duty in building the health system, in providing public health care, and in protecting people's health rights (Gao 2005).[1]

---

[1]The authority and laws do not specify what type of health care people are entitled to as a basic human right, but in the new health reform agenda, there are very specific plans about what health care services should be universally provided to people free of charge (for example, public health services like vaccinations to children under age of 5). The list is increasing over the years, and has the tendency to change from selective primary health services to comprehensive health services.

© Springer Nature Singapore Pte Ltd. 2019
J. Tu, *Health Care Transformation in Contemporary China*,
https://doi.org/10.1007/978-981-13-0788-1_3

The official discourses of people's health (care) rights also have limitations. First, Chinese people do not share an equal health care right. The first healthcare guidelines laid down in 1950 after the funding of PRC suggest health work is oriented towards 'workers, peasants and soldiers' (Wang 2010), which subtly exclude some people, such as those labelled as 'bad classes'. The 1954 Constitution also stipulated that 'working people of the People's Republic of China have the right to material aid in old age, and in case of illness and disability', in another word, only the 'working people' have the right to such material assistance as health services, although working people include the majority of the population/labourers (Yang 2017: 13). Even today social welfares like health care are tied to an individual's (rural/urban) household registration, work status, political background, and employment status and so on. People are attributed different entitlements according to their social characters (also see Chap. 4). In another words, their health care right is not citizenship-based. Second, there is no special law about people's rights and entitlements in terms of health and health care, and the state has never promised free health coverage to its citizen.[2] The discourses about people's health (care) rights are briefly mentioned in some general laws above, which have never guarantee free health care (but only material aid to help people receive care) and have not specified the state and medical institutions' responsibilities to ensure people's health (care) rights. The occurrences of letting die incidents recorded in the last chapter are also partly due to the absence of such a law that specify health care to citizen at whose expense.

Besides, the discourse of health care rights is also influenced by the Chinese tradition and the CCP's strategies of linking rights with socio-economic needs. Chen (2012: 6) writes that since the imperial era, the emperor's obligation to provide for the economic well-being and livelihood of the people under his rule constituted the bedrock of the dynasty's legitimacy. In socialist China, people's welfare is one of the pillars of political legitimacy. The party-state actively encourages a conceptual linkage between 'livelihood' and 'rights', putting the Chinese conceptions of 'rights' as a socio-economic concern, rather than a political concern (Keane 2001; Perry 2008). The state promotes the right to subsistence (*shengcun quan*) and the right to development (*fazhan quan*) as the prime human rights (NPC 2005). Basic needs such as health care are framed as the right to subsistence. The Constitution of the Chinese Communist Party (*dangzhang*), amended and adopted on 14 November 2012, remains committed to catering for people's growing 'needs' (CPG 2012b), although efforts have been tempered in the market era. The meaning of needs and the satisfying of such needs as health care are significant in understanding China's governance. The inability to meet these needs continually challenges the legitimacy of the authority.[3]

---

[2]A basic health and health promotion law is drafted and under review (see http://health.people.com.cn/n1/2017/1223/c14739-29724759.html, retrieved 31 March, 2018).

[3]When writing this part about needs and rights, I have got inspiration from reading 'Exit, or Evict: Re-grounding Rights in Needs in China's Urban Housing Demolition' by Ho (2013) and from discussion with the author.

The content of health care rights as regulated by the law needs to be directed by local content, historical change, and lived experience. This chapter investigates the historical and discursive shifts in people's health care responsibilities, rights and needs. It centres on the 'care of the self', in which health care responsibility increasingly transfers to individuals, the 'entrepreneur of the self', in which individual patients are required to become active consumers in the market, and patients' recent rejection of the state framing of individual responsibility by articulating their rights to basic needs. The ideas of the 'care of the self' and 'entrepreneur of the self' are frequently related with neoliberal subjectivity. Market reforms have convinced many researchers of the emergence of neoliberal subjectivity and neoliberal citizenship in China (Anagnost 2004, 2008; Keane 2001; Yan 2003; Ren 2010). Nevertheless, this chapter questions the neoliberal vision of health care among Chinese patients. It shows that the situation in the post-reform Chinese health sector is more complex than just the emergence of neoliberal subjectivity and neoliberal citizenship.

3.1 The Individualisation of Health Care Responsibility

Beck and Beck-Gernsheim (2002) write, in modern society, the modes of public provision have become more and more fragile and individuals have become primarily responsible for their own livelihood. They use the phrase 'institutionalised individualism' to denote that the institutions of modern society are increasingly set up for the individual rather than for the group. In recent years, the rise of the individual and the consequential individualisation of society in China have also been noted by scholars (Hansen and Svarverud 2010; Hansen 2013; Yan 2010a, b). However, unlike Western countries, where the market is the primary force behind the rise of the individual, in China, it has been the party-state which has initiated such changes by enforcing a number of top-down institutional reforms through two processes: first, the dis-embedding of individuals from traditional collectives (such as kinship) and re-embedding them in the socialist collectives during the Mao era; second, the 'untying' of individuals from various collectives of state socialism and re-embedding them in the stratified order of the market society in the reform era (Yan 2009, 2010a). In the post-reform Chinese health sector, the cut in healthcare spending by the state and the institutional changes over recent decades have gradually devolved responsibility of health care to individual citizens. The steady erosion of collective institutions, such as urban work units and rural production collectives, which provided key social goods, has pushed more people into the market. Social organisations that traditionally engaged in welfare provision (such as religious organisations, lineage societies, benevolent associations, occupational guilds, and merchant associations) were weakened during the Maoist period and have not yet recovered in the market era.[4] The state withdraws its responsibility, many collectives either vanish or become non-functional, and the civil society has not sufficiently developed. The family then becomes the main site and even the sole source of social support.

3.1.1   Health Care as a Moral Responsibility of the Family

The shifting health care responsibility shows the increasing importance of the family in health care provision. Over recent decades, there has been a redrawing of the family boundary, from the involvement of the state in what appears to be purely private matters of family life in the collective era, to the retreat of the state by returning the space as well as welfare responsibility to the individual family in the post-reform era. In the market era, the household production system makes the family the central unit of production, labour disposition, consumption, and care taking. The family becomes the most important moral framework in people's life.

For the family, health care is some form of moral responsibility. The elderly rely on their adult children for health care. The adult children buy medical products, pay medical fees, provide daily care, and handle the 'complex' hospitalisation and insurance reimbursement procedures when their parents are sick. The elderly refer to the provision of these medical products and expenses by their adult children as the children's concern for them. My research shows that help in health care between family members becomes the criterion to define *xiaoshun* (filial piety) between elderly parents and adult children, *zong* (loyalty) between wives and husbands, and *ciai* (love and benevolence) between adult parents and young children. One of my interviewees, Auntie Lou (Interview P12), told me her relative's story. The husband, in his late 40s, suffered a cerebral haemorrhage. The family tried all kinds of treatment for him, transferring him from one hospital to another. Although months of treatment exhausted most of the family savings, the husband's condition continually worsened with little hope of recovery. The wife and son planned to take the husband back home for terminal care. The proposal was violently rejected by the husband's brother, under the pressure of whom, the wife and son could do nothing but keep the dying patient in hospital. The moral responsibility obliged the family to continue seeking medical care under great financial pressure, even when the patient's condition became hopeless. Prolonging life regardless of the realistic effect of continuing medical intervention works as a way to prove filial piety (from the son to the father) and loyalty (from the wife to the husband) among family members, especially when the patient is the dominant member of the family. At the end of Auntie Luo's story, two elderly women nearby, who had provided long-term

---

[4]There are rising numbers of NGOs, charities, and religious groups in the post-reform era, which are regarded as a necessary supplement to the work of the state. However, there are few social organisations serving in the health care sector, except some targeting particular illnesses such as HIV-AIDS and tuberculosis, but their impacts are limited (see Duckett 2008).

care for their chronically sick husband respectively, showed great sympathy for the wife and son. The family bears the cost of medical treatment and provides long-term daily care. In the family, woman plays the crucial caregiver role. Long-term illness poses challenges not only to the patients, but also to the family members who provide care when other care institutions and medical support are not available. Health care thus places a heavy burden on the family, economically, physically, emotionally and morally.

The Chinese government in recent years has reemphasised the traditional value of filial piety.[5] The affective relationship among family members is mobilised by the state to reduce its responsibility. However, the capacity of the family to constitute a protective capsule is varied and the family cannot always effectively take health care responsibility. Many families are fragile in front the catastrophe of major illnesses and may even turn into a 'site of triaging abandonment' (Biehl 2005). Local people told me many stories about unfilial adult children who disregarded their elderly parents' illnesses. In one case (from Interview P39), an old widow suffered a broken knee and her kneecap needed to be replaced, which would cost tens of thousands Yuan. However, none of her three daughters or one son was willing to pay for the surgery. After several days' wait in hospital, the widow was sent back to her home in the village by one of her children and left alone without any further treatment. Such stories told by the local elderly reveal the grave concerns generally held among these elderly, who envisage similar incidents happening to them in the future, though many believe that their adult children would be more filial. Single elderly parents who depend on their adult children for health care face greater uncertainty. The elderly's loss of power and exclusion within the family in contemporary Chinese society has been recorded by many literatures (Shen 2011; Yan 2003). Traditional family values have encountered challenges as young people partake in social mobility and exhibit increasingly individualised values. The traditional mechanism of intergenerational reciprocity has broken down with the introduction of values associated with the market economy (Yan 2003). The rise of the nuclear family, in which old parents live separately from their adult children, also makes daily care become more difficult. The rising private responsibility of health care entangles with the changing family structure, sometimes making it difficult for the elderly to exert a moral claim of care. Lacking effective social support structures, many elderly people easily fall into a miserable life, being 'abandoned' once the family is unable to take health care responsibility.[6]

---

[5]Based on the Confucian virtue of filial piety, elderly parents should have a right (although the term of 'rights' was not used) to receive care from their adult children, which has also been incorporated into the civil law of both the Republic of China (since 1911) and the People's Republic of China (since 1949) (from Fan 2010: 59–60). Since 1996, the government has further put the duties of adult children to take care of their elderly parents into the law—'Law of the People's Republic of China on Protection of the Rights and Interests of Elderly People' (CPG 2005).

[6]Besides the many accounts by the people in my field site, the media have also reported stories about elderly people who could not get sufficient health care when their family was unable to shoulder health care responsibility. Also see Wu (2010) research about suicide in China which recorded cases of sick elders committing suicide due to the absence of state and family support.

The more that health care becomes a private family matter, the more it relies on the financial ability of the individual household and mirrors the inequality in the market economy. Without a proper health insurance system and social support structure, China has seen high out-of-pocket payments in health care and high rates of household saving for medical care. People save money for their whole lives for potential major illnesses, but when devastated by an illness, many still quickly get into difficulties facing high medical fees. The disengagement of the state in key areas such as health care makes it necessary for individuals and families to fend for themselves, leaving the imbalances in redistribution untouched, sometimes even exacerbating socio-economic inequalities. As Fan (2008) writes, family-based care provision is not based on a right to claim social welfare entitlement; it is offered out of sympathy, love or charity between family members, and is essentially non-egalitarian.

3.1.2   The Remaking of Traditional Self-Cultivation and Socialist Self-Reliance

Chinese patients have long been responsible for their own health care. The Confucian traditions of *xiushen* (cultivating the self or life) and *yangsheng* (nurturing life) emphasise the responsibility of self-cultivation and self-responsibility in keeping healthy. In the imperial era, there was no systematic public health care provision for the general public. The traditional nuclear, joint or extended family was the main or only rational source of support for family members in times of illness. The situation continued in the Republican period (1912–1949), despite the fact that the Nationalist government had made some efforts to initiate the setting up of a public health system.[7] Generally, state provision appeared limited in the area of health care before the founding of the PRC (Wong 1998). Local elderly recalled the disastrous flood and the subsequent outbreak of cholera in Riverside city in 1945. Over 450 people were drowned in the flood, but much more people lost their lives in the break out of cholera.[8] The government then, under unstable political circumstance (at the end of Sino-Japan war while the domestic war was about to start), had little power and limited resources to deal with the epidemic. People relied on their own responses (for instance, escaping the epidemic area, personal hygiene) and the limited local social forces (private doctors, chemists, and medical guild, etc.) to counter the epidemic. Recalling this historical public health incident, local

---

[7]In the late Qing and early Republican era, the health of the nation was largely the responsibility of the citizen, instead of the responsibility of the government, although some new discourses that relate population health with the strength of the nation-state began to emerge with the introduction of 'hygienic modernity' (see Rogaski 2004).

[8]The number of 450 was obtained from a local government official. But there is no accurate number of the people who died in the cholera after the flood, although the local elderly estimated that there were tens of thousands of deaths.

elderly I met generally admitted that the CCP government after liberation functioned much better than the Nationalist government in public health and social services.

Yet, even in the collective era when the state provided public services and social welfare, it still emphasised individual responsibility. The national pursuit of 'self-reliance' (*zili gengsheng*) under Mao's leadership promoted the notion that Chinese people could create a unique bright future by their own efforts. This 'self-reliant' policy influenced the health sector in that it mobilised people to solve their own health problems (Chen 2001). For some people (such as the *danwei* workers), health care was understood to be the responsibility of the state or collective and its provision was relatively good. However, the majority of the population outside the government and *danwei* system, especially those in the rural areas, were excluded from receiving equal benefits. The Cooperative Medical Scheme, a system in which people organised themselves to help each other in the rural areas, was also based on the self-reliance ideal to avoid becoming dependent on the state. In this period, the family still played an important role in caring for its members (Chan and Chow 1992; Wong 1998). In the rural areas of Riverside County, many people's health care experiences in the collective era show that they relied heavily on themselves and their families and friends to secure health care, which frequently could not be met sufficiently in an era of scarcity. Besides, many welfare and aid programmes in this period have been opened only to the elderly, orphans, the weak, infirm and disabled, and to those solitary people without families to rely upon (the 'three-no').[9] Such programmes have sought to encourage self-reliance and self-enterprise in those who are the 'abled' and 'healthy'. The research of Chen (2012) on the urban poor in China notes that, in the early socialist era of the PRC, the new state developed 'active production' to improve the livelihoods of the poor, instead of making provision for 'passive relief'; the 'glory of labour' and the 'shame of relief' was emphasised in an attempt to create new citizens out of 'useless' people by training and mobilising the poor for productive labour. The ability and willingness to work and earn one's own entitlement to become qualified labour have become a condition of social citizenship. The benefit of welfare and aid has been based on the 'reciprocity principle' that claimants would 'contribute' back to society and the state with their hard work and labour.

In the post-reform era, the health care burden was further shifted from the state to individuals. The contribution of individuals to the total health expenditure increased from just over 20% in the late 1970s to almost 60% by 2000 (Cai 2009). People are further encouraged to become self-responsible and self-managing subjects in the context of the state's withdrawal from welfare provision. Concerns over health have turned public spaces like parks and squares into the spaces for engaging in health practices and medical product sale. In Riverside, medical product stores and

---

[9]See Article 45 of the Constitution of the People's Republic of China (CPG 2004). It is also in correspond with traditional welfare value that the *guan* (widower), *gua* (widow), *gu* (orphan) and *du* (single men) were regarded as deserving of charity (Wong 1998: 30).

chemist shops have been mushroomed around the county; health improvement books and magazines are sold in every market, square and bookstore; people regularly practise household treatment and food therapy; the middle-aged and elderly gather in public parks and community centres every sunny day, partaking in all kinds of health practices, such as fitness dance and swordplay. Recently, self-tracking devices such as health apps installed in smartphones and other wearable devices are widely adopted by people from all ages to monitor their body and health. People rely on these indigenous practices for self-management and show a remarkable sense of personal responsibility in health maintenance. The rise of self-care and self-diagnosis is not only because of the individualisation of health care responsibility, but also due to the lack of affordable and reliable health care. Chen (2003) research shows that *qigong* practice in post-Mao China has become popular because it provides a relatively cheap and accessible form of alternative healing; the self-cultivation and self-discipline of *qigong* practice constituted a form of oppositional politics framed in terms of the management of health at a time when China was shifting from state-subsidised medical care to for-profit market medicine. The research of Farquhar and Zhang (2012: 19) on *yangsheng* activities similarly shows that these activities proliferated in 'the context of the State-driven biopolitical reorganisations of the social'. They find that elderly practitioners considered *yangsheng* activities to be healthy practices, a medium for play, and a means to increase personal power as well as for the collective crafting of the good life; these activities were also considered by practitioners as a matter of civic duty to avoid becoming dependent on their family and the state. People display a remarkable sense of individual health care responsibility. When posed the question of 'should health care responsibility be taken by the state or the individual', the locals made remarks like the following:

> Logically, the responsibility should be taken by the individual self. Because illness is an individual private matter, disease and disaster are individual private matters. If the state can share some of the responsibility, it's the state's concern for us mass populace. In the past, before the Liberation, who came to take care of you! The new society still has its advantage. (Interview P36)

In local people's logic and reasoning, illnesses, diseases and disasters have always been private matters that should be taken care of by people themselves. They belong to the self-bounded private unit (of family). Obtaining sufficient resources to satisfy physical needs and counter disasters is traditionally privately bounded within groups of families and close kin. The taking of some health care responsibility by the state in the collective era demonstrated its concern for the mass populace. When the state retreated from welfare provision in the market era, it did not take away what was inalienable from the populace, but reduced its 'grace' to the people and asked them to be self-responsible as before. As a result, the change did not trigger a strong rejection from the people when the market reform began because many people were enjoying an improvement in their material lives and medical prices had not then sky-rocketed.

The individualisation of health care responsibility and 'care of the self' in the post-reform era are different from neoliberal technologies. Keeping healthy and taking care of oneself and one's family are promoted by the media and official discourse as a moral responsibility between family members, and a civil duty from the individual to the state. They serve a collective end. Sigley (1996: 463–4) notes that Confucianism links individual self-cultivation to the good management of family, and further to the effective governance of the state in a continuous social hierarchy. Traditional self-cultivation serves to naturalise or preserve certain moral, social and political order, it is marked as 'hierarchical rather than liberal' and 'authoritarian rather than neoliberal' (Kipnis 2007: 393). Besides, self in the Chinese 'cultivation of the self' is not an independent self-contained individual of Western civilisation that have a clear boundary between one and other, but an 'interdependent self defined by one's social role and relationships' (Hwang 1998: 21).[10] The historical concept of individual or self is grounded in the notion of a common good. In the socialist collective era, the state again emphasised individuals' roles to serve a common good of the collective and state. In the post-reform era, individuals follow the time-honoured traditional value system to serve a collective end, which, however, does not exist in the neoliberal discourse of individual (that is not based on the premise of a common good, but serves to improve economic efficiency, productivity and profitability). The ideas of individual health care responsibility are widely accepted in the post-reform era precisely because they resemble the pre-socialist practices of *xiushen* and *yangsheng*, and the socialist discourse of self-reliance. However, market reforms do add a new layer of requirement on individual patients, who are required to become not only self-responsible, but also active consumers in the market.

3.2 Patient-Consumer: The Neoliberal Subject?

In the market era, health care activities have increasingly become consumption activities. Patients become clients and consumers in seeking proper medical products in the market. This section outlines how patients partake in consumption activities to protect and improve their health care, and how consumption is used by the state to encourage a new subjectivity that fits the requirements of the market economy.

---

[10]Hwang notes the 'ensembled individualism' of the Oriental tradition includes 'physical self', which is dependent upon others, and a 'social self' embedded in a stable social network. The physical self is usually named as 'small self' while the social self is termed as 'great self'. In many cases, the 'small self' has to make compromise in front of the 'great self'.

3.2.1 Patients as Consumers Negotiate Medical Care

In the post-reform era, health care has increasingly become a commodity purchased in the market. Patients in my field frequently compare medical services as commodities and want to choose and bargain for the best products. The new consumption discourses, to a certain extent, empower the customers of health care and give rise to more 'service-oriented' health care. Patients become more informed with multiple health care options, but also face an ever more complex consumption circumstance. They are bombarded by various health services, medical products and health information. Patients have to draw on an increasing array of information in order to make the right decision. In the booming market of medical products and services that promise effectiveness and immediate availability, patients actively try all kinds of medical services, use mixed therapies to maximise the effects, visit various medical institutions, seek multiple doctors, consume a variety of pharmaceuticals, and quickly abandon the ineffective treatment. The underlying fear of illness and exorbitant costs associated with health care also fuel the consumption of pharmaceuticals (Chen 2008: 127). Patients' medical consumptions are not always rational, according to those with biomedical expertise. Nevertheless, they constitute people's strategies to counter the uncertain medical market.

Patients face many uncertainties over medical charges. Under the fee-for-service payment plan, hospitals maximise their profits by measures such as over-ordering high-tech tests, prescribing expensive drugs, and prolonging the length of hospitalisation. Overcharges, fabricated charges, and charges for items patients have not used are frequently exposed by the media. The case study by Liu and Mills (1999) found that in appendicitis and pneumonia treatment, one-third of drug expenditure was considered unnecessary, more than 50% of examination expenditure was clinically unnecessary, the length of hospital stay could be cut by 10–16% without influencing the health outcome, and around 20% of all medical expenditure could be reduced. The locals express their feelings regarding hospital expenditure, commenting that in hospital 'the money is like water in a loose tap, running away fast without stopping', which easily drains a family's life savings. Many began to take actions to bargain medical prices in the same way as they buy other commercial products:

> That day I was in xxx' clinic, I told him [the doctor] 'I didn't want to eat your medicine anymore', he asked me why, I said your medicine was too expensive. After this talk, he charged me several Yuan less. I think I should still bargain a little bit, I told him I couldn't afford to eat your medicine, it was too expensive, and I was old without any pension… (Interview P39)

The subtle choice of reason—'old without any pension'—gave 69-year-old Mrs. Deng, a local resident, the moral standing to argue for lower fee. The private doctor, who opened his own clinic, frequently provided services to customers according to their financial circumstances. He made a compromise by reducing the charge by several Yuan. The patient felt satisfied while the doctor did not lose much but kept a loyal customer. Similarly, 71-year-old Mr. Dai (Interview P42) told me that he once intentionally asked the doctor in the People's Hospital why the drugs from the hospital pharmacy were much more expensive than those in the chemists outside the hospital. The doctor later gave him the prescription note allowing him to buy medicine outside the hospital. Instead of directly negotiating the drug price, the patient tactically questioned the price difference between the hospital and the chemists. The doctor made a concession by skipping the hospital code that prohibited patients from buying medicines outside the hospital, which saved Mr. Dai some money. Mr. Dai felt satisfied and praised the doctor's consideration for the patient, while the doctor did not lose much personally and gained respect from the patient. Sometimes when the negotiation attempt fails or the situation makes it too difficult to negotiate, patients may just change to another doctor. Local doctors similarly talked about increasingly active patients who, on arrival at the hospital, would tell the doctors their difficult financial situation and request that the doctors find a way of reducing costs. These patients would check every item on the medical bill and might violently complain if something went wrong. One of my interviewees, Teacher Yang (Interview P30), told me that when her mother was diagnosed with cancer and was enrolled in the hospital, her father carefully made a record of the drugs used and compared it with the receipts. One day he found that the hospital was overcharging for a particular kind of drug that cost 500 Yuan a bottle. Later, an investigation exposed that the nurse and head nurse had taken away the 'extra' medicines from the patients and reselling them to the chemist for profit. Like Teacher Yang's father, many patients in Riverside rely on themselves to make plans and calculate medical costs.

The market environment and uncertain health sector have forced patients to become 'calculative'. In the market, 'calculation' is a virtue, a technique of self-preservation and a strategy to avoid being defrauded. Besides calculating the cost efficiency for themselves, patients also consciously calculate health professionals' incomes and hospitals' profits. 'Calculations' lead to 'suspicions', and people consequently question the legitimacy of the incomes of health professionals and hospitals. People feel suspicious about the invisible structure that they cannot penetrate and have suggested ways to change the situation. Many of my interviewees talked about how to label drug prices clearly in order to make patients fully informed. Their practical calculations and considerations have gone far beyond their individual concerns and have shown their willingness to contribute to the system's construction. However, there is a lack of opportunity for them to express their views or participate in the system's construction, except for their individual measures to calculate and negotiate medical prices. Even for these individual measures of bargain, their effects are limited. Many doctors would make concessions in response to patients' bargain only when their own interests were not seriously jeopardised. The flexibility that enables negotiation is restricted to some basic treatments. For emergent or major illnesses that require large sums of money, patients have little negotiation power and have to shoulder the heavy burden of medical costs themselves.

In the market, health care is incorporated into individual consumption behaviour, requiring individuals to monitor and safeguard qualified products. Patients are deemed to be rational economic actors to exercise choice and calculation in shopping for medical services. Questioning, bargaining, passively refusing, actively requesting and calculation are measures used by patients to resist the unequal and unsatisfactory health system in which 'only the doctors have a say'. The market has rendered individual patients in a productive way, making them conduct their own lives according to economic rationales. It produces new forms of self-reliance which is different from the traditional self-cultivation and socialist self-reliance. The new forms of self-reliance are also shown in the rising consumer rights that encourage patients to solve their issues and protect their interests within the consumer rights framework in the market, rather than relying on the state.

3.2.2 Assert Consumer Rights Vis-à-Vis Medical Institutions and Professionals

Consumerism influences patients, who are increasingly concerned about their rights as consumers in relation to the medical products they purchased. In post-Mao China, the state itself has promoted consumer rights as part of its economic reform agenda, creating the 'consumer citizen' by introducing legal and other formal appeal avenues and mobilising consumers to assert their rights (Hooper 2005). Rising consumer rights are evident not only in patients' multiple choices and greater participation in healthcare decision making, but also in patients' acts to resist unsatisfactory health care and protect their entitlement to good care. 'We often encounter people who feel unsatisfied with our services …. They feel they spend money thus should get certain kind of service …' (Interview D28), complained a local doctor, who at the time of interview was working in a local hospital's Medical Affair Department, specialising in solving medical complaints and disputes. The rising consumer rights consciousness has added new elements to medical disputes. More and more patients have begun to complain to hospital administrators and ask for compensation when medical services are not in accord with the costs. Another doctor expressed:

> They [the authorities] instil the '3.15' consumerism to patients. Although health care is a kind of consumption, it's a special consumption. However, they still put this [medical dispute] within '3.15' [consumer rights protection framework] to solve. When medical accident happens, it's the hospital's responsibility. (Interview D76)

'3.15' indicates 15th March, the 'World Consumer Rights Day', which the Chinese government has instituted since 1987 to tackle commercial fraud and propagate consumer rights. Since then, a relatively well-organised consumer protection movement, consumer associations, and a completed legal framework have emerged. Chinese consumers with increasing buying power are becoming a powerful force, if not politically, in articulating their rights. The commodification of medical services has led to patients frequently putting medical disputes within the consumer rights protection framework while laws and regulations on medical dispute resolution are incomplete and inconsistent.

Consumer rights argue for the interests of patients against health professionals and hospitals—the interests of the customers versus those of the providers. However, health professionals do not agree with the consumer rights protection framework. They argue that health care is a special product, different from an ordinary commercial product. Scholars' opinions on this are not in consensus, and the courts and local governments employ the consumer protection law differently. Patients as consumers do have more of a say in deciding what services they receive, especially for those with purchasing power. However, health care 'consumption' is different from ordinary consumption. Expertise gives medical providers more opportunities to exploit their knowledge monopoly and reap more rewards in the Chinese health market. Besides, although patients creatively adopt the consumer rights discourse to protect their interests, their arguments and actions can hardly go beyond the state-framed structures. People assert interests or entitlements not vis-à-vis the state, but vis-à-vis the medical institutions and professionals that provide care. The government, which seems to 'empower' patients with consumer rights, actually transfers healthcare responsibility to individuals, who are asked to safeguard quality health care and secure consumer rights by themselves. It also shifts the blame of poor health care from the state to medical institutions and professionals that provide care. Consumer rights are employed not to achieve patients' inalienable social rights, and have little possibility to change the differentiation of health care access created in the market economy.

3.2.3 Differential Consumption and the Reconfiguration of Neoliberal Subject

The market shapes individuals to be self-responsible citizens and consumers. Yet, many people's efforts to refashion themselves into successful consumers end up with failure. While some patients seek quality health care and have strong desires for imported products and special services, others are still striving for basic and sufficient care. However, in the market, patients, both rich and poor, have rising aspirations for qualified health care. Patients experience pressures of the market economy to fashion themselves and their families as modern subjects in consuming the right products but, for those with less financial ability, fewer chances exist to consume the qualified products and humane care. The overburdened health professionals and commercialised hospitals are unable to provide emotional support to every patient, but reserve it for the privileged few. Health care has become an ambiguous commodity in the 'service sector', and human-oriented (*yirenweiben*) care is targeted at the middle-income citizens and the rich, who can afford (Zhan 2013). The advanced ward is created to produce a spatial segregation and 'distinction' (Bourdieu 1984) in the crowded hospital environment. Exorbitant fees are exercised as a form of exclusion; only the rich and insured cadres are able to avail themselves. The interaction of poverty, marginality, and the daily practices of concrete care reinforces people's subjective sense of inequality, as shown in the following conversation:

> Resident A: If you do have power, he [the doctor] will treat you nicely and carefully.
>
> Community Guard B: If you do have money, you may not necessarily go to his place for treatment [but go to a better one].
>
> Resident A: That's true...The people who have power may even be received by the hospital head in person, those doctors and nurses surely treat you very well...The person, who has money, can go to a higher-level hospital instead of staying in the lower-level hospital... Only we normal people have to listen to whatever they [doctors] say. No matter we live or die, we need to be responsible by ourselves. (Interview P37)

The locals mentioned that medical accidents and mistreatment frequently happened to the poor rather than the rich and powerful. The health market has produced a new sense of vulnerability at the intersection of inequality and care. In medical consumption, purchasing the right medical products and qualified health services has increasingly become a technique of self-management. The ability to consume the right products becomes an outward sign of successful agency. However, technologies of the self in consumption are constrained for the poor, who are most easily exposed to counterfeit medicine, suffer from poor quality care, and encounter indifferent attitudes, ignorance, and discrimination.

Consumption is viewed as a 'social palliative', promoted by the government to keep the population docile during the transformational period and to fill the large ideological void following the death of Mao (Latham 2002; Elfick 2011). However, health care, that increasingly becomes a form of consumption, produces further differentiation, resentment, and 'symbolic violence' towards those who cannot pay. Cartier (2009: 385) rightly notes that in China 'for the vast majority of people, symbolic and media consumption are more realistic than the acquisition of actual goods'; those who have consumption awareness and desires but cannot realise them feel more social differentiation and division. The market reform has compromised the symbolic socialist order of equality and common wealth, created new economic hierarchies among the populace and correspondingly introduced new orders of health care access. It becomes a threat to the party-state's legitimacy and endangers the very stability that the government promoted consumption for.[11]

The promotion of self-responsible consumer-patients tends to individualise and marketise health care problems. People feel the pressure to get sufficient health care and consume the right products. The impoverished are increasingly held accountable for their 'failure' in the consumption of qualified products. Patients also blame the professionals and hospitals for their provision of differentiated health care, instead of the government. Yet, when the medical price became unbearably high and health care consumption becomes increasingly differentiated, people began to

---

[11]That is why in recent new healthcare reforms the authorities began to reemphasize the public welfare nature of health care.

question the responsibility of the authorities. Involved in the people's discourse is their protest against being dehumanised in the commercialisation of health care, and their quest for an equal right to qualified care. They still expect the government to react in the case of public health care, and argue that health care should be based on the bodily needs not solely on the purchasing ability.

3.3 Negotiate Health Care as Basic Needs and Government Responses

Patients' acceptance of self-responsibility and self-care is only to a certain extent. When health care becomes increasingly unaffordable, patients began to reject the state's framing of individual responsibility, refuse to refashion themselves as neoliberal consumers, and demand the right to basic needs as promised by the party-state since the collective era.

The way that the Chinese government actively relates needs to rights provides people the chance to contest and negotiate their entitlement to basic needs. The government has put its political legitimacy to govern on satisfying and improving people's livelihoods. The discussions of reforms over recent decades have always involved the ideas that the state bears the responsibility for ensuring people's livelihoods, and people have the right to a minimum standard of living. However, the recent market reform has made the official discourse untenable. The delicate relationship between individual needs and social structure indicates that the current health system cannot sufficiently satisfy people's health care needs.

3.3.1 Unmet Health Care Needs and State Legitimacy

In 2006, Premier Wen Jiabao visited some peasant families in the municipality of Riverside County. On the way, he was surprised to be stopped by a little girl. The little girl told 'Grandpa Wen' that her grandfather was sick in bed, but the family was too poor to seek health care. Wen, an affectionate guardian of the underclass, paid heed to the case and persuaded local officials to send the little girl's grandfather for medical care and to provide a subsidy to the poor family. The case was reported by the local media and widely talked about by local people. After the premier's visit, the grandfather was sent to the best hospital in the municipality for free treatment. The local government refurbished the family's dilapidated house and allocated them a monthly subsidy. The little girl is one of the few lucky ones who have succeeded in attracting the attention of a high level official and obtained certain resolution of their family problems. The leader of the central government showed benevolence towards people's difficulties. The central government represented itself as the protector of people's needs. It redistributed responsibility to the local government, which then directed the local hospital to give free care to the old man. However, nothing was mentioned about payment. The hospital which had suffered losses due to this special case would try to recoup the money from other ordinary patients (from Interview 40). It would finally encroach upon other people's needs.

Unlike the little girl, many poor and disadvantaged people have little opportunity to make their presence felt and have their needs heard in such a unique way. In May 2014, a Chinese farmer in Anhui Province cut off his own feet when they deteriorated into severe necrosis, causing unbearable pain (Luo 2014). The patient did not have health insurance and was unable to pay the high medical fees. In 2012, a peasant in Hebei province amputated his festering leg using a saw and a fruit knife (Xinhua Net 2013). The peasant could not find sufficient financial support from any party, including his rural health insurance, thus had to rely on himself to survive. Miserable stories like this routinely appear in the media, signifying a much broader issue of unmet health care needs in post-reform China. The market reform has changed the state's promise of shared prosperity to a scenario of individual survival. Without money, patients do not dare to go to hospital, but seek to self-medicate or manage at home. Within families, when it is impossible to relieve suffering of every case at once, family members have to make difficult decisions on which service to purchase and which family member to save. In my field, a 'worthy' hierarchy is frequently shaped by such factors as life quality, the probability of survival, the cost of treatment, or the productivity of a patient. A poor family tends to save the young instead of the old, and the abled instead of the disabled. The young male, as the family bread winner, tends to be more 'worthy' than the unsound and unproductive member. It is not uncommon to hear cases of patients have to forgo care because of unaffordable medical costs, or committing suicide (in many cases sick elderly family members) because they do not want to become a 'burden' to their family in terms of high medical fees (see Wu 2010).

The evaluation of the worthiness of life and letting the unproductive elderly die are frequently forced life choices for poor families. The family worthy hierarchy has a different texture of feeling compared to the neoliberal value, but the market reform does add a neoliberal layer of values to health sector, where medical providers make judgements about the worthiness or deservedness of patients in terms of their ability to pay and the contribution they can make to the profit-gaining hospital (Chap. 2). The body with less 'value' (profits) may be brutally ignored. The state has implemented a variety of regulations to establish equal rights for patients and prohibit discrimination in health care.[12] However, in practice, notions of (patient) freedom and autonomy are used not only to legitimate the market mechanism

---

[12]Such as the code of conduct for health professionals requires health professionals to 'respect patients' right of being saved, treat patients equally regardless their ethnicity, religion, place of origin, financial condition, status, disability, illness, etc.', from Article 2 of the 'Code of Conduct for Medical Institution Professionals' released by the Ministry of Health (MOH 2012).

whereby people can choose services freely, but also by professionals and hospitals to shirk their care obligations for poor patients, and by the government to reduce its 'burdens'.

Prior to the market reform, the state played a central role in determining distribution and consumption. The research of Linda Wong on social welfare in China notes that according to socialist values, 'the ultimate goal of social distribution is allocation according to need, rather than merit and ability' (1998: 1), but before the advent of communist society, the socialist principle was 'distribution according to work' (ibid.: 191), thus although the regime claimed to satisfy needs, it could not realistically do so. In the post-reform era, distribution according to needs has been superseded by distribution according to capability in the market economy. The market economy with 'Chinese characteristics' encourages ever-rising desires alongside the promotion of domestic spending. State legitimacy is increasingly related to the provision of commodities and the satisfaction of consumer desires in the market. Being economically successful and having buying ability in the market become conditions for realising social rights. Meanwhile, the state constantly promises to satisfy people's needs in the official discourse. However, welfare provisions formerly considered as basic needs provided by the socialist state, such as health care, become largely a matter of personal and family responsibility to be fulfilled in the market. Everyday life with regard to health care is experienced with a heightened sense of uncertainty and feelings of inadequacy. People's claim of needs in terms of health care services becomes increasingly inconsistent with the authorities' resources distribution and health system's provision of health care. Individuals are torn between the neoliberal idea of individual responsibility to satisfy needs and the socialist legacy of demanding existence needs from the state.

3.3.2 Rights to Basic Needs

Needs are the preconditions for human action and interaction. The lack of resources to meet people's needs may impede their participation as a full member of society to achieve valued goals (Doyal and Gough 1991: 49–59). 'Needs' are absolute, imperative, and objective, which differ from 'wants' that are perceptions, fleeting, and subjective. People who claim their needs are actually in shortage of necessary resources, which are essential to live and prosper. (Reisman 2007: 39) Physical health is one such need that requires the resources of health care. In the Chinese context, needs are used situationally by patients to seek health care, aid and compensation. People sometimes intentionally expose their bodily injuries or illnesses: the two self-amputation farmers above were photographed by journalists, who transmitted images of the broken leg and amputated feet directly to the public; patients unsatisfied with poor quality care photographed their inflamed wounds and put these images on the internet; an injured worker exposed his illness to claim medical and financial compensation from a private company[13]; beggars on the streets exposed their sores, ulcers, broken legs, or described family members' illnesses with picture proofs to elicit public sympathy (see Fig. 3.1). The exposure of somatic suffering and the display of bodily injury express the biological needs of bare life. The pubic feel uneasy about these exposures, because the seriously broken body should belong to the spatial context of the hospital, not a rural house or street. The exposure of corporeal injuries and suffering challenges the psyches of the public, who increasingly questions the government's ability to protect people's health. The strong emotion attached to these pictures and words suggests individuals are not just neoliberal subjects, but also concrete persons who have basic needs. The damaged body then becomes the basis to claim citizenship in the face of reduced protection from the state, the irresponsibility of private enterprise, and the impingement of the profit-motivated hospitals and professionals.[14]

Needs pose a moral imperative and form a foundation for the people to conceive their entitlement to health care. Concrete needs transform into an abstract sense of rights that drive people's actions. The linking of needs and rights has been a persistent official discourse, and has also been used in people's practical actions and contestations of their benefits. People have recourse to imperative needs and argue for a need-based right of health care. They contend that public services like basic health care should be organised and allocated by the state on the basis of needs. People also appeal to the socialist principle and the collective era for a more responsive welfare structure. Although local people admit that there are many problems with health care in the collective era, they argued that they were at least secure in receiving preliminary care.[15] Many disadvantaged groups in the market era, who have lost their basic healthcare coverage, share the sense of violation and outrage, and frequently look to reinvigorate a subsistence ethic as the state's governing principle of social life. They appeal to the rhetoric of socialist citizenship to legitimate their health care needs. The socialist past is thus both the source of individual responsibility (as shown in this chapter earlier) and the source of criticism of the neoliberal-inspired changes.

The territory of unfulfilled needs and people's individual, sometimes extreme actions to defend their needs put symbolic pressure on the government, and continually challenge the moral legitimacy of the party-state. Recently the new healthcare reform reemphasises health care as one of the basic needs of living that the state should secure. Needs are catered for in the form of universal basic insurance, basic health care services, preventive care and public health. The health

---

[13]Such as the well-known case in 2009 about a migrant worker, Zhang Haichao, who took thoracotomy lung examination to prove he got pneumoconiosis in order to defend his right for compensation (see Xinhua Net 2009).

[14]Even in the 1990s and early 2000s, the broken body entitles the disabled people to claim certain benefits from the government, such as free body check, the subsidy for taking out medical insurance, and the exemption of taxes when doing business.

[15]Generated from many interviews and conversations with local people when asking them to compare health care in the past and that now.

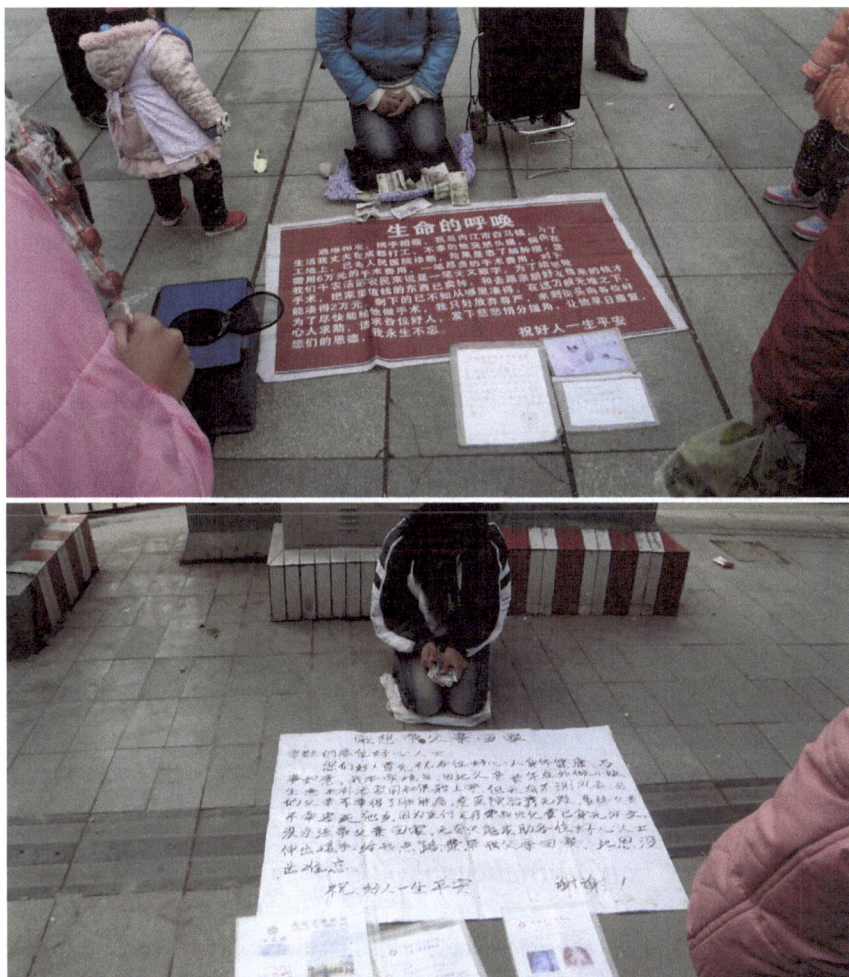

Fig. 3.1 Begging with the 'Excuse' of unaffordable medical fees ('excuse' because many people suspect some cases may not be real)

insurance scheme, co-paid by the government and the individual, indicates a shift in responsibility for health care. Those people, who were left without any safety net in the market reform, now began to receive some social security. However, despite the improved insurance coverage, the rapid increase of overall medical costs still prevents many people from getting the needed health care. A recent study found that the percentage of households suffering 'catastrophic' health expenses barely changed between 2003 and 2011 (from Economist 2012). The conflicts between needs and supplies, the expectation of good care and financial constraints continue to be experienced by many. In Riverside County, several years after the new healthcare reform, the locals were still telling many gloomy stories about poor patients who could not access the necessary health care.

After ascending to power in 2012, the new Xi-Li leadership has demonstrated its commitment to people's needs. In the Third Plenum of the party's Central Committee in 2013, the communiqué calls for the deepening of healthcare reforms so that all citizens have good access to healthcare, and also for an improvement in social security programmes to better meet people's needs (CPG 2013). The ongoing reform shows efforts to expand the scope and scale of medical assistance and to increase insurance subsidies, with special attention given to those who have been rejected for health care previously, such as migrant workers, the employees of private enterprises, self-employed people, and the employees of poorly-performing or bankrupt companies.[16] The state set up a system that tries to meet people's needs in a more equal and appropriate way, but its implementation is embedded in the local political economy, which frequently compromises its realisation. With a rapidly ageing population, China will face enormous challenges in providing adequate health care for its people. The state provisions are still a long way off being fully sufficient to meet people's rising needs. Even the state began to retake health care responsibilities, it continues encouraging self-reliance and self-help. It encourages the public to purchase extra commercial insurance for major illnesses, in facing the catastrophic health expenditures. It also encourages the social and market forces to provide alternative solutions, such as crowd-funding (*zhongchou*)—the internet based public donation system, to help poor families support its seriously ill members.

3.3.3 Need-Based Care as 'Grace' from the State, Rather Than an Inalienable Right

Nevertheless, as the socialist state establishes its legitimacy by welfare reform, the claim of certain social citizenship by the people is made possible. However, health care rights in China, unlike that in the social democratic context, are not bound to the transnational discourse of human rights, and are not determined by the criteria of biological needs alone. Nikolas Rose uses the concept of 'biological citizenship' in the developed Western context, emphasising that the 'bare life' of human beings is the basis of citizenship claims (Rose 2007; Rose and Novas 2005). Biological citizenship in Petryna's research (2002) in Ukraine after the nuclear disaster at Chernobyl is about demanding redress and recognition from the state for certain

---

[16]An article 'Deepening Health System Reform' (Li 2013) written by an official of the NHFPC at the end of 2013 admits that the total medical resources were still insufficient to meet health care needs. It notes that the future healthcare reform aims to reach more fairness and justice by prioritising basic health care, putting major investment in the rural areas, communities at the bottom, difficult localities, and the middle and western regions of China. Also see 'Chinese government to raise health insurance subsidies' (CPG 2012a).

body damage, for obtaining treatment, and for welfare benefits. Chinese patients, by exposing their biological injuries, also struggle for the recognition of their injuries and strive to achieve proper health care. However, in contrast to the people in Chernobyl and the Western context that there is a system for them to make claims, Chinese patients frequently do not have access to a system within which they can make claims to basic needs. Many of the collectives, through which people made claims of needs in the collective era, have already disappeared in the market era. Individual responsibilities and rights are frequently defined against medical institutions and professionals, defined in terms of individual families, not vis-à-vis the state. The state-framed rights such as consumer rights still require people to secure their own care, rather than have the inalienable rights to demand from the state. Patients' families sometimes directly ask for help from the state, such as the little girl who stopped the eminent official on his visit. However, these claims of 'rights to basic needs' show their arbitrariness that success or failure is determined by factors such as the ability to attract media attention and public sympathy, or the occasional interventions from high level officials. These acts to negotiate health care needs succeed only occasionally. They are 'passive dispositions to suffer certain harms because of certain lacks' (Thomson 1987: 100, cited in Ho 2013: 145). When the government shirks its responsibility, many cannot effectively obtain their needs. Besides, although politicians from the central government always give symbolic recognition to people's needs and show determination to meet the people's rising needs, the local governments that have their immediate priorities of mandates (targets like political stability and economic development) frequently ignore people's certain needs.

In addition, many people continue to conceive the new welfare benefits they received in recent years as 'graces' from the state rather than inalienable rights. For instance, local elderly people above the age of 60 have received a basic pension of 55 Yuan per month from the state since 2009. Instead of regarding the pension as a right, many regard it as an act of grace by the central government. Local elderly people repeatedly compare the 55 Yuan pension from the state with the responsibility of their adult children who should support them. For thousands of years, elderly family members have put their care expectations upon their adult children. Now that the elderly receive some support from the state without investing anything, they feel grateful and regard the state to be more accountable than their unfilial or poor adult children who are unwilling or unable to provide support. Similarly, peasants got the land tax abolished and began to get subsidies for farming in the Hu-Wen period. Instead of regarding the subsidy as a right, local farmers regarded the land tax that had lasted for thousands of years since the imperial era as an obligation, and the new regime that not only abolished the land tax but also subsidised farmers was a benefactor greater than the emperors. The minimum life allowance, which is only a few hundred Yuan per month, has also met with positive responses from the rural poor. Many ordinary Chinese, especially those in the rural areas, received little from the state in the past and had few illusions in the first place;

now the government at least subsidise them with something. People at the bottom,[17] especially the elderly, show gratitude to the central government and the CCP, which have improved their material life and made it possible for some of the basic entitlements to be realised, a situation unparalleled in China's long history. The discourses are in accordance with the party-state's official discourse that always puts the people as the beneficiaries of government agendas. The new healthcare reform, together with a series of other welfare schemes, to some extent, improve the moral image of the party-state among the large populace, who feel that they are being considered and cared for by the state instead of being ignored and neglected (as in the 80s and 90s). Nevertheless, the newly-gained benefits are still 'grace' from the state rather than inalienable rights.

As a conclusion, since the market reform, China has seen the individualisation of health care responsibility that people are required to take responsibility for their own care. The state and collective institutions withdrew from welfare provision. Individuals also lack the support and protection available in more traditional settings. Health care becomes individual's responsibility, framed as a moral responsibility between family members, and a civil duty from the individual to the state. The private responsibility of health care in the post-reform era is not simply due to the withdrawal of state and collective protection, instigated by the penetration of the market. For many locals, it is also a remaking of the Confucian self-cultivation and collective self-reliance. This individual health care responsibility corresponds with the collective idea of civic duty that encourages individuals to stay healthy and avoid becoming a burden to the state. It follows the time-honoured traditional value systems to serve a common good (of the family, collective or state), which does not exist in the western neoliberal discourse. Meanwhile, market reforms do add a new layer of requirement on individual patients, who are required to become active consumers in the market. The patients-consumers make choices among multiple medical products, actively negotiate medical prices, and assert their consumer rights. The market reform is changing health care provision from the socialist ideals of a basic service for all, to the provision of opportunities to access good services for all, although the actual availability is limited to those who can pay. Having the ability to care for oneself and for one's family, and being able to secure qualified medical products in the market constitute a new moral subject in the market era. The promotion of self-responsible consumers converts health care issue to individual problems. When satisfactory health care cannot be obtained, blame is attached either to health care providers (who are accused of providing differentiated and discriminatory care) or individual families (that fail to take care of their members). It transfers attention from the failure of the healthcare delivery system and the state. At the meantime, people's views regarding health care are complex, contradictory, and changing over time. Facing increasing inequality and unmet

---

[17]Han (2012) shows that disadvantaged groups feel more satisfied than privileged ones in China. She explains that it results from the complex interactions of a host of socio-economic, experiential and social cognitive factors, and suggests that life satisfaction is influenced more powerfully by dynamic life experiences and subjective evaluations than by objective status.

health care needs, many people began to question the individual responsibility of health care. They defend health care as a basic need. The morality underpinning the need-based requirements is universality. In other words, not just those who can pay should get health care, but everyone should get certain basic and emergency care. In the market era, people embrace market values, but also defend their subsistence rights. Patients sometimes regard themselves as the beneficiaries of government welfare programmes, but also value themselves as clients or customers who make choices between multiple medical products, yet, at other times, they are citizens who actively make claims for qualified care and strive to secure their health care entitlements.

The largely unmet healthcare needs have challenged the authority's moral legitimacy, forcing the government to improve health care provision in recent years. The new healthcare reform, together with a series of welfare programmes to rebuild a safety-net, shows the state's resurgent commitment to meet people's needs. However, huge gap still exists between the rising needs and actual service provisions. Besides, even the state began to retake health care responsibilities, it continues encouraging individual self-reliance. Many people still regard the newly-gained benefits as 'graces' from the state rather than inalienable rights. They defend their health care by performing to be the needy one. Their actions are struggles for passive inclusion, thus may not fundamentally improve their citizenship rights. The realisation of health care entitlements is not solely based on needs or rights, but also determined by factors such as who can attract more media attention and public sympathy, by the occasional interventions from high level officials, and by the categories and qualifications regulated by health insurance policies (see Chap. 4). Overall, the changes in recent decades show as double processes of individuals being dis-embedded from and (re-)embedded in some forms of protection: the shift from the 'community person', who was traditionally surrounded by the extended family, community, and social forces for welfare, and the 'work unit person' (*danwei ren*), who relied on the state and collective for social services in the collective era, to the 'social person' (*shehui ren*), who was responsible for one's own welfare in the market, and the recent reintegration of individuals into public welfare programmes. The fusion of socialist ideology, neoliberal values, traditional self-cultivation, and recent welfare ideas is reconfiguring people's sense of responsibilities, needs and rights.

References

Anagnost, Ann. 2004. The Corporeal Politics of Quality (suzhi). *Public Culture* 16 (2): 189–208.
Anagnost, Ann. 2008. From "Class" to "Social Strata": Grasping the Social Totality in Reform-Era China. *Third World Quarterly* 29 (3): 497–519.
Beck, Ulrich, and Elisabeth Beck-Gernsheim. 2002. *Individualization: Institutionalized Individualism and Its Social and Political Consequences*. London: Sage Publications.
Biehl, Joao. 2005. *Vita: Life in a Zone of Social Abandonment*. Berkeley: University of California Press.

Bourdieu, Pierre. 1984. *Distinction: A Social Critique of the Judgement of Taste*. Cambridge, MA: Harvard University Press.

Cai, Yong. 2009. Regional Inequality in China: Mortality and Health. In *Creating Wealth and Poverty in Postsocialist China*, ed. D. Davis and F. Wang, 143–155. Stanford, CA: Stanford University Press.

Cartier, Carolyn. 2009. Production/Consumption and the Chinese City/Region: Cultural Political Economy and the Feminist Diamond Ring. *Urban Geography* 30 (4): 368–390.

Central People's Government, PRC. 2004. *The Constitution of the People's Republic of China* [Zhonghua renmin gongheguo xianfa]. Retrieved 2 June, 2013 (http://www.gov.cn/gongbao/content/2004/content_62714.htm).

Central People's Government, PRC. 2012a. *Chinese Government to Raise Health Insurance Subsidies*. Retrieved 3 Mar, 2012 (http://english.gov.cn/2012-02/22/content_2074190.htm).

Central People's Government, PRC. 2012b. The General Principle of the Constitution of the Chinese Communist Party [Zhongguo gongchandang dangzhangcheng], Retrieved 28 Oct, 2013 (http://www.gov.cn/jrzg/2012-11/18/content_2269219.htm).

Central People's Government, PRC. 2005. *Law of the People's Republic of China on Protection of the Rights and Interests of Elderly People* [Zhonghua renmin gongheguo laonianren quanyi baozhang fa]. Retrieved 20 July, 2013 (http://www.gov.cn/banshi/2005-08/04/content_20203.htm).

Central People's Government, PRC. 2013. *CCP Central Committee's Decision on Many Significant Issues concerning Comprehensively Deepen Reform* [Zhonggong zhongyang guanyu quanmian shenhua gaige ruogan zhongda wenti de jueding]. Retrieved 17 November, 2013 (http://www.gov.cn/jrzg/2013-11/15/content_2528179.htm).

Chan, Cecilia L.W., and Nelson W.S. Chow. 1992. *More Welfare after Economic Reform? Welfare Development in the People's Republic of China*. Hong Kong: Hong Kong University Press.

Chen, Nancy N. 2003. *Breathing Spaces: Qigong, Psychiatry, and Healing in China*. New York: Columbia University Press.

Chen, Janet. 2012. *Guilty of Indigence: The Urban Poor in China, 1900–1953*. Princeton, NJ: Princeton University Press.

Chen, Meei-Shia. 2001. The Great Reversal: Transformation of Health Care in the People's Republic of China. In *The Blackwell Companion to Medical Sociology*, ed. W.C. Cockerham, 456–482. London: Wiley-Blackwell.

Chen, Nancy N. 2008. Consuming Medicine and Biotechnology in China. In *Privatizing China: Socialism from Afar*, ed. L. Zhang and A. Ong, 123–132. Ithaca, NY: Cornell University Press.

Doyal, Len, and Ian Gough. 1991. *A Theory of Human Need*. London: Macmillan.

Duckett, Jane. 2008. Health NGOs: a Second Generation of Policy Advocates? *China Review* 42 (6): 16.

Economist. 2012. *Health-care Reform: Heroes Dare to Cross*. Retrieved 22 July, 2012 (http://www.economist.com/node/21559379).

Elfick, Jacqueline. 2011. Class Formation and Consumption among Middle-Class Professionals in Shenzhen. *Journal of Current Chinese Affairs* 40 (1): 187–211.

Fan, Ruiping. 2008. A Reconstructionist Confucian Approach to Chinese Health Care. In *China: Bioethics, Trust, and the Challenge of the Market*, ed. J.L.P.W. Tao, 117–133. New York: Springer.

Fan, Ruiping. 2010. *Reconstructionist Confucianism: Rethinking Morality after the West*. London: Springer.

Farquhar, Judith, and Qicheng Zhang. 2012. *Ten Thousand Things: Nurturing Life in Contemporary Beijing*. Cambridge, MA: MIT Press.

Gao, Qiang (The Minister of the Ministry of Health). 2005. 'Developing Medical and Health Work, Making Contribution to Build a Socialist Harmonious Society' [Fazhan yiliao weisheng shiye, wei goujian shehuizhuyi hexieshehui zuo gongxian]. *People's Net*. Retrieved 13 Apr, 2011 (http://politics.people.com.cn/GB/1027/3590082.html).

Han, Chunping. 2012. Satisfaction with the Standard of Living in Reform-era China. *The China Quarterly* 212: 919–940.

Hansen, Mette Halskov. 2013. Learning Individualism: Hesse, Confucius, and Pep-Rallies in a Chinese Rural High School. *The China Quarterly* 213: 60–77.

Hansen, Mette Halskov, and Rune Svarverud. 2010. *iChina: The Rise of the Individual in Modern Chinese Society*. Copenhagen: Nordic Institute of Asian Studies Press.

Hooper, Beverley. 2005. The Consumer Citizen in Contemporary China. Working Paper No. 12 in Centre for East and South-East Asian Studies, Lund University. Retrieved 12 Dec, 2013 (http://lup.lub.lu.se/luur/download?func=downloadFile&recordOId=951451&fileOId=3128706).

Ho, Cheuk Yuet. 2013. Exit, or Evict: Re-grounding Rights in Needs in China's Urban Housing Demolition. *Asian Anthropology* 12 (2): 141–155.

Hwang, Kwang-Kuo. 1998. Guanxi and Mientze: Conflict Resolution in Chinese Society. *Intercultural Communication Studies* 7 (1): 17–38.

Keane, Michael. 2001. Redefining Chinese citizenship. *Economy and Society* 30 (1): 1–17.

Kipnis, Andrew. 2007. Neoliberalism Reified: Suzhi Discourse and Tropes of Neoliberalism in the People's Republic of China. *Journal of the Royal Anthropological Institute* 13 (2): 383–400.

Latham, Kevin. 2012. Rethinking Chinese Consumption. In *Postsocialism: Ideas, Ideologies and Practices in Eurasia*, ed. C.M. Hann, 217–237. New York: Routledge.

Li, Bing. 2013. *Deepening Health System Reform* [Shenhua yiyao weisheng tizhi gaige]. Retrieved 5 Dec, 2013 (http://www.moh.gov.cn/xcs/wzbd/201312/94aa978156224464b827fea5b71bef25.shtml).

Liu, Xingzhu, and Anne Mills. 1999. Evaluating Payment Mechanisms: How Can We Measure Unnecessary Care? *Health Policy and Planning* 14 (4): 409–413.

Luo, Chris. 2014. Farmer Cuts off His Own Feet after Being Unable to Afford Frostbite Treatment. *South China Morning Post*. Retrieved 22 May, 2014 (http://www.scmp.com/news/china-insider/article/1512067/anhui-farmer-unable-afford-medical-expenses-amputates-own-feet).

Ministry of Health, PRC. 2012. *The Code of Conduct for Medical Institution Professionals* [Yiliao jigou congye renyuan xingwei guifan]. Retrieved 10 Mar, 2013 (http://www.moh.gov.cn/mohjcg/s3577/201207/55445.shtml).

National People's Congress, PRC. 2000. *The General Principles of the Civil Law of the People's Republic of China* [Zhonghua renmin gongheguo minfa tongze]. Retrieved 3 June, 2014 (http://www.npc.gov.cn/wxzl/wxzl/2000-12/06/content_4470.htm).

National People's Congress, PRC. 2005. *Rights to Subsistence and Rights to Development are the Prime Basic Human Rights* [Shengcun quan he fazhan quan shi shouyao de jiben renquan]. Retrieved 16 Dec, 2013 (http://www.npc.gov.cn/npc/xinwen/rdlt/fzjs/2005-06/27/content_338893.htm).

Perry, Elizabeth. 2008. Chinese Conceptions of "Rights": From Mencius to Mao—And Now. *Perspectives on Politics* 6 (1): 37–50.

Petryna, Adriana. 2002. *Life Exposed: Biological Citizens after Chernobyl*. Princeton, NJ: Princeton University Press.

Reisman, David. 2007. *Health Care and Public Policy*. Cheltenham: Edward Elgar.

Rogaski, Ruth. 2004. *Hygienic Modernity: Meanings of Health and Disease in Treaty-Port China*. Berkeley: University of California Press.

Rose, Nikolas. 2007. *The Politics of Life Itself: Biomedicine, Power, and Subjectivity in the Twenty-first Century*. Princeton, NJ: Princeton University Press.

Rose, Nikolas, and Carlos Novas. 2005. Biological Citizenship. In *Global Assemblages: Technology, Politics, and Ethics as Anthropological Problems*, ed. A. Ong and S.J. Collier, 439–463. Malden, MA: Blackwell.

Ren, Hai. 2010. *Neoliberalism and Culture in China and Hong Kong: The Countdown of Time*. London: Routledge.

Shen, Yifei. 2011. China in the "Post-Patriarchal Era" Changes in the Power Relationships in Urban Households and an Analysis of the Course of Gender Inequality in Society. *Chinese Sociology and Anthropology* 43 (4): 5–23.

Sigley, Gary. 1996. Governing Chinese Bodies: The Significance of Studies in the Concept of Govermentality for the Analysis of Government in China. *Economy and Society* 25 (4): 457–482.

Thomson, Garrett. 1987. *Needs*. London: Routledge & Kegan Paul.

Wang, Shaoguang. 2010. China's Double Movement in Health Care. *Socialist Register* 46: 240–261.

Wong, Linda. 1998. *Marginalization and Social Welfare in China*. London: Routledge.

Wu, Fei. 2010. *Suicide and Justice: A Chinese Perspective*. London: Routledge.

Xinhua Net. 2009. *Recent Update of the "Thoracotomy Lung Examination" Incident: Expert Confirm Zhang Haicao got Pneumoconiosis* [Kaixiong yanfei shijian zuixin jinzhan: zhuanjia quezhen Zhang Haicao huan chenfei bing]. Retrieved 6 June, 2013 (http://news.xinhuanet.com/employment/2009-07/28/content_11783387.htm).

Xinhua Net. 2013. *Man unable to Pay Medical Fee, Cut Off His own Right Leg* [Nanzi youbing wuqian zhi zi ju huanbing youtui]. Retrieved 22 May, 2014 (http://news.xinhuanet.com/health/2013-10/11/c_125511492.htm).

Yan, Hairong. 2003a. Neoliberal Governmentality and Neohumanism: Organizing Suzhi/Value Flow through Labor Recruitment Networks. *Cultural Anthropology* 18 (4): 493–523.

Yan, Yunxiang. 2003b. *Private Life under Socialism: Love, Intimacy, and Family Change in a Village, 1949–1999*. Stanford, CA: Stanford University Press.

Yan, Yunxiang. 2009. *The Individualization of Chinese Society*. London: Athlone Press.

Yan, Yunxiang. 2010a. The Chinese Path to Individualization. *The British Journal of Sociology* 61 (3): 489–512.

Yan, Yunxiang. 2010b. Introduction: Conflicting Images of the Individual and Contested Process of Individualization. In *iChina: The Rise of the Individual in Modern Chinese Society*, ed. M.H. Hansen and R. Svarverud, 1–38. Copenhagen: Nordic Institute of Asian Studies Press.

Yang, Jingqing. 2017. *Informal Payments and Regulations in China's Healthcare System: Red Packets and Institutional Reform*. Singapore: Springer.

Zhan, Mei. 2013. Human Oriented? Angels and Monsters in China's Health Care Reform. In *Health Care Reform and Globalisation: The US, China and Europe in Comparative Perspective*, ed. P. Watson, 71–92. London: Routledge.

Chapter 4
Health Insurance Regime
as Differentiation and Discipline

Before the market reform, health care was mainly publicly or collectively provided, and consisted of health care for workers under the Labour Insurance Scheme (LIS, *laobao yiliao*),[1] public health care for government employees through the Government Insurance Scheme (GIS, *gongfei yiliao*),[2] and the rural Cooperative Medical Scheme (CMS, *hezuo yiliao*) for peasants.[3] In the 1980s, the collective production system that supported rural health care was replaced by the household production system. The rural CMS and collective medical facilities could not be sustained anymore.[4] Besides, the role of 'work units' in providing health insurance to urban employees has been greatly weakened as they were required to become more efficient in the market. Many public employees 'dove into the business sea' (*xiahai*) or were laid off by their work units,[5] becoming responsible for their own health care. Together with the collapse of rural cooperative medical insurance

---

Part of this chapter was published in *Hygiea Internationalis* 2016, 12(2): 51–72 as an open-access article (Tu 2016).

---

[1]It was mainly funded by the welfare funds of enterprises, providing employees and their immediate family members with full or partial medical care coverage.

[2]GIS was financed directly by governments at various levels, provided to people working in government and public institutions, including the staff of cultural, educational, health, and research institutes, and students at colleges and universities.

[3]It was funded by contributions from participants and heavily subsidised by the rural collective welfare funds and government.

[4]Since the early 1980s, the rural cooperative medical insurance system has collapsed, only 5.4% of China's 940,000 villages had cooperative medical care in 1985 and 15% in 1994, though this figure was approximately 90% in the late 1970s (Wu 1997: 148).

[5]From 1995 to 2002 alone, about 60 million employees were cut from state or collective enterprises (Ying 2010: 3).

© Springer Nature Singapore Pte Ltd. 2019
J. Tu, *Health Care Transformation in Contemporary China*,
https://doi.org/10.1007/978-981-13-0788-1_4

scheme, health insurance coverage in China has decreased to the minimum, leading to a rapid increase in direct out-of-pocket payment (Grogan 1995; Gu 2008).[6]

In the new healthcare reform, one of the main reform agendas is to set up a basic health insurance system that provides insurance for all. It includes health insurance for urban employees (introduced in 1998), jointly paid for by governments, employers and employees; health insurance for unemployed urban residents (since 2007), mainly paid for by residents and subsidised by governments; and a new cooperative medical insurance scheme for rural residents (since 2003), co-paid by governments and individuals. The government provides subsidies for the poor to take out medical insurance. At the meantime, the GIS (*gongfei yiliao*) provided by government to people working in government and public institutions continues. The four insurance schemes coexist, covering 95% of the Chinese population by the end of 2011, up from less than one-third in 2003 (Gao et al. 2014). Yet, people with different insurance scheme are reimbursed differently: GIS has the best reimbursement rate, LIS follows, and insurances for rural and urban residents have relatively lower reimbursement rates. In Riverside County, many patients have benefited from insurance programmes. Health insurance programmes have also been proclaimed by local health professionals as the most, or even the only, successful part of the new healthcare reform. Nevertheless, this chapter holds a more critical view to analyse the function of health insurance as a mechanism of governance and differentiation.

From the perspective of governmentality, insurance can be considered as a 'technology of risk' (Ewald 1991: 197) that organises people to share the burden of risks involved in life. Francois Ewald (1991: 206) notes that insurance as 'a distributive sharing of a collective burden' contains a social rule of justice and a principle of social solidarity, which is different from the judicial idea of deciding accident compensation following an investigation of the cause of injury. However, the new health insurance schemes in China contain contradictory and competing ideas. Health insurance is organised with the hope of improving social justice through the distribution of health care burden collectively. Yet the implementation of China's insurance schemes follows the judicial model. Insurance reimbursement is linked with the investigation of the cause of injury—the evaluation of whether the illness or injury was due to natural causes (in that case the insurance will cover the medical bill) or due to the behaviour of individuals (in that case the individual should bear the medical costs). The definition of 'qualified' patients in the health insurance regime serves as the gatekeeper to safeguarding the insurance funds targeting the needy people, but it also produces new differentiation, discrimination, and inequality among patients. Health insurance policies combined with other state policies (for instance household registration, population control, and employment status) produce categories and qualifications that subject patients to a structure of selection and means-testing. It also provides the authority with new mechanisms of

---

[6]In the mid-1990s, approximately 95% of rural residents were paying for their own care (Grogan 1995). Even with the government's efforts to change the situation since the late 1990s, the Third National Health Service Research in 2003 still showed that about 65% of the population (45% of urban population, and 70% of rural population) did not have any insurance (Gu 2008: 60).

surveillance and control, and enables more efficient governance. Health insurance regimes form the basis of biopower and constitute the power/knowledge in Foucauldian sense to monitor, shape and control the behaviour of individuals as well as the conduct of the population. This chapter explores how health insurance regimes constitute regulatory devices, enable the evaluation of the qualification and worthiness of patients, and correspondingly serve to extend the state control and surveillance of individuals and the population. It also examines the ways in which health insurance brings life into economic calculation and is used by profit-driven hospitals and professionals to maximise profits, and, in the process, produces new discriminations and inequalities among patients. The follow up study also displays the government's effort to correct the above issues by further reducing the differences and segregations within insurance schemes, and in the process improving its moral legitimacy.

4.1 Health Insurance as Segregation: The Exclusion of Migrants

Rural-to-urban migrant workers have been widely researched in China. Migrant workers take the dangerous, difficult and dirty jobs that the urban residents are not willing to do. They have low social status and unequal access to public services in the city, and are referred to by scholars as the 'second-class citizen' (Solinger 1999; Whyte 2010). When migrants work in the city, only some well-functioned companies provide health insurance, which is co-contributed by workers and employers. Many migrants cannot get health insurance in their working place and, as a result, confront serious health care exclusion. A 40-city survey conducted by the State Council in 2004 shows that only 15% of migrant workers participate in social security schemes and only 10% have medical insurance (from Lee and Shen 2009). In the new healthcare reform, the state has developed health insurance for urban employees, insurance for unemployed urban residents, and cooperative medical scheme for rural residents, but no suitable insurance programme is available to migrant workers, among whom, many are peasant workers living cities. The health insurance system is coordinated within the jurisdiction territories of each municipality and is linked to people's household registration (*hukou*). The use of health insurance is restricted to assigned hospitals and pharmacies in places where people's *hukou* is located. If patients seek health care in other places, they either pay out-of-pocket or go to the assigned hospitals outside their municipality with a low reimbursement rate. The segregated and fragmented health insurance system cannot meet the demands of the increasingly mobile population. In 2012, the number of migrants in China was 236 million (NHFPC 2013b). In Riverside County, about one fourth of the population, over 250,000 people, annually migrate to seek job. The market economy creates these free floating workers, but the existing system does not provide a portable or national level medical scheme to protect them. By examining this marginal group in the current health system, this section tries to understand how the health insurance scheme shapes and facilitates a process of exclusion in health care governance.

4.1.1 The Migrant Worker Who Got a Brain Tumour

In September 2012, during my week-long observation in the rehabilitation department of the TCM Hospital, I met a brain tumour patient, a young migrant worker in his early 30 s, who was being treated in this department. I talked with him over the week and got to know his story. In April 2012, the migrant worker had fainted at the construction site he worked at, in Henan province. His colleagues called the ambulance. In the hospital, the MRI scan showed a tumour in his brain. He got emergency treatment in Henan province, which cost him over 10,000 Yuan, several months of his salary. Soon after the emergency treatment, he migrated back to his home province Sichuan. He registered in *Huaxi* Hospital, the best hospital in the provincial capital. The main site of the hospital was full and could not accommodate any more patients, so he was accommodated in the hospital's newly-built sub branch situated in the suburb. Doctors from the main hospital came to operate on him several days later. After the operation, he stayed in the hospital for about a month. Later on he was transferred to the Provincial Tumour Hospital, another top level hospital in the provincial capital, where he got regular medical checks and radiotherapy for two months. The tumour hospital was also full. The department he visited only had 50 beds, but there were more than 80 inpatients. 'How expensive health care is in those big hospitals!' he exclaimed. The operation in *Huaxi* Hospital cost him more than 36,000 Yuan. Each time he visited the Tumour hospital, the MRI scan would cost more than 2000 Yuan and radiotherapy cost more than 4000 Yuan, not to mention other expenses. The overall medical expenditure since his first hospitalisation had already surpassed 100,000 Yuan, a huge amount for most Chinese families, let alone for a peasant like himself. He had bought rural health insurance annually, but he predicted that he might only claim back about 20–30% of his expenditure. Most of his treatments were in places outside Riverside County (the Henan province where his tumour was diagnosed and the provincial capital where he got operation and radiotherapy). The insurance scheme encourages patients to seek health care in low level medical institutions before going to higher level hospitals by giving higher reimbursement rates for hospital care at the bottom level. In 2012, the reimbursement rate of rural CMS in Riverside County was 90% for medical expenditure beyond 100 Yuan in township level hospitals; 80% for costs that exceeded 200 Yuan in county level hospitals; 60% for expenditure beyond 600 Yuan in municipal level hospitals; 55% for costs beyond 700 Yuan in provincial level hospitals and approved hospitals outside the province; and for treatment in other hospitals, the reimbursement rate was 45% for costs beyond 800 Yuan (see Table 4.1). The tumour patient would be reimbursed at the lowest rate for his treatment in Henan province and the provincial hospitals, because he did not know that he should have obtained a hospital transfer reference from his local county hospital first. Doctor Chen in the rehabilitation department commented that many patients in serious and emergency situations, like this tumour patient, would go directly to high level hospitals or hospitals near their work places, and therefore would not be able to obtain the transfer reference from their hometown hospital in the first place. Besides, the health insurance only covers

Table 4.1 CMS reimbursement at different levels of hospitals in 2012

	Reimbursement for costs exceeded (Yuan)	Reimbursement rates (%)	Reimbursement ceilings (Yuan)
Township hospitals	100	90	120,000
County hospitals	200	80	120,000
Approved municipal hospitals	600	60	120,000
Approved provincial hospitals and approved hospitals outside the province	700	55	120,000
Other (non-approved) hospitals outside the municipality	800	45	120,000

the items on the name lists of drugs, treatments, and medical facilities. In the tumour patient's case, many expensive drugs and tests were not covered by his insurance. The tumour patient's prediction of 20–30% reimbursement is consistent with other patients' experiences. In the field, I collected dozens of lists (displayed in local hospitals I visited) of patients who had received reimbursements between 2010 and 2012. Rural CMS patients on these lists, who had sought health care outside the local municipality, were generally reimbursed around, or less than, 30% of their overall medical expenditure.

After treatment in the provincial capital, the migrant worker came back to Riverside. He came to the TCM Hospital daily for acupuncture and rehabilitation. Although he had been registered as an inpatient, like many other inpatients whose homes were not far from the city, he came to the hospital for treatment in the morning and went back home in the afternoon. In this way, he could be covered by his insurance that targeted inpatient care mainly. The hospital could save the hospital bed and accommodate more 'inpatients' than its actual bed capacity. During the week I observed at the hospital, the tumour patient constantly asked the doctors about his medical expenditure. In the long acupuncture process, he frequently lamented that only his elder brother was earning money to support the family since he got sick. His previous treatments had already cost more than 100,000 Yuan and he needed more money for the ongoing rehabilitation and further radiotherapy. Other patients in the same ward often gave him suggestions on what social assistance was available and how to apply from the government. I suggested that he should apply for the medical aid for major illnesses. He told me that he needed to wait until the Health Insurance Bureau approved his reimbursement, only then could he take the insurance reimbursement documents to apply for further medical aid from the Bureau of Civil Affairs. 'I might get 2000 to 4000 [Yuan medical aid]', he predicted. The medical aid aims at helping poor families to counter major illnesses. Being mainly funded by the local level governments and supplemented with subsidies from the central government and social donations, the capacity of medical aid is limited. A report from the Riverside County Bureau of Civil Affairs showed that in 2010 it had given medical aid to 16,484 people in the urban area, which amounted to 3,466,800 Yuan. However, when this was distributed to individual patients, each patient received on average about 210 Yuan in aid. Since the setting up of rural CMS in Riverside, the Bureau of Civil Affair initiated a 'second medical aid' for poor rural families to get up to 20,000 Yuan aid in cases of major illnesses. The official data though, show that the total amount used in second aid was 138,000 Yuan in 2005, 600,000 Yuan in 2006, 1 million in 2007, and 1,137,015 Yuan in 2009. In 2006, the 600,000 Yuan aided only 136 patients, giving less than 5000 Yuan on average per patient. In 2009, the 1,137,015 Yuan aided 415 serious patients (whose medical fee surpassed 30,000 Yuan), but each patient on average only got about 2700 Yuan in aid. In a local town, I collected a list of about 70 patients who got the 'second medical aid' in 2008, which showed that most of them only received 1500 Yuan in aid, although all of these patients' medical expenditure surpassed 20,000 Yuan.[7] Without any special connection, the tumour patient had good reason to predict that he might only get a few thousands Yuan in aid, merely a drop in the bucket of the total expenses.

4.1.2   Bureaucratic Regulations, Social Separation and Exclusion

The tumour patient's case reveals the many obstacles migrant workers face in general in order to get health care. These include a fragmented health insurance system, the *hukou* system that ties health care and other social services with people's place of origin, overcrowded hospitals, exorbitant medical charges, low insurance reimbursement, complex and unclear policies, and so forth. The different insurance schemes that organise people together in the sharing of risks also produce separation among patients who are divided into different patient statuses. While people now have more access to social assistance, the rural population are still extremely vulnerable when facing major illnesses. Even for those who receive insurance reimbursement, the funding is frequently inadequate. People's financial burden for medical care is still excessive, and protecting vulnerable groups from health-care-related impoverishment remains a challenge, albeit with insurance coverage (Li et al. 2012; Fu et al. 2018). Moreover, various rules and policies constitute a corpus of insurance knowledge, which people are not familiar with. The information billboards displayed around hospitals and insurance bureaus only provide a general introduction about health insurance policies. There is no detailed insurance regulation (such as insurance coverage item list, reimbursement procedures) available on-line or given to the public, and local reimbursement policies change from year to year. The locals have to go to the insurance office to enquire in person. The migrant's case also points towards the overly bureaucratic approach of

---

[7]On the list, only one patient received 4500 Yuan in aid, the highest amount, but his overall medical expenditure was 88,825 Yuan.

insurance administration. Health insurance schemes are administered by several departments separately. Health insurance for urban employees and urban residents are administered by the Social Insurance Department at different levels of government under the Ministry of Human Resources and Social Security. The rural CMS is administered by the Rural Health Insurance Bureau under the Ministry of Health. Medical aid is under the administration of yet another department—the Ministry of Civil Affairs. The overly bureaucratic arrangement makes reimbursement procedures lengthy and complex. Patients have to pay medical fees out of pocket first, and get reimbursed after their treatment. The reimbursement process involves many procedures and a mass of paper work. After several months from his first hospitalisation, the migrant worker had not received any benefit. The over-bureaucratic arrangements sometimes deter people from seeking proper health care and insurance benefits.

In China, the urban areas for a long time have been the privileged sites of medical services and facilities, which, however, are not available for migrant workers. Many literatures have recorded the poor access to proper health care for rural-to-urban migrants, and the health risks of these migrants, including infectious diseases, maternal health, occupational disease and injuries, psychological distress and mental health problems, and poor long-term health (Chen 2011; Hesketh et al. 2008; Hu, Cook, and Salazar 2008; Milcent 2010; Peng et al. 2010). The combination of health insurance schemes and the *hukou* system produces exclusions for migrant workers, disabling them from receiving affordable health care in the city. The return of migrants to their hometown to seek health care may overwhelm the newly-built rural insurance system (Hu, Cook, and Salazar 2008). Xu (2009: 40) argues that 'the governmental attitude towards migrant workers was not to 'let' them 'die', but it was more about letting them "move" rather than making them "live". My research on health care access suggests that migrant workers are either 'let' to die in the city (see the migrant's case in Chap. 2) or expected to 'move' back to their hometown to 'live' (such as the tumour patient above). The labour of these young, healthy migrant workforces contribute to the improvement of living conditions in the urban areas and to the economic prosperity in China. The city also provides millions of migrant workers with a chance to earn more, and thus improves the lives of migrants and their families, but only when they are healthy. When illness comes, the city fails to provide them with protection. Referring to Foucault, Gay Becker writes that marginality reflects 'the biopolitical division between those whose lives are managed with the goal of enhancement and those whose lives are judged as less worthy and who are allowed to die' (2007: 300). Lacking education and 'quality' in the neoliberal market, migrant workers rely mainly, even solely, on their 'healthy' bodies to support their lives in the city. When they become sick and (temporarily or permanently) lose their 'productivity', they become 'valueless', experience indifference, and are driven away from the city back to their hometowns in order to survive. The movement of goods and labours in the market economy is not matched with the flexibility of social services. Public services are framed by the rigid separation between localities, between rural and urban areas, that has been in place since the collective era. These fragmentation and segregation impair labour mobility (which is fundamental to China's economic development) and social solidarity.

4.2 Health Insurance as Regulatory Technology

Health insurance schemes have specific regulations for the categorisation and qualification of patients. These regulatory rules vary from place to place, but generally there are several shared categories of illnesses or treatments that are not covered by the three main insurance schemes: injuries caused in traffic accident, medical accident, or other accident due to negligence[8]; injuries caused by one's drug-taking, fighting, or other illegal behaviour; treatment due to individual self-harm, suicide, alcoholism, etc.; medical treatment sought by oneself (a patient does not go to the appointed hospital or does not get a transfer reference before going to a high level hospital); drugs or treatments outside insurance coverage; medical treatment for cases that are not in accordance with birth planning policies.[9] These regulations construct a 'grid of abstract categories' that works as normative rules and judgements. They encourage people to be responsible subjects, not to hurt themselves intentionally, and take responsibility themselves or seek compensation from the person who caused their injuries rather than rely on the public insurance. They also produce the 'civic worthiness' of health care according to individual's conduct. Injuries caused by irresponsible or 'immoral' acts, such as fights, alcoholism, and criminalities, are 'unworthy' of state covered health care. The individual is 'objectively' evaluated by these criteria which constitute a punitive gaze, surveying individual behaviour, but frequently failing to acknowledge individual's entitlement.

4.2.1 The 'Unqualified' Patient Under Population Control

In Riverside, I recorded many cases of insured people who were only partially-qualified or unqualified for health insurance coverage. The pre-marriage birth is one of the unqualified categories. One such case involved a 19-year-old who

---

[8]This regulation is especially unfavourable for migrant workers. The rural CMS, the insurance most rural-to-urban migrant workers have, does not cover industry injuries—injuries caused during work, because it presumes that the industry injuries will be covered by the labour insurance. However, it ignores the large numbers of migrant workers, who take dangerous work in the city and have high possibility of getting injured during work, but frequently do not have labour insurance.

[9]The lists are based on the local health insurance reimbursement regulations and the internet search results about health care that is not covered by various insurance schemes.

gave birth to a baby by caesarean in the county hospital in 2012. After the birth, the preterm baby was sent to the municipal hospital for intensive care. The overall medical costs of the mother and baby were over 10,000 Yuan, but neither of them could get any reimbursement, although the mother had joined the CMS. The CMS proclaims that it covers all the fees of a natural delivery and part of the costs of a caesarean. However, in order to get the benefit, the birth must take place in the appointed medical institution with a birth permit (*zhun shengzheng*). The birth permit is a certificate obtained by married couples to legitimate a birth, a policy related with the population control currently carried out in China. Only those who abide by state birth policies (married couples, one child in most cases) can obtain medical insurance reimbursement. The young mother, unmarried, could not get the birth permit. Her pregnancy thus became 'undesired' and the baby was a result of an 'unwanted birth' according to the state policy. The young mother was not entitled to insurance coverage for the birth. The baby, born out of marriage, would encounter more difficulties to obtain a *hukou*, without which he would not be able to get the new-born baby medical insurance. Thus, the baby had no coverage for his earlier treatment. Besides, the ethical environment in the local community has not changed as quickly as the economic development and sexual behaviour of young people. Premarital pregnancy is still highly stigmatised and frequently becomes the target of gossip within a community.[10] The family, embarrassed by the 'dishonoured' birth, could hardly speak out in the community, let alone fight for their insurance entitlement.

Population governance in China has relied on both the cruder disciplinary practices (sometimes coercive abortion) and more subtle controls such as the link of birth with health insurance and other welfare benefits. Birth control in China has been relaxed recently. The coercive elements in population control, although still occasionally exposed by the media, have been used much less frequently over the years (Hesketh 2010). The disciplinary techniques have become more subtle forms, which work to shape and guide individual conduct (see Greenhalgh and Winckler 2005; Greenhalgh 2009).[11] The state-initiated propaganda and policies that stigmatise and discriminate unmarried birth also serve the birth control. State policies, together with social norms, construct the standards of appropriate behaviour and a moral form of self-governance where an unmarried young woman is expected to control her own reproductive activities. The link of social welfare to birth behaviour

---

[10]I first heard about this case through the gossip by a group of elderly women in a local community in DY town. Later I got more information about this case through informal talk and interview (Interview P39) with several community members. But when discussing this case, all of them immediately lowered their voices.

[11]Greenhalgh and Winckler (2005) find, in China's population control, the neoliberal biopolitics emerge in the people's effort to produce the 'quality child'. They note that the reproductive self-discipline is a kind of regulated freedom, guided by powerful logics of science and technology, the market, and the transnational consumer culture; it is produced by forces seeking to shape individual desires and behaviour to their own ends. Greenhalgh (2009) further notes that bio-governance in China aimed at the management of the vital characteristics of human populations, and exercised in the name of optimising individual and collective life, health, and welfare.

materialises this control.[12] When an 'illegal' birth occurs, the health insurance exposes the patient to new punitive regulatory techniques, adding embarrassment to the already embarrassed family. Health care thus facilitates the surveillance and control of the population.

Greenhalgh (2003) suggests that China's population-planning creates legal 'non-persons' out of those born 'out-of-quota'. The unplanned births give rise to 'unplanned persons' who have no access to schools, village land, etc., and thus in essence creates 'stratified citizenship'. In health care, these 'unplanned babies' and women with 'unplanned pregnancy/birth' are excluded from health care entitlement. Children and women, who come from more economically vulnerable families and need insurance reimbursement more than others, tend to be more affected by these policy 'penalties', because they have less resources and connections to overcome policy obstacles. Health insurance produces a diffuse apparatus of power/knowledge with normative power that endorses certain values and behaviour while rejecting others that are not in accordance with the government's aims. The health care right—the right to get insurance benefits here—is a matter ratified by the state, rather than a right given at birth. The actual entitlement is based on neither need nor right, but on rule abidance. Through the deployment of insurance regulatory, the individual and social body become more pliable and amenable. Insurance enables the beneficiary's 'voluntary' compliance. However, people often subtly negotiate their insurance entitlements.

4.2.2   Becoming Qualified Patients: Negotiate Insurance Reimbursement

Insurance qualifications form a controlled sphere of 'normal' and 'abnormal' illnesses. People respond by seeking to become the 'qualified' or legitimate patients. Aunt Wen, a local resident in her 60 s, broke her collarbone in May 2011, when she fell from her husband—Uncle Wen's motorbike. Uncle and Aunt Wen recounted to me in detail how Aunt Wen was hospitalised and reimbursed:

> Uncle Wen: We were opportunistic this time. When she broke her bone, we hadn't bought health insurance yet. I went [to the community office] to ask whether health insurance was still for sale, he [the staff] told me it was. I asked that if I bought the insurance could I use it immediately, he said it could cover hospitalisation that happened from January this year. On the second day I bought insurance for both of us, and then we went to the hospital [laugh]…Later we got more than 60 percent reimbursement. Before reimbursement, they would come to investigate the case, inquiring how she got hurt. When we just went into hospital, I said she fell down from my motorbike, but falling down from motorbike wouldn't be reimbursed, thus I said she fell down from the stair when going downstairs to shopping.

---

[12]The link of social services with social-control mechanism has long been used by the party-state since the Maoist period.

JT: How did you know motorbike accidents wouldn't be covered?

Aunt Wen: They told us. When we just went into hospital, the other patients nearby [in the same ward] asked us how I broke my bone, we told them I fell off from motorbike, they told us we wouldn't be reimbursed if we wrote falling off from motorbike. My eldest daughter hearing this immediately threw the [insurance claim] form she had already filled, she did business and was very 'cunning'. Later she asked the doctor for another form. She said she forgot where the first one was. (Interview P11)

Aunt Wen was an urban resident and could join the health insurance for urban residents by paying an annual fee, which would cover hospital care occurring within a year period (not for accumulation). In 2011, it cost 170 Yuan to join the insurance scheme. The health insurance specifies that injuries directly caused by individual actions of the patients or others would not be covered, such as transport accidents. Instead of getting this information from the hospital or health professionals, Aunt Wen learnt this from other patients in the same ward, who frequently shared information with each other. Her family then made another excuse for her injury. Later on, the insurance bureau came to investigate Aunt Wen's case. Aunt Wen made up a detailed story about how she fell down from the stair outside her home when going out for shopping. In Aunt Wen's treatment, an expensive steel plate was installed to fix her broken bone. The whole medical expenditure was about 10,500 Yuan. Aunt Wen claimed back 6700 Yuan from insurance, and thus paid only about 3800 Yuan out of her own pocket. Aunt and Uncle Wen felt happy about this result and proclaimed that the insurance scheme was great. 'You pay a little but get a lot', Uncle Wen commented. We all laughed when Uncle Wen said humorously that they were speculators who went to the hospital immediately after purchasing their health insurance. Patients like Uncle and Aunt Wen pragmatically took advantage of the policies and adapted to the circumstance to gain benefits. The definition of 'qualified' and 'unqualified' patients is a subtle negotiation process that both the insurance bureau and the patient take part in, rather than simply a label allocated from above.

Nobody felt that it was 'illegal' to 'make the story up' and 'take advantage of the policy', but rather, everyone felt happy for the result that Aunt Wen finally got reimbursed. Their 'opportunistic' action was morally justified, considering that normal patients frequently endured heavy financial burdens in the commercialised health care sector. As Ong and Zhang write, increasingly, in contemporary China, 'individuals are obliged to exercise diligence, cunning, talents, and social skills to navigate ever-shifting networks of goods, relationships, knowledge, and institutions in the competition for wealth and personal advantage' (Ong and Zhang 2008: 8). Individual patients rationally assess situations and act prudently. They negotiate quietly, and creatively challenge the official rules with their value framework and practical actions. These subversive, indirect actions by patients to circumvent or resist state rules are widespread. Although these daily 'resistances' cannot directly change the rules, they do, to some extent, push back the policies that people think did not serve them well. They allow individuals to temporarily seize control of their own situations, and to secure health care access and benefits within the changing system.

4.2.3 Using Guanxi to Gain Benefits: The Unequal Insurance Reimbursement

People display an agentive ability to accommodate to existing policies. Local patients also widely use connections to obtain benefits from health insurance and aid programmes. Yet, these individual agentive efforts make insurance compensation and medical aid inconsistent. The 'honest' and less connected patients may easily lose out. The cases of Mrs Lou and Mrs Huang below, demonstrate the huge difference in compensation for similar treatments in the same hospital:

> Mrs Lou, a local resident in her 30 s, broke her leg in 2011. She was taken into the TCM Hospital soon afterwards. The financial condition of Mrs Lou's family was average. Her husband was working as a porter for a furniture store with a salary of just over 2000 Yuan a month. Her son was studying in a local middle school. Mrs Lou was a worker in a local textile company, earning merely over 1000 Yuan per month. The company offered employees medical insurance, co-paid by the company and employees. However, Mrs Lou declined the insurance in order to save her portion (dozens Yuan a month) of contribution, because she knew her job was unstable and the insurance would not be lifelong if she left the company before the retirement age (55 years old). Moreover, she thought she was young and healthy and would not need medical insurance. As a result, when she got injured in 2011, she did not have any insurance. Luckily, her sister was working in a local health office. The sister helped Mrs Lou register under the name of a relative, who had rural CMS. This well-connected sister also found an acquaintance in the hospital and arranged an experienced senior doctor to operate for Mrs Lou. A steel plate was installed in Mrs Lou's leg. She stayed in the hospital for 19 days. The whole hospitalisation cost over 20,000 Yuan, almost ten times her husband's monthly salary. This huge amount of money was borrowed from relatives. Later, through her sister's connections, she was reimbursed more than 10,000 Yuan, and thus only paid several thousand Yuan out-of-pocket. 'It's lucky we got the reimbursement, otherwise, we would be in a very difficult situation. We repaid the borrowed money after receiving the reimbursement'. She told me that now many people were like her, borrowing money for major surgery and repaying the debt after getting reimbursement. 'The state policy is good, [it would be better] if there was less corruption at the bottom', she concluded. (From Interview P6 and field notes on 4 January 2012)

> 68-year-old Mrs Huang broke her arm in 2010. She and her husband went to the TCM Hospital, and registered under the doctor who they had known for decades. Through this doctor, Mrs Huang was able to register as an inpatient with a hospital bed ready on the day. 'If it was not for him, I would not be hospitalised that soon. I might have stayed in the [hospital] corridor waiting for a bed. There were no more beds available. Without connections or extra money, they would not have allowed me to go into hospital', Mrs Huang stated these words with gratitude to her doctor. Later on, in surgery, a steel plate was put in Mrs Huang's arm, and she stayed in the TCM Hospital for over 20 days. Her total medical expenses were over 20,000 Yuan. Mrs Huang had rural CMS, but she claimed back less than 4000 Yuan. 'The [imported] steel plate couldn't be reimbursed, the anaesthetic couldn't be reimbursed, the bedding fees were not covered…' Mrs Huang counted to me in detail the items not covered in her case. Her husband, Mr Huang, told me that he learnt from the insurance bureau that injury (*shang*) received much less reimbursement compared with illness (*bing*). In Mrs Huang's case, she had been injured. Mr Huang explained that the reimbursement process was related with *qing* (affection or relationship). 'If we have a good relationship, I [the health insurance administrator] will reimburse you [the patient] for those drugs that are not specified by the insurance policy. If we don't have good relationship, I won't reimburse you for these items. You know our family's condition. We didn't have any

connection, therefore claimed back only a little', Mr Huang sighed. (From Interview P1, Interview P27, and field notes on 17 December 2011 and 26 September 2012)

The differentiation of *shang* (injury) and *bing* (illness) is a simplification of insurance rules by local insurance officers. The different compensations on injury and illness are based on the division of health care responsibility. While many injuries are directly caused by patients or other individuals' actions, illnesses in many cases are beyond one's control. However, this differentiation is not in accordance with people's conception and lived experience of illnesses which include all symptoms and injuries requiring medical care. The implementation of insurance policies thus frequently causes misunderstandings and doubts from patients. Individuals like Mr and Mrs Huang suspect that the disparities in insurance compensation among patients were due to *guanxi* connections. 'No matter what you do, you need *guanxi* and *renqing* [relationship, affective tie] in this small county', Mr Huang lamented. The staff at the insurance bureau have power to interpret policies according to individual cases. The interpretation and implementation by local administrators have certain arbitrariness and leave space for well-connected individuals to benefit more. In the cases above, Mrs Lou and Mrs Huang had similar injuries, were enrolled in the same hospital, had about the same overall medical expenditure (over 20,000 Yuan), used the same insurance scheme (the rural CMS), but were reimbursed greatly different amounts (more than 10,000 Yuan for Mrs Lou and less than 4000 Yuan for Mrs Huang). The difference, without denying the impact of the official reimbursement rate that was slightly (5%) higher in 2011 than in 2010,[13] was largely because of Mrs Lou's sister, who worked in a local health office and had insider knowledge about how the system worked. With good connections to the doctor, Mrs Lou's sister could ask the doctor to use more medicines that were covered by insurance; with good connections to the health insurance bureau, the items that were not specified by the insurance policy could also be reimbursed. The locals I met invariably agreed that knowing someone in the local medical 'circle' was fundamental in getting reliable health care and favourable reimbursement. By using *guanxi*, Mrs Lou and Mrs Huang were enrolled in the overcrowded hospital in a timely fashion. With good connections, Mrs Lou could use a relative's insurance to receive higher compensation for health care; without connections, Mrs Huang, even with insurance, got a much lower compensation. While on the surface it seemed that Mrs Huang's low reimbursement was due to her mismatch of reimbursement criteria, it was actually due to their lack of connections. Through connections, the state-subsidised health care became available for people who was not entitled but was well connected. Without connections to overcome official rules, Mr Huang felt discriminated against, and could only respond by complaining about local implementation and corruption. Even Mrs Lou, who

---

[13]Local official reimbursement rate of the rural CMS in the county level hospital was 60% for medical expenditure beyond 400 Yuan in 2010, and 65% for medical expenditure beyond 300 Yuan in 2011.

personally benefited from health insurance, consciously criticised corruption at the bottom.

Overall, the new insurance scheme serves as a mechanism of control, making people more 'governable'. Yet the 'governance' is always open to manoeuvre in local context. In health care access, patients draw upon different forms of capital to secure qualified health care and get insurance benefits. Patients' informal measures to accessing health care and their taking advantage of current policy were morally justified, which helped the 'weak' patients benefit in the imperfect system. These actions constitute ordinary peoples' 'creative compliance' in daily life when facing social structures that they cannot participate in or cannot reject directly. Agency, though, is always unequally distributed among people, who are embedded in specific social relationships and power structures. The frequent use of *guanxi* and *renqing* to take advantage of the 'grey area' that is not specified by the policy, contributes to an abundance of arbitrary cases and potential corruption. The new health insurances, that should improve health care equality, contrarily create new injustice and predicaments. The locals question the varied insurance benefits and seek individual channels to overcome obstacles if possible, but can hardly argue against the system arrangement itself. They seek to meet the regulations and standards to become the 'qualified' one who is entitled. They creatively use the rules and regulations that already exist in the system, adjusting themselves to strive for inclusion, creating a new dependency that leaves them vulnerable to arbitrary interpretation (by the local administrative agencies). Even though they raise questions regarding the official rules, and sometimes act to circumvent them, they seldom act to challenge the rules directly. In many cases, what patients employ are just 'tactics' rather than 'strategies', to use De Certeau's terms (1984). A tactic is 'a calculated action determined by the absence of a proper locus', 'must play on and with a terrain imposed on it and organized by the law' of an exterior power, and must operates in isolated actions and seizes control only momentarily; it is defensive and opportunistic, functions limitedly, and is 'an art of the weak' who does not 'have the options of planning general strategy' (1984: 37). In the health sector, the all-round strategies of the authorities and the manoeuvres of hospitals and professionals could function more subtly and powerfully than the 'tactics' of the patients, as shown below.

4.3   Health Insurance for Profit

4.3.1   Defraud the State's Money: A Zero-Sum Competition for Resources

Since the new healthcare reform, government spending on health care has increased rapidly, mainly through fiscal transfers from the central government to boost public spending on health care at the local level. However, most of the money goes on health insurance, public health, community and township medical institutions, and not directly to public hospitals at or above the county level. Public hospitals without sufficient investment from the state still have to work under the business model, focusing on maximising profit. The profit-motivated hospitals make money on the newly-promoted insurance programmes. In Riverside County, patients were encouraged to go into hospital even for minor illnesses; doctors were motivated to prescribe heavily for insured patients; hospitals made claims for services that were medically unnecessary or never provided; lacking an established referral system, higher level hospitals sometimes 'bought' insured patients from lower level hospitals (by paying a so called 'referring fee'); private hospitals even directly contacted well-connected people to 'act' as patients and made profits from these people's insurance. The over-medication and higher charge for insured patients have long been noted in the Chinese health sector, but the recent wider insurance coverage has made the situation even worse.

Health insurance allows for patients' medical fees to be partly covered. Recent research shows that, in the new healthcare reform, the total payment from health insurance programmes was estimated to account for over 50% of provider revenue, and over 25% of total health expenditure (Gao et al. 2014). However, this same research, alongside another recent study (Li et al. 2012; Liu et al. 2014),[14] shows that the new health insurance schemes have limited effect in reducing patients' medical expenditure, because the overall health care expenditure has escalated exponentially. In Riverside County, many informants reported that the overall medical fees for some illnesses had been doubled or tripled since the implementation of new insurance schemes. Surgery to remove an appendix cost less than 2000 Yuan in the local county hospital five years ago, now it easily surpassed 5000 Yuan. The rapid increase of overall medical expenditure, to some extent, offset the effects of medical insurance. The locals vividly described: 'If you [the patient] said you had insurance, they [doctors would over-prescribe to generate profits] just like rob your money with a hammer', and 'we dare not go to the People's Hospital, guns and cannon are installed at the gate of the People's Hospital, who dares to walk in?' (Interview P43) Hammers, guns and cannons are metaphors for the exorbitant medical charges that scare people away. Many locals commented that hospitals and doctors just *zheng* (defraud) the state's money. *Zheng* in local dialect is defined as money being taken away illegally. Medical insurance enables hospitals to reap money from the state investment, instead of from patients directly. The profit is aggressively pursued by hospitals and doctors, who know how to capitalise on the new insurance programmes. The insured patients then become a new asset (a source of income) to (be chased by) the commercialised hospitals and clinics.

Doctors are easily caught in an ethical dilemma: they are instructed by their hospital to induce patients' medical consumption, at the same time, they are

---

[14]Zhu, Hengpeng. 2018. 'After Eight Years' Health Reform, Do You Have a "Sense of Gain"?' (*yigai banian, ni you huodegan ma?*). *Caixin Net.* (http://m.opinion.caixin.com/m/2018-02-09/101209601.html). Retrieved 12 Mar 2018.

concerned about the very sustainability of health insurance schemes. Nevertheless, as long as the money is earned from the public fund, not directly harming individual patient's interests, many feel more justified in doing so. Besides, doctors argue that they have no assurance that if they saved the insurance fund it would remain in the system to be used by more patients rather than be squandered by corrupt officials. With little trust towards the system, they too exploit public resources for personal benefits. In the collective era, public interests were morally superior to private interests, but there seems to be a moral reverse in the market era. People have less collective concern, and stealing from the state has become too normal to be regarded as immoral. As a young hospital administrator reasoned:

> It's the state's money anyway, as long as you take 'reasonably', as long as you have a way to get it, as long as you do not compromise patients' interests [directly] or make up [fake] clinic record, you can get more money from it. (Interview D25)

The young hospital administrator showed a high degree of understanding and willingness of making money from the state investment, albeit rejecting certain blatant measures. However, in the long run, it may finally hurt the public interest. The locals complained endlessly about the abuse of state investment and ironically commented on the loss of collective spirit. Health professionals and hospitals were depicted by patients as opportunists who take advantage of the state policy. Local people showed a general worry that these new insurance schemes would not be sustainable. While older generations experienced the state investment in public services such as health care as part of a collective unity, people in the market era have experienced it increasingly as part of a zero-sum competition for resources. Hospitals and doctors profit from the state investment, defending that it otherwise would be taken away by corrupt officials. Patients too, hurry to use the state-subsidised health care while it is still available. Everyone competes to reap more benefits, with little sense of the collective and of solidarity.

4.3.2 Budget Audits and Counter-Strategies

Over the past few years, the possible overuse and waste of medical insurance funds,[15] alongside growing health care demands,[16] are endangering the sustainability of health reform programmes. Local levels of government are responsible for

---

[15]The information is provided by health professionals and administrators in the field. In Riverside County, the rural CMS started in 2005. Although the local authority has always attempted to control the use of the CMS fund, several years later, the money was said to be overused so much that the insurance bureau owed the county hospitals large amounts of remuneration that should be paid by the CMS fund. For instance, local doctors reported that, in 2012 alone, the rural CMS bureau had owed the People's Hospital over 20 million Yuan reimbursement.

[16]The sustainability issue links not only to the surging health care expenditure, but also to the changing demographic structure with a rising proportion of elderly population.

financial shortfalls of health care funding, and thus face great pressure to strive for a balance between contribution and expenditure. Following the central government's proposal to control medical expenditure and to experiment with alternative payment plans (MOHRSS 2011), local authorities also introduced relevant measures. In 2013, the local municipality released a 'Reform Plan for County-level Hospitals in the Next Five Years'. The plan proposed that clinical pathways would be experimented in county hospitals to standardise the treatment of over ten kinds of illnesses. It also guided the health insurance bureau to evaluate and monitor local hospitals' stock and use of drugs, and the cost and length of a patient's hospitalisation. The payment plan of rural CMS was changing from a 'fee-for-service' model (that medical services are unbundled and paid for separately) to a 'global budget' (that the governing agencies determine the total budget) and 'prospective payment system' (that insurance reimbursement based on predetermined prices, including giving capitation to certain treatment).

In 2013, the local health insurance bureau set fixed annual budgets for hospitals and initiated a capitation experiment to budget medical treatment for each CMS inpatient within 4200 Yuan. Responding to these limits, local hospitals required their departments and doctors to 'adjust' budgets accordingly. Those who surpassed budget limits would be deducted bonuses. Public doctors began to hesitate to accept insured patients, and would refuse serious patients who may have used up large amounts of the budget or exceed the budget limit. Since 2013, some rural patients found that it became difficult to be hospitalised in county hospitals if they wanted to use their insurance. It is similar in other parts of China. In 2012, the official media reported the story of a cancer patient, a retired cadre with labour insurance in Hebei province (People's Net 2012b). The patient was rejected by all the hospitals in his city and could not use his insurance, specifically because of the budget limitations. His expensive cancer treatment would use up a large portion of, even exceed, the budget quota of local hospitals. The patient was just one of the many labour insurance holders in Hebei province who were rejected by their local hospitals as a response to the budget audit. The policy that aimed at the macro goals of reducing medical costs ironically led to the neglect of patients' actual needs. The serious patients, who were refused by their local hospitals, would face more difficulties in seeking health care outside their localities.

Besides direct budget restrictions, in Riverside County, since 2013, a strict ceiling has been set for prescribed drugs and tests outside the insurance coverage list (Fig. 4.1). This is a measure designed to make more treatment items covered by insurance and thus reduce patients' burden in overall medical expenditure. The doctors, who overprescribed uninsured drugs and tests for inpatients, would be fined. Adapting to these regulations, local doctors began to ask patients to seek health care in outpatient departments first. Patients were told to take a variety of physical examinations and medications in outpatient departments by paying out-of-pocket, and then being hospitalised if necessary. A doctor in the People's Hospital helped me understand why he and his colleagues did so:

> By asking a patient to go to the outpatient department for treatments and tests, our hospital can earn the money, it is cash money [paid by patients directly], and it is irrelevant to the Health Insurance Bureau, [it's] very good [for us]...The patients pay their own money for tests. It costs hundreds, even thousands Yuan, but cannot be reimbursed. Calculating the result, it's still the patients who lose.[17]

Moreover, with the introduction of clinical pathways that assume a 'single disease' model, doctors found that patients with multiple illnesses and complications were not fit for pathways. It gave further justification for doctors to ask patients to get treatments that were not covered by insurance. When health bureau controls the total budget of hospitals and puts a strict ceiling on the medical cost of insured patients, hospitals and doctors respond by adjusting the intake of patients, the quality of care, and the drugs used for patients. In the last decade the Ministry of Health has ordered hospitals to reduce prices of specific drugs 23 times, however, hospitals have responded, in part, by ordering higher-priced alternatives (LaFraniere 2010). Over the years, the authority has gradually cancelled the commissions for selling drugs, first in community health care institutions, then in public hospitals, most hospitals respond by prescribe more clinical tests and checks, and increase the charges on other items. Facing every policy change, hospitals and health professionals can always develop counter-strategies to secure their interests, even though they may not be able to reject the government protocols directly. The recent regulations that aim at making health insurance sustainable, instead of giving doctors and hospitals incentives to control costs by reducing over-prescription, have again resulted in the increase of patients' out-of-pocket payments. Empirical research (Gao et al. 2014) in other parts of China also found that in recent healthcare reforms, the out-of-pocket ratio, length of hospital stay, the total inpatient costs, drug cost ratio, treatment effect, and patient satisfaction exhibit little difference between the fee-for-service and capitation models. Although the payment reform was associated with some reduction of the inpatient out-of-pocket costs, it did not reduce overall inpatient expenditure, and health care providers respond to capitations by shifting to outpatient utilisations.

Health professionals clearly realise the possible burden patients may take. Many of the doctors I encountered would reduce the costs for the patients that pay out-of-pocket expenses, while earning money from the insured patients. They give cheaper medicine to poorer patients, appropriately using the system and policies to reduce the burden of certain impoverished patients, while earning money from other 'ordinary' patients. Doctors need to balance new regulations, hospital's interests, their own interests, and patients' interests. They face various constraints in medical practice, have few alterative choices but have 'to write more [clinic notes], hand more [prescriptions] for approval, communicate more information [with patients and hospital leaders], spend more time on document writing', a doctor from the People's Hospital complained. Doctors spend more time on documenting to pass

---

[17]This is a follow up interview with one of the local informants, whom I kept in contact with after the fieldwork. The new budget control started from 2013, by then I have already left the field. This informal interview happened in July 2013.

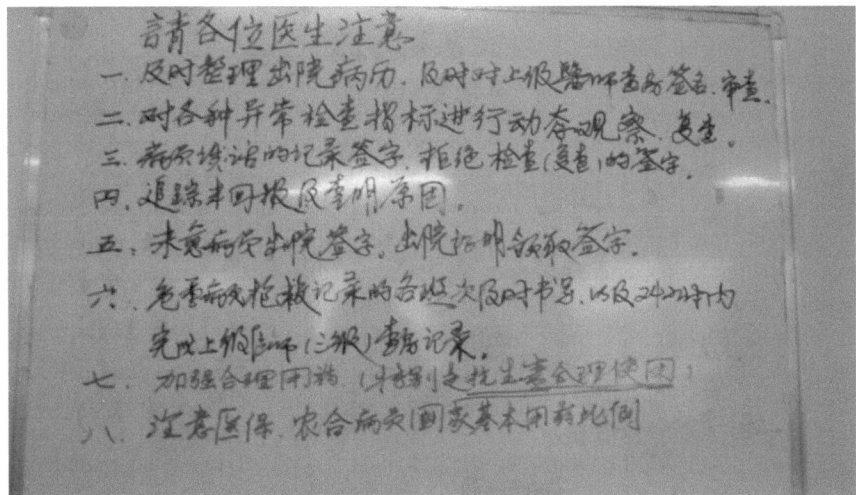

Fig. 4.1 'Notices to Doctors' in a doctor's office of an inpatient department: the last two notices concern the regulations on the use of drugs

the audits of administrative agencies, yet the time left to take care of patients is reduced. In a system that frequently puts patients' and professionals' interests in conflict, health professionals may preserve their own interests by sacrificing patients' needs. Protesting their innocence, public doctors argued that their counter-actions were just survival techniques in a system that has placed increasing demands and constraints on them. The administrative agency increases its control over doctors and hospitals by regulating who they treat, what medicine to use, how much to charge, and what procedures to take. Hospitals and doctors resist the new budget audits by carrying out their own projects. Doctors feel powerless to change the situation, but place blame on the government who initiate a variety of inconsistent policies. They claim that it is the corrupted insurance bureau and local governments who have caused the shortage of insurance funds, as opposed to them. Insurance funds are administered by insurance agencies at local municipalities. This decentralised administration gives the local government both power and responsibility for the operation of health insurance schemes. When insurance funds become deficient, health professionals thus attribute blame to the local corruption in a system lacking transparency.

The reform policies, such as the financial scrutiny, have been put in place to achieve statistical improvements or government performance, but are not designed from the perspectives of patients and doctors. The new financial scrutiny and audits, unlike neoliberal techniques, do not lead to more efficient management or contribute to economic efficiency. They operate not through autonomy, but involve compulsory rules, which make the health professionals audited feel pressured and alienated. They encounter silent resistance from hospitals and health professionals who develop new, efficiency-hindering practices from below. These procedures of examination and assessment also expose patients to more complex hospital experiences. Patients have little say in the process. There is no systematic arrangement for public participation in the surveillance of medication and insurance fund use. During my fieldwork, the information about medical cost and reimbursement of every rural CMS patient began to be displayed regularly in each hospital for public surveillance. Yet, the public, who lacks expert knowledge, cannot easily identify problems from simply the cost and reimbursement numbers. The newly-obtained entitlements for patients, such as the entitlement for insurance reimbursement, encounter the quiet encroachment by hospitals and health professionals, who develop their own protocols to counter new reforms.

As a conclusion, the new health insurance schemes induce excessive use. Hospitals and health professionals capitalise from the state-subsided insurance programmes. Hospitals compete to attract insured patients and generate profits from their insurance. Instead of acting as the mediators between preserving the state interests and satisfying patients' needs, hospitals and professionals take advantage of their intermediate roles to profit from both the patients' private payment and the state's investment (which are supposed to mainly benefit patients). The sense of uncertainty concerning the sustainability of insurance schemes makes those who have 'skin in the game' to resort to whatever it takes in order to benefit from the system as much as possible. The state attempts to safeguard insurance funds through financial scrutiny and audit. It promotes standardisation in medical practice, and uses insurance to budget and constrain hospitals and doctors' behaviour. However, these measures encounter silent resistance from healthcare providers. Profit-motivated hospitals and professionals can always develop counter-measures to preserve their own interests, and 'creatively' circumvent the state policies that they are unsatisfied with. Yet, in the process, patients become renewed objects of profit-generation and budget calculation by medical institutions and professionals, and would be easily denied officially granted benefits. In the competition among doctors, patients, medical institutions, and government agencies, patients' claims over health care are easily held 'hostage' by the commercialised hospitals and profit-driven professionals to defend their own interests in the face of government administrations.

4.4 Health Insurance for Governance and Legitimacy: The Making of Governable Subjects and the Consideration for Social Equality

The setting up of health insurance is based on the notion of social equality and solidarity. It aims to improve equality through the distribution of health care burden collectively. Recent reform efforts have increased the coverage of health insurance and included the formerly uninsured population. The government invests heavily in the previously neglected rural areas, particularly in the form of subsiding rural population's health insurance. It also provides subsidies for the poor to take out medical insurance. Besides, there is a medical aid system for patients with 'major illness' or those facing financial difficulty. All these show the social justice commitment of the party-state that aim to build a health system to provide essential health services to every citizen. Over the years, it has already built up the world's biggest health insurance network, covering more than 1.3 billion population.

However, from a critical point of view, current health insurance arrangements also function to segregate and differentiate the population. The existence of four insurance schemes separates people into four groups with different entitlements: rural residents, urban residents, urban employees, and government employees, although the separation is historically based. At the meantime, it marginalises and excludes certain population that cannot be categorized into the four, such as the migrant workers who come from rural areas but work in the city. Besides, the implementation of insurance schemes follows the judicial model, that it imposes various regulatory rules and criteria to individuals, and those patients who cannot meet or satisfy these criteria are marginalised. The normative categories of insurance recognise some patients' needs but remain blind to others'. Moreover, insurance policies still contain rationalities and mechanisms produced in the collective period (that health care was determined by one's place of residence, *hukou* registration, employment status, etc.), which coexist and conflict with the rationalities of the market era. The over-bureaucratic insurance arrangement and reimbursement procedures exclude certain groups and discourage some patients from obtaining much needed medical aid. Besides, the eligibility tests of insurance claimants leave space for arbitrary interpretations, leading some people to benefit disproportionally. The inconsistent criteria and categories produce a deepening sense of injustice.

The new health insurance schemes constitute biopower, subjecting patients to a structure of selection and means-testing. Governance is embedded in the health insurance regimes to shape and reshape the conduct of individuals and the population. Insurance policies not only generate 'positive and productive forces for the compliance and regulation of the body' (Hewitt 1983: 72), but also produce subtle, punitive techniques to refrain people from violating normative rules. The insurance bureau that determines the qualification of patients is 'biobureaucracy' (Kohrman 2005), which exposes people to a set of knowledge, criteria and identifications. Although the deserving/undeserving distinction has a long history in the party-state's welfare allocation (as shown in Chap. 3), the new insurance schemes further categorise patients as being deserving or underserving, qualified or unqualified. There is also a clear division of state and individual responsibilities that it is an individual's responsibility for illnesses and injuries caused by suicide, accidents, fighting, alcohol consumption, criminal actions, etc. The insurance schemes underlie values of self-responsibility, that patients are required to conduct themselves in a responsible manner and to become qualified subjects. These insurance schemes are used by the state as surveillance measures and disciplinary norms to control the population, birth, and individual conduct.

Health insurance schemes are central in shaping people's experiences under the new healthcare reform and are critical in shaping the public's perception of the authority. The issues involved in current insurance arrangements certainly pose challenge to the moral legitimacy of the authorities. Over the years, the authorities are continuously correcting and reshaping current system to meet people's health care needs in a more equal and appropriate way. In early 2012, the central government released a series of new health reform targets for the following years, including giving migrant workers more equal access to medical services (CPG 2012a). Some local governments have also experimented in supplying social security programmes for migrant workers.[18] At the meantime, insurance coverage and reimbursement for people seeking health care in other cities and provinces have been improved, which are especially good for mobile populations like the migrant worker above. Furthermore, in August 2012, several state departments issued a guideline to setting up an insurance system for major illnesses, targeting to reduce rural and urban residents' financial burden in front of major illnesses. The insurance for major illnesses is mainly subsided by the government, embedded into current insurance schemes and automatically allocated to those insured people without extra fees. It promised to cover over 50% out-of-pocket payment after the reimbursement of the basic health insurance.[19] Following the state's guideline, health insurance for major illness has also been provided in Riverside by local authority from October 2013.[20,21] Besides, the state subsidy for people to purchase insurance has increased over the years, and reimbursement level is increasing gradually. Medical aid system is being improved. Commercial insurances are also encouraged by the government to complement the state health insurances. Recently, the government made efforts to integrate the three major insurance schemes into a coherent one, albeit leaving out the GIS for government employees. A coherent insurance scheme covering most Chinese population (except government employees) will be implemented nationwide in the following years. Accompany that, since 2018, an all-in-one National Medical Security Bureau (*guojia yiliao baozhang ju*) is being set up to reduce the over-bureaucratic management of health care (insurance) that separate people and prevent them from obtaining medical reimbursement and

---

[18]However, without proposed funding mechanism, most local governments are not willing to provide migrants with appropriate public services that need to be supported by the local finance.

[19]Central People's Government, PRC. 'Guideline on the Development of Insurance for Major Illnesses of Urban and Rural Residents by Six Ministries' (*Liu bumen guanyu kaizhan chengxiang jumin dabing baoxian gongzuo de zhidao yijian*). (http://www.gov.cn/gzdt/2012-08/31/content_2214223.htm). Retrieved on 11 Nov 2017.

[20]In 2013, local policy regulated, the insurance for major illnesses will cover part of the out-of-pocket expenditure after basic health insurance reimbursement. It will cover 50–55% of the out-of-pocket if it is between 5000 and 20,000 yuan, 60–65% if it is between 20,000 and 50,000 yuan, 70–75% if it is between 50,000 and 100,000 yuan, and 80–85% if the expenditure is over 100,000 yuan.

[21]Yet, in a context where many items for major illnesses are not on the insurance list and where the overall medical expenditures increase rapidly for catastrophic illnesses, the implementation and effect of major illness insurance need to be carefully evaluated.

aid.[22] The state on the one hand addresses the financial access barriers facing vulnerable groups, on the other hand further develops cost-control measures. New reform efforts have been made to contain medical practitioners' behavior and medical fees[23] (e.g. the Healthy China Plan has set targets for the percentage of out-of-pocket payment in total health expenditure) (Fu et al. 2018). All these aim to improve equality and prevent people from falling to impoverishment due to illness. Although its effect needs to be carefully evaluated, it suggests the government's emphasis on equality and its efforts to ensure people having equal health care entitlements.

Overall, from the analysis of China's health care insurance, we see the conflicting logics and rationales within the government's arrangement of health insurance: the use of insurance for governance of the population and for legitimacy; the values of deservedness and self-reliance, and the value of equality and justice. It is noticeable about the authority's efforts to correct the problems within the insurance system: from insurance as segregation to insurance for equality; from insurance for profit by health care providers to the containment of profit-making behaviors by the authorities. The reforms and corrections the party-state made suggest its contingency in governance and its efforts to continually working to solve new problems and reinventing itself in the process. In the following years, the definitions of eligibilities and qualifications, the values of deservedness and equal entitlement will be ongoing contentions in the unfolding of the new healthcare reforms among patients, health professionals, medical institutions, insurance managing bodies, and the government that oversee the direction of health reforms. The definitions of qualification, expenditure, and allocation are still determined by the administrative authorities, and by the profit-motivated medical institutions and professionals, but seldom by the users—the ordinary patients. The insurance benefits in the current healthcare reform still show the state's acknowledgement of individual needs and claims, which are 'granted' rather than entitled. Health care that is not based on inalienable rights cannot prevent individual existential needs being encroached upon by political and economic needs, by commercial interests

---

[22]As early as 2013, the State Council has released a 'State Council Institutional Reform and Functional Transformation Plan' in 2013 (CPG 2013c), including integrating the separated health insurance administrations into a coherent one. In early 2018 during the Chinese National People's Congress, all these reform efforts start with the announcement of setting up the National Medical Security Bureau (*guojia yiliao baozhang ju*) (see http://www.gov.cn/zhuanti/2018lh/2018zfgzbg/zfgzbg.htm, retrieved 15 Mar 2018).

[23]"The medical fee containment' becomes one of the major reform targets as the new health reform progresses. In 2015, five ministries issued guidance to contain the unreasonable increase of medical fees in public hospitals (see http://www.mohrss.gov.cn/SYrlzyhshbzb/shehuibaozhang/zcwj/yiliao/201512/t20151208_228150.html, retrieved 12 March, 2018). In 2017, seven ministries again issued document to guide public hospital reform, one of the aim is to contain the increase rate of medical fees in public hospitals nationwide below 10% (http://www.nhfpc.gov.cn/tigs/s3581/201704/0563e06eff4441ffa9772dc30b487848.shtml, retrieved 12 Mar 2018).

and profit driving behaviours, and by officially sanctioned programmes. It is worthy to see how this will change as the basic health and health promotion law is being developed in China[24] and as the party-state continually reinvents itself.

References

Becker, Gay. 2007. The uninsured and the politics of containment in U.S. health care. *Medical Anthropology* 26 (4): 299–321.

Central People's Government, PRC. 2012a. Chinese government to raise health insurance subsidies. (http://english.gov.cn/2012-02/22/content_2074190.htm). Retrieved 3 Mar 2012.

Central People's Government, PRC. 2013c. State council institutional reform and functional transformation plan (Guowuyuan jigou gaige he zhineng zhuanbian fangan). (http://www.gov.cn/zwgk/2013-03/28/content_2364821.htm). Retrieved 29 July 2013.

Chen, Juan. 2011. Internal migration and health: Re-examining the healthy migrant phenomenon in China. *Social Science and Medicine* 72 (8): 1294–1301.

de Certeau, Michel. 1984. *The practice of everyday life*. Berkeley: University of California Press.

Ewald, Francois. 1991. Insurance and Risk. In *The Foucault Effect: Studies in Governmentality with Two Lectures by and an Interview with Michel Foucault*, eds. G. Burchell, C. Gordon, and P. Miller, 197–210. Chicago: University of Chicago Press.

Foucault, Michel. 1972. *The archaeology of knowledge*. New York: Pantheon Books.

Fu, Wei, Shuli Zhao, Yuhui Zhang, Peipei Chai, and John Goss. 2018. Research in health policy making in China: Out-of-pocket payments in healthy china 2030. *BMJ* 360: k234.

Gao, Chen, Xu Fei, and Gordon G. Liu. 2014. Payment reform and changes in health care in China. *Social Science and Medicine* 111: 10–16.

Greenhalgh, Susan. 2003. Planned births, unplanned persons: "Population" in the making of Chinese modernity. *American Ethnologist* 30 (2): 196–215.

Greenhalgh, Susan. 2009. The Chinese biopolitical facing the twenty-first century. *New Genetics and Society* 28 (3): 205–222.

Greenhalgh, Susan, and Edwin A. Winckler. 2005. *Governing China's population: From Leninist to Neoliberal biopolitics*. Stanford, CA: Stanford University Press.

Grogan, Colleen M. 1995. Urban economic reform and access to health care coverage in the People's Republic of China. *Social Science and Medicine* 41 (8): 1073–1084.

Gu, Xin. 2008. *Towards universal coverage of healthcare insurance: The strategic choices and institutional frameworks of China's new healthcare reform (Zouxiang quanmin yibao: zhongguo xin yigai de zhanlue yu zhanshu)*. Beijing: China Labour and Social Security Publishing House.

Hesketh, Therese. 2010. China's one-child policy is slowly being eased. *The Guardian*. (http://www.theguardian.com/commentisfree/2010/oct/24/china-one-child-policy-eased). Retrieved 5 May 2014.

Hesketh, Therese, Ye Xue Jun, Li Lu, and Hong Wang Mei. 2008. Health status and access to health care of migrant workers in China. *Public Health Reports* 123 (2): 189–197.

Hewitt, Martin. 1983. Bio-politics and social policy: Foucault's account of welfare. *Theory, culture & society* 2 (1): 67–84.

Hu, Xiaojiang, Sarah Cook, and Miguel A. Salazar. 2008. Internal migration and health in China. *The Lancet* 372 (9651): 1717–1719.

---

[24]A basic health and health promotion law is drafted and under review (see http://health.people.com.cn/n1/2017/1223/c14739-29724759.html, retrieved 31 Mar 2018).

Kohrman, Matthew. 2005. *Bodies of difference: Experiences of disability and institutional advocacy in the making of modern China*. Berkeley: University of California Press.

La Franiere, Sharon. 2010. Chinese Hospitals are Battlegrounds of Discontent. *New York Times*. (http://www.nytimes.com/2010/08/12/world/asia/12hospital.html). Retrieved 28 July 2014.

Lee, Ching Kwan, and Yuan Shen. 2009. The paradox and possibility for a public sociology of labor in China. *Work and Occupations* 36 (2): 110–125.

Li, Ye, Qunhong Wu, Ling Xu, David Legge, Yanhua Hao, Lijun Gao, Ning Ning, and Gang Wan. 2012. Factors affecting catastrophic health expenditure and impoverishment from medical expenses in China: Policy implications of universal health insurance. *Bulletin of the World Health Organization* 90 (9): 664–671.

Liu, Kai, Wu Qiaobing, and Junqiang Liu. 2014. Examining the association between social health insurance participation and patients' out-of-pocket payments in China: The role of institutional arrangement. *Social Science and Medicine* 113: 95–103.

Milcent, Carine. 2010. Healthcare for migrants in urban China: A new frontier. *China Perspectives* (2010/4): 33–46.

Ministry of Human Resources and Social Security. 2011. Opinions of MOHRSS on advancing the health insurance payment method reform (Renli ziyuan he shehui baozhang bu guanyu jinyibu tuijin yiliao baoxian fufei fangshi gaige de yijian). (http://www.mohrss.gov.cn/yiliaobxs/YILIAOBXSzhengcewenjian/201105/t20110531_83732.htm). Retrieved 22 Sept 2013.

National Health and Family Planning Commission, PRC. 2013b. Summary of the 2013 reports on the development of China's migrant population (< Zhongguo liudong renkou fazhan baogao 2013 > neirong gaiyao). (http://www.nhfpc.gov.cn/ldrks/s7847/201309/12e8cf0459de42c981c59e827b87a27c.shtml). Retrieved 10 Oct 2013.

Ong, Aihwa, and Li, Zhang. 2008. Introduction: Privatizing China: Powers of the Self, Socialism from Afar. In *Privatizing China: Socialism from Afar*, 1–20. Ithaca, NY: Cornell University Press.

Peng, Yingchun, Wenhu Chang, Haiqing Zhou, Hu Hongpu, and Wannian Liang. 2010. Factors associated with health-seeking behavior among migrant workers in Beijing, China. *BMC Health Services Research* 10: 69.

People's Net. 2012b. Promoting global budget, public hospitals reject labour insurance holder (Tuixing zhonger yufuzhi, gongban yiyuan jushou zhigong yibao huanzhe). (http://js.people.com.cn/html/2012/04/23/102395.html). Retrieved 4 July 2012.

Solinger, Dorothy. 1999. *Contesting citizenship in urban China: Peasant migrants, the state, and the logic of the market*. Berkeley: University of California Press.

Tu, Jiong. 2016. Health insurance regime as differentiation and discipline: The Chinese health insurance reforms. *Hygiea Internationalis: An Interdisciplinary Journal for the History of Public Health* 12 (2): 51–72.

Whyte, Martin King (ed.). 2010. *One country, two societies: Rural-urban inequality in contemporary China*. Cambridge, MA: Harvard University Press.

Wu, Yanrui. 1997. China's health care sector in transition: Resources, demand and reforms. *Health Policy* 39 (2): 137–152.

Xu, Feng. 2009. Governing China's peasant migrants: Building Xiaokang socialism and harmonious society. In *China's Governmentalities: Governing Change, Changing Government*, ed. E. Jeffreys, 38–62. London: Routledge.

Ying, Xing. 2010. Barefoot lawyers and rural conflicts. In *Reclaiming Chinese society: The new social activism*, eds. Y. T. Hsing and C. K. Lee, 64–82. New York: Routledge.

Chapter 5
Gift Practice in the Chinese Health Sector: Inequality, Power and Governance

Chinese patients frequently give 'gifts' to health professionals in order to get better care. Social scientists for a long time have been concerned about the symbolic value of gifts that 'there is much more in the exchange itself than in the things exchanged' (Levi-Strauss 1969: 59, cited in Yang 1989: 38). Malinowski finds the system of exchange in the Trobriand Islands was based on the principle of reciprocity. He shows that gifts and counter-gifts, giving and taking comprised 'one of the main instruments of social organisation, of the power of the chief, of the bonds of kinship, and of relationship in law' (1922: 167). Mauss (1954) emphasises the tripartite obligations to give, receive, and reciprocate, by repetition of which social relationships are made and maintained. Gift-exchange, like the potlatch in his analysis, is an economic phenomenon, also a phenomenon of social structure, a moral economy of redistributing resources that promote social integration and cohesion. He makes a differentiation between gift and commodity in which exchanges range from purely instrumental transaction to purely altruistic gift, which are premised on opposing principles. Gift exchange is regarded as safe and good, while commodity exchange is threatening and morally bad (Gregory 1982). Cheal (1988: 19) frames the concept of 'gift economy' as 'a system of redundant transactions within a moral economy, which makes possible the extended reproduction of social relations'.[1] However, this concept is based in the Western context (such as Christmas gifts). These researchers tend to emphasise gifts' roles in sustaining social structure and stability, promoting social relations and cohesion. What about gift practice in a society that has experienced great transformation?

Many scholars have researched on gift exchange in the Soviet context (Kornai 2000; Ledeneva 1998; Rivkin-fish 2005; Stan 2012). Some view gifts as the legacy of state-controlled bureaucracies (Kornai 2000; Ledeneva 1998); others view gifts as a direct consequence of the political and economic transformations after the fall

---

[1]With regard to the redundant, Cheal means that gifts add nothing to their recipients, bring no net benefit to their recipients, are often things that the recipients could have provided for themselves, and are ritual offerings for the purposes of interaction courtesy.

© Springer Nature Singapore Pte Ltd. 2019
J. Tu, *Health Care Transformation in Contemporary China*,
https://doi.org/10.1007/978-981-13-0788-1_5

of the Soviet Union (Kornai 2000; Stan 2012; Yurchak 2002). Studies record the change of gifts in health care of the post-Soviet context from a part of the moral economy of the ideal socialist medicine to the emerging market economy of short-lived exchanges (Andaya 2009), from a part of the personal relations of reciprocity to the market-like exchanges (Rivkin-Fish 2005). The neoliberal transformation in the post-socialist context increases social inequalities and competition, thus further heightens the predatory side of informal exchanges (Stan 2012). Similar to the post-socialist countries, China has experienced great transformation from a planned to a market economy over the past several decades. However, different from the former Soviet countries, China remains socialism and communist rule. To what extent is gift-exchange in the Chinese society relevant, similar or different from gift-exchange in these previous studies? Gifts have been researched by many Chinese scholars (e.g. Yang 1994; Yan 1996). Yang (1994) situates gift in the larger context of the socialist state redistributive economy, and shows how people use gift to overcome socialist bureaucracy. Yan (1996) correlates gift-exchange with *guanxi* (relationship) and *renqing* (favour or human affection), and outlines the changes of gift practice in a village from the reciprocity exchange to the upward flow of gifts along with the radical social changes in China. Recently, Yang Jingqing's research (2017) on gift-giving (red-packet in particular) in China's health sector situates gift practice in the changing institutional context amid China's social-economic transition. It holds the persistence of socialist health ideology, the continuity of bureaucratic organization of the medical profession, and the commercialization of healthcare have jointly created an institutional setting in which the red packet has become a tenacious ailment of the healthcare system (Yang 2017: 19). Still, gifting in the Chinese health sector has not received enough academic attention and critical review from sociological and anthropological perspectives, although it has been widely practiced and reported.[2]

Gifting in the health sector has deep cultural and social roots in China. Its practice has experienced many changes during the dramatic market transformation over recent decades. Market economy has disrupted both the traditional practice of gifting, and the socialist gift practice under Mao. Patients and doctors negotiate the new ethics of health service, money and gifts in a broad context of the commercialisation of the health sector and the individualisation of health care responsibility. This chapter explores the subtle power dynamics involved in the changing gift practice among patients, health professionals, hospital administrators, and governments. Section 5.1 outlines the changing gift practices and principles that govern gifts, and how patients use gifting and its principles to seek reliable care and hold health professionals accountable. As I will show below, gifting touches upon

---

[2]There are some researches about 'red-packets' and kickbacks in the Chinese medical sector, but mostly in the area of ethics and philosophy (Qiu 2006; Wang 2005a, b). There is a lack of empirical research and the research from the sociological and anthropological perspectives, due to the difficulty to carry out research and obtain relevant data. Gifting in the health sector is carried out behind closed door or under the table, thus it is difficult to quantify gift practice and its efficacy. However its prevalence in people's accounts of health care makes it unignorable.

the emotional component of relationship. Gifts from patients elicit a doctor's responsibility and obligation to reciprocate, thus improve the trustworthiness of the doctor and his or her treatment. However, the commodification of the health sector changes the moral economy of gift, and alters the moral constraints patients imposed on health professionals through gifting. Section 5.2 analyses how gift practice opens up avenues for profit-generation by health professionals who hold expertise. Gifts, instead of promoting social solidarity, increasingly contribute to deepening inequality and stressful relationships. Patients, in turn, use gifts to counter domination by reporting gift-taking behaviour, attacking gift-takers, or resisting gift practice if they feel unsatisfied with health care received. In the process health professionals become as vulnerable as the patients. Section 5.3 illustrates how the practices of gifting constitute part of the informal practices of local governance while the authorities also contain these practices to sustain party legitimacy. The conflicts between the informal practice of gifting in local governance and the containment of gift practices to improve legitimacy produce many dilemmas for people within the health system. Overall, gifting in China's health care sector is used for circumvention, domination, extraction, and contestation by different players. It reconfigures the power dynamics between patients, professionals, and governments, which this chapter presents.

5.1 Gifting: An Individual Technique for Better Care

5.1.1 Changing Gift Practice[3]

Traditionally, patients would send gifts to doctors after treatment to express satisfaction of good care, and to show their gratitude of being cured from a difficult illness. In Riverside County, the gifts could be home-made food, local products, plaques (*paibian*) or silk pennants (*jinqi*), with patients' appreciative words accompanying them. Patients' families sometimes set off firecrackers in front of doctors' clinics as thanks, which recognise a doctor's professional skills and ethics, and also broadcast his or her good name in the community. Gifts such as plaques and silk pennants, hang on the clinic wall (see Figs. 5.1 and 5.2), are like licences, awards, or certificates doctors display in their clinic, retaining an aura of cultural legitimacy and 'an echo of the symbols with which figures of traditional authority surrounded themselves' (Giddens 1994: 89). These gifts, a mixture of material and symbolic rewards, serve as an expression of gratitude and recognition, and play an important role to connect *guanxi* and *renqing*—the long-term cultivation of

---

[3]The description of the changing gift practice in this section is a generalisation of local's accounts (especially local elderly's accounts) when they compared gifts in the past and that now in the medical sector. Although I followed locals' accounts and depicted the change of gift in a linear way, I do admit that the change of gift overtime is not linear, and the changes of gifts in the rural and urban areas are also different.

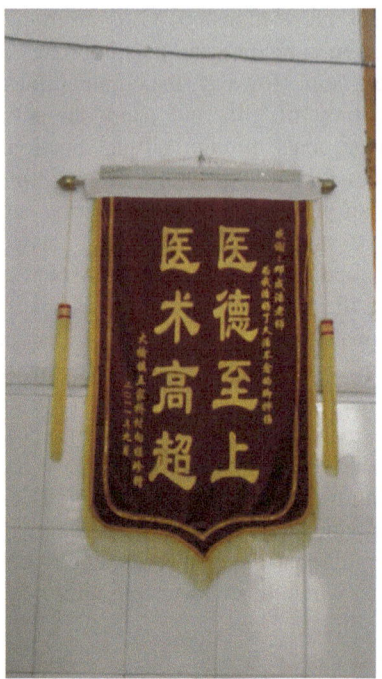

Fig. 5.1   Gift from patient—red silk banner (*jinqi*)

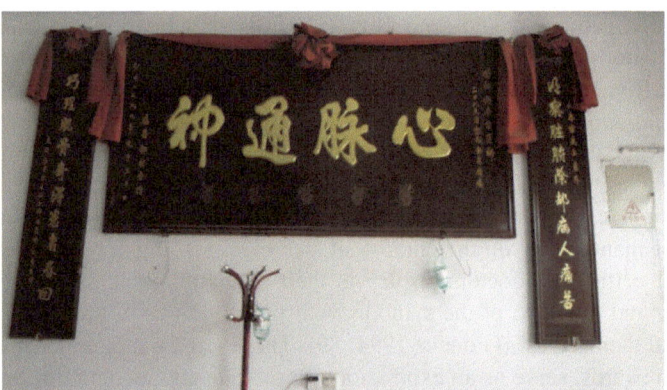

Fig. 5.2   Gift from patient—plaques (*paibian*)

relationships in a local community.[4] There were few cash gifts from patients to doctors. Sometimes even medical fees were paid in the form of red-packets in which patients' families put money according to their economic condition. Poor families gave material products (such as rice, grain, and noodles) to substitute for the medical fee. In the local *renqing* society, doctors were regarded as morally responsible and having obligations within the moral economy of gift. Gifting in the traditional context constituted a part of moral economy, a system that was 'embedded' (Polanyi 1944) in a local society, allowing people both rich and poor to get certain health care.

In contrast to the earlier period, the collective era after the founding of the PRC was short of both cash and material products. Gift exchange was greatly reduced, but did not disappear. People, especially peasants, maintained the tradition of giving something to doctors (such as home-grown vegetables, fruit, noodles, and eggs), although the practice was publicly prohibited. In the command economy where one needed to wait for a long time to gain hospital admission or special services, some gave gifts to doctors or administrators to jump the queue, seek diagnoses from doctors with a good reputation, or obtain special services (Bloom et al. 2001: 29). Gifting in the collective era, albeit on limited scale and practised secretly, enabled ordinary patients to get relatively better health care in an era of shortage. Again, there were few cash gifts. Doctors received their salary from the state or the collective, their incomes did not directly come from patients, and gifts were extra expression of gratitude from patients.

In the post-reform era, people continue giving material and symbolic gifts to doctors. During my observations in local community clinics, patients frequently came to give small gifts to doctors. By regularly sending these small gifts, local patients set up long term *guanxi* with doctors in their community, and accumulated *renqing* for the future so they could obtain free health advice and reliable health care at a reasonable price. The process of gifting nurtures intense feelings of mutual indebtedness and obligation, and forms the continuous accumulation of a supportive network. However, in public hospitals, gifts gradually change from small products to expensive commodities, from material to monetary form (especially in major illnesses and surgeries). A retired doctor from a local hospital recounted this change:

> With the progress of [market] reform, people's living standards increased, their health consciousness also increased. Deng said 'Let some people become rich first'. When seeking health care, those who became well-off first, wanted to see a better doctor. They began to give gifts to doctors: some soybeans, some eggs, some beef…more and more. Later, 'Who need your beef, cash money is better', thus red-packets became popular…At the beginning only rich people gave red-packets. As time went by, ordinary patients also gave red-packets in order to see a good doctor, but this became somewhat difficult [for the poor]… (Interview D59)

---

[4]This does not mean that the exchange of material and symbolic gifts in the traditional context does not involve calculation. The emotional indebtedness and reciprocity in traditional gift practice also involve a calculation of contributions, but this calculation has a different texture of feeling than the market calculation. The universal capacity to calculate should not be confused with the market calculation that subjects everything into economic evaluation.

'Let some people become rich first' is what Deng Xiaoping, the state leader in the 1980s and 1990s, said in his 1992 southern tour to speed up market reforms. The changing forms of gift correlate with the deepening of market reforms, the wide availability of both commodities and cash, and the increasing importance of money in daily consumption. The change from material to monetary gifts is also due to numerous practical reasons, for instance, monetary gifts are more tangible, their anonymous nature make tracing them more difficult, and choosing a proper gift is difficult.[5] Material goods become less attractive in gifting practice, as these goods could be easily acquired on the market in the post-reform era. Over time patients have begun to opt to give cash equivalents to the amount of an intended gift.[6]

These monetary gifts are generally named *hongbao* (red packets or envelopes containing money). Red packets, which have a long tradition in the Chinese society,[7] emerged in the health sector (in large scale) only since the 1980s, and got increasing public and government concern in the 1990s and 2000s (Li and Su 1997; Yang 2008: 46). It is defined by the authority as inappropriate or illegal benefits (Yang 2008: 44), has been incorporated in the corruption study (Fan 2010). As the doctor above expressed, the red-packet, given by the rich to distinguish them so they could receive better services, later became a common practice among patients and placed a heavy burden on the poor. Later this chapter will show that the large amount of informal payment in the form of red packet has been increasingly regarded as bribery. It is viewed by the people I met as the pathological issue introduced by the advent of the market economy.[8]

5.1.2 'Compulsory' Gift-Giving

Previous surveys show that over 50% patients (even more inpatients) in Chinese hospitals have given red-packets or other informal payments to doctors, mostly for doctors' reciprocity (Bloom et al. 2001; Yang 2017: 7). Although it is impossible to

---

[5]The rising consideration about health, food security, product quality, etc. makes giving a suitable material gift difficult.

[6]Material gifts are still given by patients sometimes, but frequently accompanying cash gift.

[7]Red packets were traditionally used in occasions like festivals, weddings, and birthday celebrations to convey good wishes. Red packets were also used as bribe in the past. However, most of these practices were taken within the relations of certain proximity or in the officialdom. Red packets were seldom used in the health sector, where most doctors worked privately in traditional society.

[8]Following the locals' accounts, I put red-packets (money) into the broad discussion of gifts, although I am conscious about the difference between gifts and red-packets (as informal payments). In my field, both patients and health professionals categorise red-packet as gift. For doctor, it helps them to justify their red-packet receiving behaviour (because it is within the traditional gift practice), therefore disguises red-packets' extortion nature. For patients, it helps them to compare red-packets now with material gifts in the past, to reveal their change and extortion nature, and therefore criticise red-packets.

obtain exact information about how common gift practice is now, anecdotal evidence abounds. Almost every patient I encountered in Riverside County would emphasise to me the importance of gifting in health care. Mr. Xie, in his 70s, told me of his experience of gift-giving when his son was hospitalised:

> About 6 years ago, my oldest son was found to have a stomach illness and sent to the People's Hospital for surgery. We had to give roosters [to the doctors]. Besides, we had to entertain them [the health professionals who carried out the surgery] with meals, which cost hundreds Yuan. Normal meals didn't work... I bought the chickens in person, three roosters, more than 15 *jin* [7.5 kg]. I took them to him [the doctor]. He told me clearly that only because an acquaintance had introduced me [to him], had he accepted [the gift]. Later he even complained that the roosters' colour wasn't good... (Interview P43)

Mr. Xie's account was complicated by the death of his son whose stomach illness deteriorated to stomach cancer and he died not long after surgery. His personal suffering was aggravated by the contempt from the doctor who complained about his gift. Mr. Xie further emphasised the necessity of gift in major surgeries:

> If you didn't give gifts, you should be prepared to stay in the [hospital] bed for many days and nights [waiting to be operated on]. He [the doctor] might leave something inside you [your body during surgery], causing you to suffer a lot. This is true. Why did some doctors leave the haemostat inside [the patients'] stomachs? Why did some [doctors] leave the haemostatic cloth inside the [patients'] bodies? This is about medical ethics. I [the doctor] could do things arbitrarily to make you [the patient] into trouble, and require a second surgery. See, if the haemostat was in your stomach, how could you not have a second surgery? You still need to find him [the doctor] to take it out, and you will spend much more...In the past, I never heard of someone who was having surgery giving a gift or a red-packet to the doctors, it was never heard of. Now everyone around me tell me 'You have to give gift. Only after giving a gift, could you come down from the operating table [alive], otherwise, you wouldn't come down from the operating table, and would die'. These words frightened me... (Interview P43)

The stories widely circulated in the media and exchanged among local residents convinced Mr. Xie of the necessity to give a gift. He showed his outrage towards health professionals who received gifts, condemning them as those whose 'medical ethics are really bad'. However, he felt powerless to challenge or oppose gifting practice, thus opting to follow gifting rules to protect the interests of his family. Mr. Xie is not alone in expressing the compulsory nature of gift-giving. 68-year-old Mrs. Huang similarly told me that it was absolutely necessary to bribe doctors in childbirth:

> For those young people who go to give birth in the hospital, firstly [you] should give some [money] to them [doctors], or else, nobody cares about you. When my daughter-in-law gave birth, it was in the maternity hospital. You see, at the beginning, the doctor insisted on doing a caesarean section. She said the baby couldn't be born naturally, but her [the daughter-in-law's] mother didn't agree...Later my son went to give the doctor some money. At that time, this money was valuable, it was over 10 years ago, and he gave 200 or 300 Yuan. Then just a while later, she [the daughter-in-law] gave birth successfully...I was there with my daughter-in-law's mother. We said the natural birth would be good for both the baby and the adult. When we arrived at the hospital that day, another woman had had a

caesarean section and her baby had been born already, but, one week later when we checked out, they were still in the hospital…You see, was the money worth giving or not? (Interview P27)

A survey conducted by the WHO found that 46.2% of pregnant women in China delivered by caesarean section during the year 2007–2008, one of the highest rates in the world (Lumbiganon et al. 2010). The popularity of caesarean sections in China over recent years is promoted by various factors, one of which is the economic motivation of hospitals and health professionals (Lei et al. 2003; Guo et al. 2007; Mi and Liu 2014).[9] A caesarean section costs much more than a natural delivery. Recovery from a caesarean section normally takes longer than the natural delivery, thus post-delivery care also costs more. Hospitals can make more profits from a caesarean section than a natural delivery. Besides, the process of a caesarean section is usually quicker than a natural delivery, thus it improves the work efficiency of the overburdened obstetricians in crowded public hospitals. Doctors sometimes persuade patients to choose a caesarean section, exposing patients to the risk of needless surgery. In response, a patient's family, who do not want a caesarean section, give money to doctors to make sure that they try their best to assist a patient's natural delivery. In Mrs. Huang's account, money worked quietly and effectively. The doctor, who had been reluctant to come and had refused the family's request for a natural delivery, came soon after receiving the money and made the natural delivery successfully. Compared with the other woman who had been hospitalised earlier but was still in the hospital when Mrs. Huang's family checked out, Mrs. Huang felt the money was worth giving.

People told me various anecdotes about those who did not give red-packets being 'punished' during treatment. If the patient does not give,

He [the doctor] will leave you [the patient] there, arrange you for this and that [expensive physical] examination, examine you from head to foot [while delaying the operation]. (Interview P42)

You cry out painfully after surgery, you ask the doctors how you could feel so much pain, and [instead of comforting you] he will scold you. (Interview P37)

He won't be responsible, but you want to be alive, if you anger him, he may even leave you with some side effects, and make you get an infection later. (Interview P40)

However, if a patient does give a gift,

They [the doctors] will treat you more nicely and carefully. (Interview P49)

During rounds in the morning, he [the doctor] will first come to your bed, even if it is number three, instead of beds number one and two [because they do not give gifts]. (Interview P37)

You won't need to queue for a hospital bed [for days]. (Interview P44)

Rather than waiting to be operated on for a week, you will be operated on tomorrow. (Interview P48)

---

[9]The situation began to change recently due to the government's promotion of natural birth.

According to the local's accounts, safe or favourable treatment is increasingly accompanied by extra cash payments. The blatant discrimination between the ones who give gifts and those who do not makes people feel it is compulsory to give. Red-packets today are normally given to a doctor before a medical service is provided, in contrast to traditional gifts which were given mostly after a doctor's service. People pay red-packets in advance as a preventive measure with the hope of getting more attention from the doctor, and avoiding being prescribed unnecessary medicine, delayed treatment or hurt by a doctor. 'Red-packets' thus can be understood in the economic term of 'externality'.[10] Patients pay extra to rid themselves of negative externalities (for instance, over-prescription, over-charging, or negligence).

5.1.3 Gifting to Hold Doctors Accountable

The everyday practice of gifting is a transaction involved in the rich web of relational indebtedness and obligation. Gifts given by patients are to repay doctors who have provided treatment and care. After receiving the gift, doctors recognise the patients' request or gratitude, and have the moral obligation to reciprocate with more careful care. Gifts from patients elicit a doctor's responsibility and obligation to reciprocate, thus improve the trustworthiness of the doctor and his or her treatment. Gift can be regarded as an insurance for reliable care, when the system and institutional arrangements cannot insure qualified care. It acts like an extra contract (in addition to the medical fee) that further ensures the responsibility of doctors to provide good care and the right of patients to get quality care.

Gifting in many cases is a patient's active strategy to counter an uncertain medical environment. It enables patients to negotiate health care entitlement, to get better care and more insurance reimbursement. It imposes moral constraints on the behaviour of doctors. Many people complain about these informal exchanges. However, when they can use informal channels to overcome obstacles or benefit from informal exchange, they do not hesitate to use them.

Most doctors I interviewed proclaimed that gifts did not really matter. They offered comments such as the following:

> For the majority of us, red-packets don't really make a big difference, we'll treat [patients] in the same way [as we should do]. [If you gave a gift] we might only speak more gently, answer questions more patiently, and come to ask about you or check on you a few times more. However, patients cannot rest assured if not give [a gift], they want to give. (Interview D19)

Doctors claim gifts will not make any fundamental difference to the treatment. However, for patients, that little extra attention, more patience, and a better attitude are exactly what is missed in normal treatment and what patients want in an

---

[10]Inspiration got from 'Making Capitalism Fit for Society' (Crouch 2013).

uncertain medical environment. Patients cannot buy satisfactory health care through formal channels, and thus give gifts to obtain better service from doctors directly. The more crowded the hospital is, the longer the queue is, the more people would give red-packets to jump the queue and to shorten their waiting time.

The current health system fails to make 'fairer' allocations of medical resources to satisfy people's growing needs for quality care. The failure encourages people's own efforts to overcome structural obstacles to secure quality care. Gifting is one strategy to seek good care in overcrowded medical institutions and in an opaque system. Red-packets do not fit readily into the category of corruption and bribery. Giving 'is often an informal, if controversial, market practice that not only makes a particular clinical encounter work, but also provides partial assurance of qualified "trust" between medical practitioners and patients—albeit at a price' (Pei 2008). These daily informal exchanges enable the temporary alliance of doctors and patients, in order to subtly defuse and subvert the elaborate hospital regulations and official rules.

Gift practice is also promoted by the lack of trust from patients to doctors. When health care becomes a commercial product, its inherent moral values (to care, help, and save) are put into question. The virtues of health professionals who carry out the 'commercial exchange' are also questionable. A survey in 30 Chinese hospitals shows that only 10 percent of patients trusted in doctors (Xinhua Net 2013; CPG 2013). Gifts are the transaction cost to overcome distrust. Gifting can touch upon the emotional component of relationship. Gifting, as an expression of respect and gratitude from patients, could encourage doctors (whose work and skill are recognised and rewarded by extra gift) to work harder in providing better care. Gifting serves as a symbolic recognition from patients to doctors, and retains the subjective validity of *guanxi*, and cultivates the affective relationship within which trust is rooted. Gifts among patients and doctors were not merely a set of material or monetary exchange, but frequently infused with affections that structure the actions of people involved. It makes the otherwise ordinary medical encounter in an impersonal environment more humane, affective and personal amid the beautiful compliments and courteous words in the etiquette of gifting.[11] It is the art of gift, the ritual of giving and receiving that makes things happen and allows deals to be achieved.

However, the trust between Chinese patients and doctors has deteriorated to such an extent that gifting sometimes leads to more troubles. People presume that doctors would not treat patients carefully without receiving a gift. In other words, they presume doctors are all profit-oriented, and will not stick to their professional ethics without extra benefits. Patients narrate, imagine, and sometimes exaggerate the consequences of not giving gifts. In a period, the situation has worsened to the

---

[11]The function of gift to contribute to the humane health care has also been noted in other societies, such as the former Soviet Bloc. Research bribes and gifts in Russian Heath Care, Rivkin-Fish (2005) suggests that these unofficial payments, bribes and gifts make health care between patients and doctors become more personal and humane; they make sense as ethical forms of interaction within the broader context of institutional changes taking place in the post-Soviet era.

extent that patients will refuse to give consent for surgery until doctors accept their red-packet as a guarantee that nothing less than the best will be provided (Hui 2010). Patients would feel more reassured after paying the red-packet, and be 'relieved' only after the doctor has received their red-packet. By presuming that doctors would only treat patients carefully after receiving a gift, gift giving and receiving becomes normalised and routinized, those who do not give or receive then become abnormal. Under this logic, tragic incidents might occur, such as the doctor, who kindly rejected the 'red-packet', was attacked by the patient's family, who suspected something bad had happened to the patient.[12]

In short, transformations in the Chinese society over the past decades are reshaping the everyday gifting practice and social relationships. Under the market reforms, gifts from patients to doctors have changed from mostly symbolic and material forms to increasingly monetary form. Gifts can be sincere expressions of gratitude from patients and are used by patients to cultivate relationships with doctors in a reciprocal manner. They are also actively used by patients to overcome systemic obstacles that prevent them from obtaining quality health care. But in a commercialised health system, gifting increasingly becomes an individual technique for patients to hold doctors accountable amid the individualisation of health care responsibility and decreasing trust between doctors and patients. Besides, as shown in the next section, when gifting increasingly involves large amount of cash and constitutes part of profit-generation for health professionals, resents arouse among patients who receive unequal health care according to their gifting ability, and health professionals too become vulnerable.

5.2 Gift Practice as Profit-Generation and Mutual Vulnerability

5.2.1 Gift Practice as Profit-Generation

There are many unspoken rules of gifting. Red-packets are rendered mainly for major illnesses and surgeries, thus mostly given in (higher level) hospitals. In surgery, red-packets are given to both the surgeon and the anaesthetist, and sometimes to other relevant personnel. In the 'art of gifting', patients need to sense the situation and chance to give, passing the red-packet secretly. The amount to give is 'shared knowledge' in local society.[13] In Riverside, at the time of my fieldwork, the minimum amount of a red-packet was 200 Yuan (about £20). The more serious the illness, the higher amount was needed. One of my interviewees gave a

---

[12]See reports like Xinhua Net 2012. Similar incidents already happened in the 1990s. Bloom and his colleagues (2001: 30) record a report in 1995 about a man who attacked his father's doctor when the doctor refused his red-packet.

[13]The amounts of red-packets are higher in higher level hospitals and big cities.

600 Yuan red-packet for his hernia surgery in 2011 (Interview 40). Giving birth to a baby required at least 200 Yuan in the red-packet. For a caesarean section, the red-packet would be over 500 Yuan. In major surgeries such as brain surgery, patients' families even gave thousands Yuan. Life and illness are measured in the material form of gifts (in addition to regular medical fees) according to the seriousness of the treatment.[14] The commercialised health sector makes corporal human life and the vitality of the body a new frontier for calculation and capital accumulation.

Red-packets constitute an important part of a public doctor's 'grey' income (as shown in Chap. 2). In the beginning of the market reform (the 1980s and early 90s), hospital doctors, like many public professionals who lived on a fixed salary, found that they earned much less than those who 'dove into the business sea' (xiahai). In Deng Xiaoping's tour of southern China to further market reforms in 1992, he called for greater boldness in the market, stating 'letting some people become rich first' and 'getting rich is glorious'. These words provided the legal and moral basis for public professionals to make money. Doctor Lei, a retired county hospital doctor, told me he has begun to earn much more since 1993:

> In the previous year [1992], Deng Xiaoping said 'Be bolder, take bigger steps' (danzi da yidian, jiaobu mai da yidian) in order to speed up market reforms. These words had a profound influence on all walks of life. Patients became bold [in giving gifts to doctors for better care], and doctors too became daring and ambitious in making money. Patients gave money directly to doctors, hospital bonuses increased, drug kick-backs started… (Interview D19)

Deng's southern tour was a landmark of change. His words became a signal for health professionals to go ahead in the market to make money. Deng's saying 'black cat, white cat, the one that catches the rat is a good cat' was equivalently popular. The words conveyed a new ideology that concerned only the result regardless of means. Doctors began to accept red-packets, get drug kickbacks, and overprescribe to earn further bonuses.

Even though doctors received gifts, most doctors I met shared the idea that if their regular salary was raised to a satisfactory level, they would not accept bribes. A doctor from the People's Hospital stated: 'If we had dignified social status as well as enough income, who would trouble to do that kind of thing!' (Interview D28). 'That kind of thing' refers to the measures used to earn extra income, including bribe-taking, which was seen by doctors themselves as 'dishonoured', even 'shameful'. Many physicians are torn between their professional dignity and personal needs. Facing skyrocketing living expenses, doctors feel pressured to earn more and justify their profit-generating activities in terms of needs and deservedness. Public doctors describe their profession as 'hard work, high risk and low (formal) income'. They feel they are not fairly paid and earn less than they deserve.

---

[14]If the amount a patient's family gives is lower than usual, they should explain to the doctor a little about their difficult financial situation, but red-packet is not necessary if the patient is introduced through a close acquaintance.

The market economy is developed to encourage hospitals and health professionals to become self-sufficient, but the price control and other state restrictions under the socialist planned system still work to prevent health professionals to earn a sufficient amount. Officials are reluctant to boost public doctors' salaries, in case many other professionals on the government payroll demand pay rises, creating an unbearable financial burden to the government (Economist 2012). Health professionals, who are frequently low paid, need to find 'proxies' (*daili*) to supplement their income. Gift is one of the proxies to earn money in a controlled market. It serves as the wage supplement and constitutes the 'real price' (Zhan 2013) of a doctor's service.

Yet, gifting for some doctors is not just a 'proxy' to achieve 'sufficient' income, but capitalised on by them to extract a substantial amount of unjustified profits. Research notes that gifting practice has rapidly become corrupt, because certain health professionals expect or demand red-packets from patients before they provide critical services, and the large amount of money contained in the red-packet far exceeds its symbolic value and looks more like a bribe (Hui 2010). Blatant demanding of red-packets may only be conducted by a small number of doctors, but, in the process, the image of doctors as a whole has gradually changed from that of benevolent angels selflessly 'serving the people' to monsters in white cloth. The public hold moral judgement towards the money doctors gain, and the way through which the money is earned. 'In the past doctors made *benfen qian* [honest money], now they take such large amount [of illegal income] that it [their desire] is like the long fingernail of Empress Dowager Ci Xi' (Interview P40), Mr. Yang (in his 80s) expressed vividly. Empress Dowager Ci Xi of the Qing dynasty ruled China from the late 19th century to the early 20th century. She was famous for her long nails and known for her ruthless and vicious character. Her long fingernails symbolised her ruthlessness. Mr. Yang adopted them as a metaphor for the ruthlessness of doctors who take large amounts of illegal income. 'In the past they [doctors and officials] have cat's mouth, now their mouth is bigger than the lion's' (Interview P37), a middle-aged community guard complained. This change from a cat's mouth to a lion's mouth suggests the increasing amount of illegal income hospitals, doctors, and officials take. These metaphors echo many similar conversations with other interviewees. The moral boundaries are drawn between the honest money earned by doctors' hard work and skills, and that earned through excessive arbitrary charges and cheats. The market reform, however, increases the percentage of doctors' unjustified 'grey' income versus honest income, and correspondingly raises patients' gift burden. People's discourse of gifts is a moral evaluation that the gift in the past was relatively less exploitive and less capitalised, while the gift in the commercialised health care system of the market era violates the older, fairer moral economy, and presents people with a new sense of exploitation.

In traditional communities, a patient could be indebted to a doctor, to whom the patient would give compensation in the future.[15] *Baoda* (repayment) could be long

---

[15]This still occasionally happened in the rural areas of Riverside County.

term, without an immediate payment. In the market era, doctor-patient relationships (especially in urban areas and high level hospitals) increasingly become a commercial contract one in which patients as consumers need to give doctors something in order to obtain services, and the more one gives the better service one could get. The increasing monetary gift exchanges show the character of short-term instrumental transactions that giving and reciprocating happen in a short time and the relationship ends after reciprocating. In the health sector, red-packets are given one time before the surgery, and the doctor-patient relationship ends when the patient checks out from hospital. The relationships tend to be 'more completely dissolved and more radically terminated by the payment of money than by the gift of a specific object' (Simmel 1978: 376). The change of gifts from material to monetary form impacts the doctor-patient relationship, which is increasingly shaped by a calculative mentality and monetary exchange. Gift practice in the market era becomes more like a 'fictitious commodity' (Polanyi 1944)—an object of exchange that is dis-embedded from the social relationship, and even subordinates social relationship itself to the law of the market.

5.2.2 Mutual Vulnerability of Patients and Health Professionals

Gifting is a technique used by patients to seek reliable health care and to hold doctors accountable in a context of individualisation of health care responsibility. The marketization of the health sector increases inequality in health care access, which fuels the individual strategy of gifting to seek better care. Yet, the cumulative effects of gifting, instead of challenging the social structure, consolidate the existing inequality of health care access. People located in the socio-economic structure have unequal resources to deploy in informal exchange. As good medical resources are always insufficient to meet the growing needs, informal exchange, to some extent, compensates for the insufficiency for certain patients at particular times, but produces the exclusion of others. The rich, who are able to get expensive special care through formal channels, also have resources to give gift and create *guanxi* in order to obtain convenient health care. The poor, who have few connections and resources to give gifts, are limited to the use of the formal system, which becomes even more difficult to access. The wide practices of informal exchange seize the limited high-quality care from the formal system, strain the already stretched health system, and therefore further sacrifice the interests of those who do not have resources and connections. In addition, informal exchanges may attract skilled professionals away from poor areas where people's general gifting ability was lower compared to high income areas, thus magnifying the gap between localities. The overuse of informal exchange to jump queues, break rules, and overcome bureaucratic obstacles, may finally harm the function of the formal system, leading to further inequality.

Although many times gifting may help patients assure immediate medical services, this is to satisfy special needs of significant others instead of promoting universal equity. It is relational or interest-defined priority, not constitutionally-defined right. Health care, determined in the circuits of gifts and money, cannot secure health care as an inalienable equal right. Individual rights can easily be compromised in the face of informal exchange and *guanxi* work. Previous researches suggest red packets increase patients' financial burden and sometimes deter patients from seeking treatment (from Yang 2017: 9)

Gift practice in the Chinese health sector produces rising inequality and stressful relationships. Patients have contradictory attitudes towards gifting. They complain about it but also actively use it for individual benefits. Patients use gifts to impose moral constraints on the behaviour of doctors. When doctors cannot follow the principle of reciprocity in gift practice, it provides justification for angry patients to argue back.[16] Gifting thus also serves as a measure of counter domination that prevents doctors from demanding too many gifts or holds them to be cautious about receiving gifts, as one doctor expressed:

> Sometimes we feel scared to receive a red-packet. Even he [the patient] didn't give it to us, we would still operate carefully. If an accident happened, trouble would come to us. If patient gave us a red-packet and an accident happened, we would be in even more trouble. Most of the time, we don't want to cause trouble for ourselves... (Interview D27)

Doctors were not willing to receive gifts if a patient's condition was uncertain or if the chances of failure for a particular surgery were unusually high. If a doctor received a gift but a medical accident happened, he or she then broke the unspoken rule of reciprocity in gifting practice and would face potential blame and dispute. Sometimes doctors were not willing to take the red-packet as it increased the pressure on the surgery, but, in order to reassure the family, they would take the money first and return it to the family after surgery. Doctors dare to receive a substantial amount of red-packet only after the middleman work of a certain reliable acquaintance, which could reduce the potential of being revealed or sued after surgery. Gifting is anxiety-provoking for both patients and doctors who need to constantly speculate about whether to give and receive, the amount to give, the intentions of each other, amongst other factors. The patient calculates the expectation of the doctor and puts the reciprocal expectation of qualified care to the doctor, while the doctor evaluates the value of the gift as well as the possibility of meeting the reciprocal demand to decide whether to receive or not. If the reciprocal demand of the patient is not meet (the patient's condition does not improve or the treatment fails), resentment may grow in the patient and conflict easily break out, with the patient sometimes taking 'revenge' on the doctor with verbal or physical

---

[16]I describe the changes of gift practices overtime earlier in this chapter, but claim that the gift practice still follows the rule of reciprocity here. It seems conflicting, but what I want to show is a transitional process, an on-going changing situation. This changing tendency arouses people's resentments, that is why there are such violent reactions from patients as shown in Chap. 6.

attacks (Chap. 6). The process creates a temporary inversion of power between patients and doctors, causing doctors to become as vulnerable as patients.

Overall, in the market, gift practice enables health professionals to transfer their skills, expertise and professional power to economic profits and dominance over patients. Gifts can be regarded as an economic compensation for the low-valued labour of doctors, but when gifts are excessively demanded, they become a channel used by doctors to generate wealth. The capitalisation of gifts turns the gift relationship away from affective bonds and towards market exchanges—the instrumental one-time exchange of cash. The informal exchange of gifts while including some people in better care, further excludes others who are less connected and resourceful. It cannot secure reliable health care as an inalienable equal right. Gifts infringe on people's moral economy, when a patient's condition does not improve or the treatment fails after giving a 'gift', when the doctor does not or is not able to 'reciprocate' the patient with careful care after receiving a gift, or when the doctor demand too large a red-packet. In these circumstances, conflicts easily break out and patients sometimes take 'revenge' on doctors with verbal or physical attacks. Gifts thus also bring uncertainties and anxieties to doctors.

5.3 Gift Complicity and Governance

The informal practice of gifting exists not only between patients and health professionals, but frequently involves hospital administrators, local officials and government departments. It constitutes part of the everyday practice of governance in China's medical institutions, officialdom, and local authorities. Yet, the informal practice of gifting undermines the formal bureaucratic rationality of the state and the moral legitimacy of the party-state, hence it is officially proscribed. The conflicts between gifting in local governance and the containment of gift practices produce many dilemmas for people within the health system, as this section presents.

5.3.1 Gift Practice as Domination, Extraction and Local Governance[17]

The market reform encourages a 'competitive ideology of short term, individual, material self-interest' (Levy 2002: 53) that promotes corruption and strata rather

---

[17]Gift here is a broad concept. Although the financial contribution I discuss in this section is more like official bribe rather than a gift in more traditional sense, it has been put in the broad discussion of gifting by my interviewees. The relationships between a gift and a bribe, between gifting and corruption are obscured in official regulations, media reports and people's discourses.

than affection and solidarity. The health sector in the market era generates new forms of inequality within health professionals, and between health professionals and administrators. In defence of their 'grey' incomes, public doctors frequently revealed corruption among hospital administrators. The sense of relative deprivation permeates their words, such as the following account by a public hospital doctor:

> The hospital leaders could buy a medical device for 800,000 Yuan while the original cost was only 500,000 Yuan. They took kickbacks in such a large sum that us ordinary doctors felt it was very unfair. The money you [hospital leaders] used to buy medical devices was earned by us doctors with our labour and skills. Therefore if there was a chance, we doctors would also make extra money. (Interview D64)

Being asked about how to solve the 'grey' income issue, the doctor responded: 'If the leader's pocket was controlled from receiving kickbacks, then doctors would naturally control themselves...now the officials shield one another (*guanguan xianghu*), there is no way to deal with it'. The leaders in her words are not only administrators in her hospital, but also officials above the hospital. The leaders obtain a large amount of grey income by manoeuvring behind the scenes, and thus have a low risk of being exposed and punished. In contrast, doctors make grey incomes little by little with great risks of be exposed and penalised. In this doctor's view, doctors' illegal incomes were quite easy to control as long as the leaders set a good example and put in place stricter supervision. What is really difficult to solve is corruption within the leadership and officialdom, due to the covering up by high level officials for lower level officials. According to this doctor, as long as major corruption existed within the administration and officialdom, the ordinary doctors who actually carried out medical practices and generated hospital revenues were justified to make illegal gains.

Doctors defend their grey incomes by comparing themselves with hospital administrators who have 'major' illegal incomes. Hospital administrators similarly argue for their grey incomes by implicating even more serious corruption in the officialdom. As introduced in Chap. 2, Chinese hospitals are not autonomous from the government. Entrepreneurial bureaucrats not only reduce investment to the health sector, but also use their administrative power to reap profits from the health sector. Hospitals, like other enterprises, easily become the source of 'gifts' for the local government. Chau (2005: 238) uses the metaphor of 'channelling' to characterise state-society interaction in China: 'Through these channels the local state agencies siphon "upward" money and gifts while bestowing "downward" official institutional statuses and protection'. Wank (2001) notes the patron-client networks between local entrepreneurs and the local state agents in China, through which entrepreneurs gained information and protection from the local state in exchange for providing goods or services that generated additional incomes for these local state agencies. It is the same for the relationship between public hospitals and local authorities. Public hospitals' daily work is inseparable from the local government's support. In the reciprocal dependency between the public hospital and the local government, the hospital needs protection and approval from the local government in order to benefit from state policies (for instance to obtain state funding) and to solve medical accidents, while the local government needs the hospital for direct or indirect financial contributions. Local hospital administrators I interviewed complained at length about the predatory behaviour of local authorities. The following quote was an excerpt from the interview with a hospital director in early 2012:

> Before the New Year, the [local] government didn't have enough money to compensate the evictees during house demolition work…Some people [within the government] said the county hospital was rich, thus they [the government officials] immediately called us and asked us to take the lead [to contribute money to the government]. They didn't specify it [how much to give], but left some space for us to deliberate. We delayed [in giving] again and again, but at last, we had to act…We are a public hospital, nominally founded by the government, so if I rejected to do this for them [the government officials], they could send another person [to replace me] to do this. This is a threat. I am the deputy of the People's Congress at the municipal and provincial [level], I represent experts from hospitals, but [even with my status] the government could speak these [threatening] words to me. Our county is just one example. It is similar in many other counties…They [the local government officials] come [to ask for financial contributions] once, twice and a third time. Once they owe us money, they will give us [administrative] approval quickly [in return]. (Interview D47)

The development of a hospital, no matter public or private, needs good connections with and support from local authorities. Local authorities are the hidden power interfering with hospital administrations. In the economic and political agenda of local bureaucrats, public hospitals that make strong profits during the recent medical consumption boom easily become the target of extortion. The reciprocal dependence between a public hospital and the local government is frequently not in equilibrium. 'There is a saying that "interacting with the government is you get something from it this time while lose something more to it next time"… Our [work] spirit is really battered' (Interview D55), another hospital administrator commented. He expressed his outrage and frustration when mentioning that the money earned through hospital staff's hard work was taken away by local administrative agencies. His words echo the view of many local hospital administrators and professionals. This hospital administrator detailed the rapacious extortions his hospital encountered from local government agencies:

> Public security organs, procuratorial organs, the courts, tax offices, police offices, post offices, the environment protection bureau, and all levels of government departments – the propaganda department, the department of politics and law, the organisation department, etc. – all come to our hospital asking for money. If the hospital does not cooperate, once the hospital has a problem, they will cause trouble for us…It [the money the hospital gives] is called 'work expenses', work [solving hospital's issue] needs money. Let me count it for you, every year, there are at least 50 people or departments we need to give 'gifts' to, and each needs to be given at least 10,000 Yuan. Besides, we have large expenditure on *yingchou* [the social interactions and receptions involving feasting, toasting and entertainment]…In order to maintain a relationship with all these departments, we spend a lot on receptions [entertainment and banqueting]. Those leaders and cadres [from the government agencies], today one comes [to visit], tomorrow another will come [to inspect], the day after tomorrow yet another will come…Another issue, *bainian* [New Year greeting], *bainian* means giving money 'gifts' to each department and official…Thinking about these, I frequently feel lost! (Interview D55)

The informal practices of gift-giving and *yingchou* has a huge impact on how governance is conducted in China, and are essential for establishing and maintaining *guanxi* (relationship), (Tu 2014; Uretsky 2016). These 'work expenses', 'gifts' and '*yingchou*' serve as the 'technologies of enforced protection and insurance' (Yurchak 2002: 306) by the state agencies. Local institutions are literally 'forced' to give gifts to local state agencies in exchange for their administrative approvals and protections. If these latent 'gift' rules were not followed properly, the hospital would be easily found fault with by local administrative agencies and bureaucrats. Higher level hospitals face direct intervention from local officials; lower level medical institutions such as village and private clinics encounter similar intervention and extortion from administrative agencies at the lower level.

The necessity of gifting becomes the premise of daily work for individuals and institutions. It is a means for individuals of demonstrating loyalty and respect to their superiors, a means for medical institutions to overcome institutional bureaucracy in daily operation, and constitutes part of everyday governance of local authorities. Sometimes, the gift is not even necessary for solving an issue, but just to avoid more trouble to come. The hospital administrators giving gifts to their leaders and officials sometimes is not whole for a better chance of promotion, but also to avoid being given the 'shoes that pinch' (*chuan xiaoxie*) during work. Hospitals regularly contribute 'gifts' to government agencies and bureaucrats to ensure the smooth function of daily hospital work and to avoid being found fault with by these administrative agencies. Gifting is an individual and institution's struggle for existence in local informal practice of governance.

5.3.2 *Resistance or Complicity?*

Health professionals at the bottom are also increasingly unsatisfied with the gift practice that tarnishes their image and leads to unfair distribution. In the collective era, distribution followed the rule of welfare for all (albeit at a low level of income). In the post-reform era, distribution according to contribution is mixed with individual gains from informal channels, such as bribes, gifts, and kickbacks. Public doctors I interviewed regard their incomes as mostly earned through their hard work and medical skill, and thus more justified, while the illegal incomes of hospital administrators and officials were not based on their merits, skills, or contributions, but resulted from the abuse of official power. The growing inequality produced in the new economic order leads to moral outrage among ordinary health professionals, whose resentment is not for the corruption or illegal actions alone, but also because they cannot equally benefit from the corrupt system. Ordinary health professionals worry that the benefits would be largely taken away by higher level administrators, thus they too tend to maximise their immediate profits instead of waiting for the trickle down. Doctors' everyday work involves constant negotiations over regulations, salaries, subsidies, and opportunities to participate in informal exchange. In an environment where people have a low sense of security for policy stability and low trust towards the system, many tend to exploit opportunities to reap short-term benefits. Doctors in my field resent the grey income of those more highly placed while justifying their grey incomes to those below them. They justify the necessity of grey incomes in a system where doctors cannot earn a dignified income while feeling ashamed of using illegal measures to gain more. They express wishes of the problematic system to be improved to create fairer distribution while worrying the change would compromise their existing interests.

Many doctors do not feel they have influence over their institutions. Facing corruption within the health sector, most doctors keep silent, tolerate, and even participate in protecting their interests. Occasionally doctors stand against and expose corruption within the health sector, but these whistleblowers face an uncertain future. On 30th May 2013, a long investigative report entitled 'Crazy Doctor: You Ruin the Hospital's Reputation, the Hospital Will Make You Lose Your Job' was published by the *Southern Weekly*, a Chinese newspaper famous for its in-depth reporting (Cai 2013). The report told the story of a female doctor in a public hospital in Sichuan, who exposed overmedication, bribe-taking, and corruption within her hospital, and was removed from her position as department director. She lost her office and was suspended from work, and sat on a bench in the hospital corridor during working hours for over 14 months as a form of protest and a way of attendance in order to save her formal employee status. At first, certain colleagues showed sympathy to her, but as time went by, she was isolated and avoided by most colleagues. Sitting on the hospital bench during working hours was her visible action to humiliate the hospital, but her extreme action was regarded by many of her colleagues as improper and morally suspect. Instead of getting the issue solved, she was deemed by the hospital to be 'mad'. Some even regarded her as 'disloyal' and a 'traitor' with psychiatric issues.[18] In a system where corruption involved almost everyone, the ones who broke silence became the 'mad' abnormal ones. Like mentally ill people that were frequently regarded as a threat to social order, the 'crazy' doctor was regarded as a threat to the 'normal' hospital order. The 'crazy' doctor represents those unwilling to obey the 'unspoken rules' of the

---

[18]Searching online, I also found this doctor had written some posts on the internet to reveal the corruptions involved in her hospital and the threats and sufferings she endured during the past few years. After the media report, the 'crazy' doctor received much public sympathy and support. She was depicted by the media and public as a 'heroic' figure who defended patients' interests and upheld conscience against the corrupt health sector. In 2014, after many media reports and wide public attention, the higher level authority began to investigate the hospital. However, it triggered protest from a group of current hospital staff, who criticised the 'crazy' doctor of destroying the hospital's fame and demanded the hospital to expel her. The doctor and the hospital went into law suit for years and it ended with the victory of the hospital in 2016. However, debates surrounding the case continue.

system.[19] However, instead of changing the situation, the whistle-blowing doctors become the target of criticism. They may be dismissed, marked as troublemakers, and encounter difficulty to obtain further employment in public medical institutions. The social and systemic problems are individualised to protect the existing interests and power structure.

Compared with public doctors in the collective era who were strictly controlled under the *danwei* system and experienced political pressures in medical practices, doctors in the market era have greater autonomy and can change jobs more easily. Unsatisfied with the pubic system, some doctors choose to leave public medical institutions for private practices. However, in a system that the majority of patient visits and health professionals are in public hospitals,[20] this bargaining power is mainly held by the skilled doctors, who are able to generate tremendous followings of patients and high incomes. Even these skilled doctors will encounter many obstacles to leaving the public system. Health professionals under the socialist system were regarded as trained by the government and it was believed that they should serve the state and be loyal to their hospital. The idea still has salience in the current health system. Further, disciplinary techniques are built within social security not only for patients (as shown in Chap. 4), but also for health professionals. Health professionals who walk out from the public system will be punished with reduced insurance and social welfare. Even when they practice medicine privately, they are still under the administration of local health authorities and hold a marginal existence in the market (see Tu 2010: 45–8). Health professionals are disciplined through these micro-managements, and most of them will therefore choose the easy solution by following the daily function of the system. These docile health professionals are necessary for the profit-driven public hospitals in the market.

5.3.3 Gift Governance and the Ungovernable Gift Practices

Gifts now increasingly are exchanged outside the instant kinship and community, and follow from the lower stratum to higher stratum, serving the interests of those already dominant. It enables dominance and exploitation by the people with

---

[19]The use of a single media case here is because I cannot find more proper case from my field. However, the views and ideas expressed by this case and the following analysis are inspired by and in accordance with the views expressed by the health professionals in my field. This incident happened in the neighbouring municipality of Riverside. When this incident happened, I communicated with the health professionals in my field (who I still kept in contact) through internet, they expressed that similar incidents had happened in Riverside County too, but I could not get complete information about these similar cases because I already left the field. Besides, media reports sometimes provide compelling 'raw' accounts of traumas and tragedies of individuals, some of which may not be witnessed by researchers, such as the case I used here.

[20]In Chins, over 90% of outpatient and inpatient visits occurred in public hospitals in 2010, and 90% of health professionals were employed in the public sector (cited from Yang 2017: 13).

professional skills, power, and status. Scott notes that 'the "gift" as a disguised appropriation can be seen as the functional equivalent of commodity fetishism under capitalism', and this 'euphemization of economic power is necessary both where direct physical coercion is not possible and when the pure indirect domination of capitalist market is not yet sufficient to ensure appropriation by itself' (Scott 2008: 307). Gift in the Chinese health sector is such a 'euphemization' of economic power, and a disguised form that enables appropriation by health professionals and administrative agencies. The micro daily gift-exchange adds up to a large social pattern that impacts social stratification. Gifts increasingly flow upward from the low to high strata, from lay persons to experts, from the rural to urban areas (red-packets are concentrated in hospitals at or above the county level in the city), from patients at the bottom to high level hospital professionals, from hospital professionals to hospital administrators, from hospital administrators to government officials, and from government agencies at lower level to government departments at higher level. Gifting thus displays an upward accumulating gesture that allows people at the higher level of hierarchy to generate prosperity and maximise wealth. It works to reinforce dominance and hierarchy, and creates injustice, resentment and growing conflicts.[21] Besides, private gifting (together with *guanxi* as shown in the insurance reimbursement in Chap. 4) 'riddles the society with hidden, secret relations' (Kornai 2000: 8). Triggered by the opaque health system, it produces more secret and grey areas in the health sector that further undermine public confidence. Furthermore, the widespread gift practice, bribery and corruption undermine the effects of healthcare reform, and it is the ordinary patients who bear the costs. In the long run, people doubt the government's ability and willingness to tackle problems, leaving the legitimacy issue wide open to be questioned.

Gift practice and favourable care are in conflict with the ideology of socialist medicine and health professionals' image of selflessly serving the people that the state promoted. Over the years, the authority has always tried to contain gift practice in the health sector, especially the giving and receiving of red-packet. Especially since Xi Jinping came to power in 2012, gifts and corruptions in medical sector have become the target of serious control amid the government's anti-corruption campaigns. Gift governance combines measures of deterrence, surveillance, and moral education. Recently it also involves tentative reforms on health professionals' income by increasing their legal salary while reducing their 'grey' incomes. Cases of health professionals getting red-packets or drug kickbacks are regularly revealed by the media. Media reports and official discourses frequently link gift-taking with the moral failure of individual health professionals.[22]

---

[21]Yan's research (1996) on gifting in a rural village in China also finds that gift receiving rather than gift giving is regarded as a symbol of prestige, thus serves the hierarchy, in contrast to previous studies in other societies that find it was the giver who gains prestige and power by transforming the gift-receiver into a debtor.

[22]Other researches also find that the Chinese media frequently put blame on low-level cadres, which diverted attentions away from high-ranking party officials and the central government (see He 2000; Zhang 2006). Murphy (2007)'s research on the party education campaigns notes that the

In response, a variety of laws, regulations, and codes of conduct have been issued by the government.[23] In doctors' offices and on hospital walls, regulations on prohibition of gifts and bribes are widely displayed (see Figs. 5.3 and 5.4). When a red-packet or instance of misconduct is exposed, the administrative agency fires a few hospital staff and occasionally suspends a doctor's license. In recent years, the punishment of health professionals who receive gifts has become more serious and bribe-taking doctors can be arrested (Xinhua Net 2004; People's Net 2013). In 2014, China even asked all hospitals of level two and above to sign an agreement with inpatients within 24 h of admission to reject giving or receiving gifts (NHFPC 2014). The public display of the state's efforts to contain gifts and punish those involved dramatizes the government as the crusader against corruption. It guides people to vent their resentment towards individual professionals and hospitals, rather than question the systemic issues and government responsibility.

However, the visibility of 'forbidding' gifts within hospital is in contrast with the invisible but widespread gifting practice. Both givers and receivers are more cautious and adept at hiding 'gifts'. In a system where high quality care is in adequate, patients will still collude with doctors in gift practice to receive favourable treatment. Local hospital administrators admitted that the prohibition of doctors accepting red-packets, gifts or dinner invitations from patients has been emphasised in almost every meeting, but it did not work. They reasoned that hospitals could hardly find any proof of the secret 'bribes' doctors received, thus even though they knew it might happen, they could do nothing but ignore it. However, what they did not reveal is their tendency to cover up gift takers in order to protect the interests of their hospital, because skilled doctors (the main gift takers) are the main contributors to the hospital's profits. Another unspoken reason for this inability was that gifts involve not only hospital professionals, but also hospital administrators and leaders, the very persons who try to control gift practice. For many years, everyone (within the health sector) has known about these illegal incomes without speaking out about them (*dajia dou xinzhaobuxuan*). Doctors feel they have no way to stop their leaders' corrupt actions, thus keep silent. The leaders, in 'exchange', have to allow the minor gift-taking behaviour of doctors, who ultimately create profits for the hospital and whose cooperation is indispensable for hospital administration. Local authorities and government officials, who are widely suspected of corruption themselves and who may even benefit directly from local hospitals, have little moral authority and motivation to punish hospitals, thus tolerate the secret transactions below them. As a consequence, everyone has one eye open and the other closed (*zhenzhiyan bizhiyan*)—knows about gift exchange without saying anything about it. The 'mutual-complicity' and 'mutual-blackmail' between health professionals

---

campaigns deflect systemic critique and blame the problems of corruption on the ethical misbehaviour of individuals; the party-state instead champions itself as the defender in the crusade against failed individual ethics.

[23]Such as the one released by Sichuan province in 2004 that specifies the punishment of health professionals who take 'red-packet' or kickbacks (see Sichuan Government 2007).

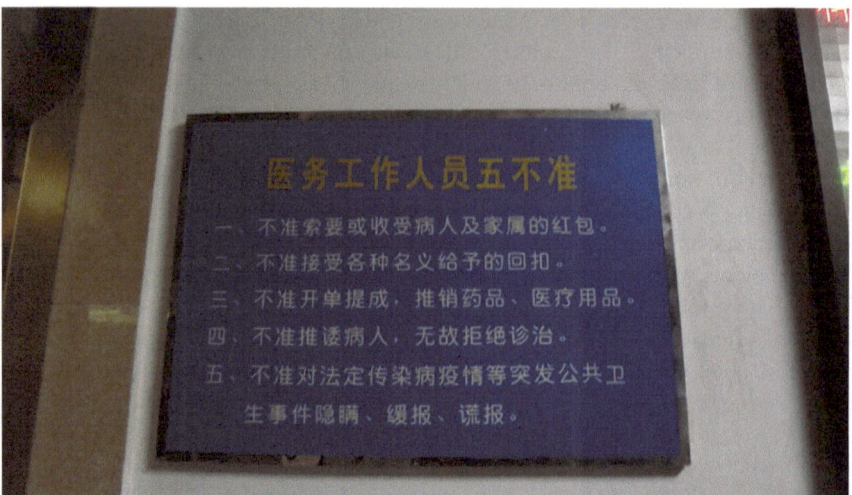

Fig. 5.3 'Five Prohibitions' on health professionals issued by the Health Department of Sichuan Province

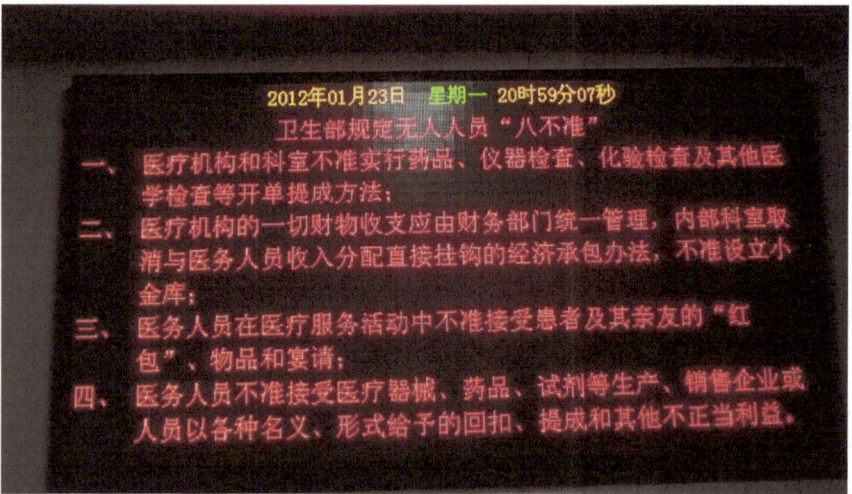

Fig. 5.4 'Eight Prohibitions' on health professionals issued by the Ministry of Health in 2004

and hospital administrators, between hospital leaders and local government officials, thus perpetuates gift practice.

Apart from the direct ban and punishment of gift-receiving, the authorities also promote ethic education and require individual health professionals to discipline themselves.[24] The promotion of self-discipline is consistent with the Confucian notions of self-cultivation that people are required to reflect on their personal ethics and cultivate themselves. It also follows the Maoist tradition of self-criticism in which the party-members and cadres are required to reflect on their own behaviour, admitting their mistakes, making corrections, and being a model for the people. Even today the communist party continues this rhetoric by requiring officials to reflect and criticise themselves in order to solve issues such as corruption. Yet few people I interviewed believe this ethically informed self-discipline will work out. In the market era, there is a lack of moral exemplar. The corrupt image of officials, hospital leaders, and medical administrators means the administrative authorities frequently lack moral credibility. As the traditional saying indicates, 'the beam at the top is crooked, the beam at the bottom will also be crooked' (*shangliang buzheng xialiang wai*). People watch rules being skirted and laws being violated by officials. Many feel that it is pointless to stick to moral behaviour. The bad example at the top enables corrupt behaviour extended to the bottom. Health administrators and officials, as the embodiment of state power, do not live up to a moral role, and are not respected by the people. When they employ moral rhetoric to justify their power and release vigorous moral codes for people below, it deviates from people's actual life experience and many are not willing to follow.

Fundamentally, it is because gift practice constitutes the everyday practice of local governance in China's health sector. Uresky (2016)'s research on Chinese officials reveals, government officials and party members who responsible for protecting the state's legitimacy and moral integrity through formal bureaucratic means also face informal expectations to engage in the very practices and behaviors (e.g. *yingchou*) that are prohibited by the state. There is a divergence between (the everyday practice of) governance and governmentaltiy (the formal government rationality), and this divergence produce dilemmas for these officials and party members. People in the health sector encounter similar dilemmas. While gift practice involves almost every actor in China's health sector and constitutes the unspoken rules of local institution management and medical governance, it is also the target of containment by the authority in order to improve its legitimacy. Reducing gifting problem to the moral failure of individual professionals serves political ends to partly transfer the state's responsibility. It not only conceals the patron-client networks between hospitals and local governments, but also justifies government agents' control of health professionals and hospitals. Yet, public and government institutions themselves are frequently ineffective representatives of popular morality. It gives health professionals standing to reject their governance.

Gift governance ignores the structural, economic, social and political foundations of gift. The informal gift-exchange plays a significant role in the routine operation of the Chinese health sector. Gifts are caught in the structural loop between the commercialised health system on the one hand and the medical pricing

---

[24]See the discussions and suggestions on medical ethic education and self-discipline to prevent corruption in medical sector in government regulations (MOH 2004, 2012).

system on the other, within which hospitals and doctors are encouraged to secure their own income but cannot earn enough through the formal channel. Gifts correlate with the individualisation of health care responsibility that patients have to secure reliable health care by themselves. Gift issue also links to the functioning of local bureaucracies and the deep pathologies of power within the authoritarian polity (that lacks transparency and surveillance) and the government (that focus on economic development, appropriate wealth from the society, and are corrupted themselves). In the social context where gifting becomes a habitual norm and functions as a necessity in every sphere, gifting in the health sector seems inevitable. Tackling the gifting problem thus requires not only regulations, but also systemic changes that reduce the necessity of 'gifts' in the first place. Besides, gifts should not be seen as completely detrimental. They relate to the culturally and historically grounded *guanxi* practice in China, and serve certain affective and social needs. Gift governance should not simply eliminate gifts, but make use of gifts and integrate them into a more transparent health system, while limiting their negative consequence.

References

Andaya, Elise. 2009. The Gift of Health: Socialist Medical Practice and Shifting Material and Moral Economies in Post-Soviet Cuba. *Medical Anthropology Quarterly* 23 (4): 357–374.

Bloom, Gerald, Leiya Han, and Xiang Li. 2001. How Health Workers Earn a Living in China. *Human Resources for Health Development Journal* 5 (1–3): 25–38.

Cai, Huiqun. 2013. "Crazy" Doctor: You Ruin the Hospital's Reputation, the Hospital Will Make You Lose Your Job ('Fengzi' yisheng, 'ni za yiyuan zhaopai, yiyuan za ni fanwan'). *Southern Weekly (Nanfang Zhoumo)*. Retrieved 1 June 2013. http://www.infzm.com/content/90898.

Central People's Government, PRC. 2013. *Why Only 10% Patients Trust in Doctors—Members of CPPCC Pay Attention on Doctor-Patient Conflict* (Weihe jin 10% huanzhe xinren yisheng – daibiao weiyuan guanzhu yihuan maodun). Retrieved 26 Aug 2013. http://www.gov.cn/2013lh/content_2349189.htm.

Chau, Adam. 2005. *Miraculous Response: Doing Popular Religion in Contemporary China*. Stanford, CA: Stanford University Press.

Cheal, David. 1988. *The Gift Economy*. London: Routledge.

Crouch, Colin. 2013. Making Capitalism Fit for Society. *Polity Blog*. Retrieved 6 Sept 2013. http://www.politybooks.com/blog/post.aspx?id=210.

Economist. 2012. *Health-care Reform: Heroes Dare to Cross*. Retrieved 22 July 2012. http://www.economist.com/node/21559379.

Fan, Ruiping. 2010. *Reconstructionist Confucianism: Rethinking Morality after the West*. London: Springer.

Giddens, Anthony. 1994. Living in a Post-Traditional Society. In *Reflexive Modernization: Politics, Tradition and Aesthetics in the Modern Social Order*, ed. U. Beck, A. Giddens, and S. Lash, 56–109. Stanford, CA: Stanford University Press.

Gregory, Chris A. 1982. *Gifts and Commodities*. London: Academic Press.

Guo, Sufang, Sabu S. Padmadas, Zhao Fengmin, James J. Brown, and R. William Stones. 2007. Delivery Settings and Caesarean Section Rates in China. *Bulletin of the World Health Organization* 85 (10): 755–762.

He, Zhou. 2000. Chinese Communist Party Press in a Tug-of-War. In *Power, Money, and Media: Communication Patterns and Bureaucratic Control in Cultural China*, ed. C. Lee. Evanston, 112–151. IL: Northwestern University Press.

Hui, Edwin C. 2010. The Contemporary Healthcare Crisis in China and the Role of Medical Professionalism. *Journal of Medicine and Philosophy* 35 (4): 477–492.

Kornai, Janos. 2000. Hidden in an Envelope: Gratitude Payments to Medical Doctors in Hungary. In *The Paradoxes of Unintended Consequences*, ed. R. Dahrendorf and G. Soros, 195–214. Budapest: Central European University Press.

Ledeneva, Alena V. 1998. *Russia's Economy of Favours: Blat, Networking and Informal Exchange*. Cambridge, UK: Cambridge University Press.

Lei, Hui-zhong, S.W. Wen, and M. Walker. 2003. Determinants of Caesarean Delivery Among Women Hospitalized for Childbirth in a Remote Population in China. *Journal of Obstetrics and Gynaecology Canada* 25 (11): 937–943.

Levi-Strauss, Claude. 1969. *The Elementary Structures of Kinship*. Boston: Beacon Press.

Levy, Richard. 2002. Corruption in Popular Culture. In *Popular China: Unofficial Culture in a Globalizing Society*, ed. E. P. Link, R. P. Madsen, and P. G. Pickowicz, 39–56. Lanham, MD: Rowman and Littlefield.

Li, Peiling, and Su Wenqiao. 1997. An Ethical Analysis of Red Packet Phenomenon (Hongbao xianxiang zhi lunli fenxi). *Chinese Medical Ethics (Zhongguo Yixue Lunlixue)* 6: 51–52.

Lumbiganon, Pisake, A. Malinee Laopaiboon, Metin Gülmezoglu, João Paulo Souza, Surasak Taneepanichskul, Pang Ruyan, Deepika Eranjanie Attygalle, et al. 2010. Method of Delivery and Pregnancy Outcomes in Asia: The WHO Global Survey on Maternal and Perinatal Health 2007–08. *The Lancet* 375 (9713): 490–499.

Mauss, Marcel. 1954. *The Gift: The Form and Reason for Exchange in Archaic Societies*. London: Norton.

Mi, Jie, and Fangchao Liu. 2014. Rate of Caesarean Section is Alarming in China. *The Lancet* 383 (9927): 1463–1464.

Ministry of Health, PRC. 2004. *The Ministry of Health's Advice on Strengthening the Construction of Health Industry's Working Style* (Weishengbu guanyu jiaqiang weisheng hangye zuofeng jianshe de yijian). Retrieved 21 Dec 2014. http://wsb.moh.gov.cn/mohjcg/s3577/200903/39740.shtml.

Ministry of Health, PRC. 2012. *Guidance on Strengthening the Prevention and Control of Corruption in Public Medical Institutions* (Guanyu jiaqiang gongli yiliaojigou lianjie fengxian fangkong de zhidao yijian). Retrieved 21 Dec 2014. http://wsb.moh.gov.cn/mohjcg/s3577/201209/55937.shtml.

Murphy, Rachel. 2007. The Paradox of the State-run Media Promoting Poor Governance in China: Case Studies of a Party Newspaper and an Anticorruption Film. *Critical Asian Studies* 39 (1): 63–88.

National Health and Family Planning Commission, PRC. 2014. *The Notice by NHFPC about Doctors and (In)patients should Sign an Agreement to Reject Red-packet* (Guojia weisheng jisheng wei bangongting guanyu kaizhan yihuan shuangfang qianshu bushou he busong hongbao xieyishu gongzuo de tongzhi). Retrieved 13 May 2014. http://www.nhfpc.gov.cn/yzygj/s3577/201402/b7f939aeaeee41c28ba80023b74c4187.shtml.

Pei, Minxin. 2008. Fighting Corruption: A Difficult Challenge for Chinese Leaders. In *China's Changing Political Landscape: Prospects for Democracy*, ed. C. Li, 229–250. Washington, DC: Brookings Institution Press.

People's Net. 2013. *Seven Doctors in Baotou Received Large Amounts of Drug Kickback being Arrested*. Retrieved 14 Apr 2013. http://legal.people.com.cn/n/2013/0413/c188502-21123200.html.

Polanyi, Karl. 1944. *The Great Transformation*. New York: Rinehart.

Qiu, Renzong. 2006. To Discuss the Conceptual and Ethical Issues of Commercial Bribery in Medicine (Lun yixue zhong shangye huilu de gainian he lunli wenti). *Medicine and Philosophy (Yixue yu Zhexue)* 27 (10): 1–4.

Rivkin-Fish, Michele. 2005. Bribes, Gifts and Unofficial Payments: Rethinking Corruption in Post-Soviet Russian Health Care. In *Corruption: Anthropological Perspectives*, ed. D. Haller and C. Shore, 47–64. London: Pluto Press.

Scott, James C. 2008. *Weapons of the Weak: Everyday Forms of Peasant Resistance*. New Haven, CT: Yale University Press.

Sichuan Government. 2007. *The Accountability System of Medical Institution Staff who Accept Red-packet and Kickback in Sichuan Province* (Sichuan shen yiliaojigou gongzuo renyuan shoushou hongbao, huikou zeren zhuijiu banfa). Retrieved 20 Apr 2013. http://www.sc.gov.cn/hdjl/jfgz/zxzl/bzzf/200702/t20070212_174973.shtml.

Simmel, Georg. 1978. *The Philosophy of Money*. London: Routledge & Kegan Paul.

Stan, Sabina. 2012. Neither Commodities Nor Gifts: Post-Socialist Informal Exchanges in the Romanian Healthcare System. *Journal of the Royal Anthropological Institute* 18 (1): 65–82.

Tu, Jiong. 2010. *Privatisation of Health Care in Transitional China: A Study of Private Clinics at the County Level*. Master thesis, Tema Health and Society, Linköping University. Retrieved 7 Apr 2013. http://liu.diva-portal.org/smash/record.jsf?pid=diva2%3A325266&dswid=6634.

Tu, Jiong. 2014. *Encountering Chinese Officials: Bureaucratism, Politics and Power Struggle*. LSE Field Research Method Lab. Retrieved 12 Dec 2014. http://blogs.lse.ac.uk/fieldresearch/2014/10/21/encountering-chinese-officials/.

Uretsky, Elanah. 2016. *Occupational Hazards: Sex, Business, and HIV in Post-Mao China*. Stanford: Stanford University Press.

Wang, Hongxia. 2005a. Analysis of the Red Packet Phenomenon in the Medical Field (Yiwujie hongbao xianxiang de zhengce duice). *Chinese Medical Ethics (Zhongguo Yixue Lunlixue)* 18 (3): 11–13.

Wang, Wenjun. 2005b. The Legal Liability of the Physicians Receiving Red Packets and Kickbacks (Yishi shouqu hongbao, huikou (ticheng) de falv zeren). *Medicine and Philosophy (Yixue yu Zhexue)* 26 (12): 52–53.

Wank, David. 2001. *Commodifying Communism: Business, Trust, and Politics in a Chinese City*. Cambridge, UK: Cambridge University Press.

Xinhua Net. 2004. *Receiving 500 Yuan Red-packet, A Doctor in Sichuan was Dismissed*. Retrieved 14 Apr 2013. http://news.xinhuanet.com/newscenter/2004-06/22/content_1539516.htm.

Xinhua Net. 2012. *Jiangxi Gaoan: Doctor Who Refused Red-Packet Being Attacked, Doctor-Patient Relationship Being Questioned* (Jiangxi Gaoan: yisheng jushou hongbao beida, yihuan guanxi zai zhao 'kaowen'). Retrieved 5 Oct 2013. http://www.jx.xinhuanet.com/news/focus/2012-07/30/c_112574325.htm.

Xinhua Net. 2013. *"Only 10% Patients Trusted in Doctors" is a Serious Warning* (Jin 10% huanzhe xinren yisheng shi ji chenzhong jingzhong). Retrieved 26 Aug 2013. http://news.xinhuanet.com/health/2013-03/11/c_124442435.htm.

Yan, Yunxiang. 1996. *The Flow of Gifts: Reciprocity and Social Networks in a Chinese Village*. Stanford, CA: Stanford University Press.

Yang, Mayfair Mei-hui. 1989. The Gift Economy and State Power in China. *Comparative Studies in Society and History* 31 (1): 25–54.

Yang, Mayfair Mei-hui. 1994. *Gifts, Favors, and Banquets: The Art of Social Relationships in China*. Ithaca, NY: Cornell University Press.

Yang, Jingqing. 2008. *The Power Relationships Between Doctors, Patients and the Party-State Under the Impact of Red Packets in the Chinese Health-Care System*. Ph.D. dissertation, Department of Social Science and International Studies, University of New South Wales. Retrieved 9 Apr 2010. http://handle.unsw.edu.au/1959.4/43116.

Yang, Jingqing. 2017. *Informal Payments and Regulations in China's Healthcare System: Red Packets and Institutional Reform*. Singapore: Springer.

Yurchak, Alexei. 2002. Entrepreneurial Governmentality in Post-Socialist Russia: A Cultural Investigation of Business Practices. In *The new entrepreneurs of Europe and Asia*, ed. V. Bonell and T. Gold, 278–324. Armonk, NY: ME Sharpe.

Zhan, Mei. 2013. Human Oriented? Angels and Monsters in China's Health Care Reform. In *Health Care Reform and Globalisation: The US, China and Europe in Comparative Perspective*, ed. P. Watson, 71–92. London: Routledge.

Zhang, Xiaoling. 2006. Reading Between the Headlines: SARS, Focus and TV Current Affairs Programmes in China. *Media, Culture and Society* 28 (5): 715–737.

Chapter 6
Power Game of *Nao*: Violent Disputes in the Chinese Medical Sector

The medical sector in China has witnessed increasing disputes between doctors and patients over the past several years. According to a 2012 report (Wang and Li 2012), medical disputes in China have increased at a rate of 22.9% annually since 2002.[1] Especially disturbing are the violent attacks, fights with and even murders of health professionals by patients. Such events are generally known as *yinao*. *Yinao*—the combination of the word '*yi*' (doctor, medical care, hospital, etc.) and '*nao*' (a disturbance or the act of speaking loudly and acting violently)—refers to the medical disputes waged by patients' families against medical personnel and medical institutions that involve violent or illegal means.[2] These disputes can take various forms, including the display of corpses at a hospital, the blockade of a hospital entrance, the destruction of property, attacks against health professionals, and in some cases, the employment of gangs by patients' families in order to pressurise medical institutions for more compensation in instances of malpractice. China's CCTV reported that in 2010 alone there were 17,243 cases of *yinao*, an increase of almost 7000 incidents from five years earlier (People's Net 2012). Statistics from the Ministry of Health show that medical violence had increased by 70% from 2006 to 2010 nationwide (CPG 2013). The official People's Net claims

---

Part of this chapter was published in *Berkeley Journal of Sociology* 2014 as an open-access article (Tu 2014).

---

[1]Chinese reports and articles gave different increase rates nationally. The rates also varied from place to place. Due to the sensitive issue of disputes and the tendency of the local government to conceal disputes, it would be difficult to find out the accurate data. The rate 22.9% is the result of a survey conducted by the Chinese Hospital Management Association, which is comparatively more official than other reports. The number is also quoted by some Chinese journal articles and media reports (all did not mention when the survey took place, but the data itself only emerged after 2012).

[2]*Yinao* can also refer to the people who use violence in medical dispute. Narrowly, it refers to the special groups of gangs employed by the patients' families to argue for more compensation. The word *nao* can be used as both a noun and a verb.

© Springer Nature Singapore Pte Ltd. 2019
J. Tu, *Health Care Transformation in Contemporary China*,
https://doi.org/10.1007/978-981-13-0788-1_6

that over 10,000 Chinese health professionals are attacked or injured every year (People's Net 2011). A ten province survey conducted in 2008 in 60 hospitals finds that more than half of health professionals had been verbally abused, nearly a third had been threatened, and 3.9% had been physically assaulted by patients or their relatives (Zhang and Sleeboom-Faulkner 2011). Research in a three-tiered hospital in Shanghai found that there were 577 cases of medical violence between 2000 and 2006, taking up 61.55% of all medical disputes that took place in this hospital during this period (Xu and Lu 2008). Besides these recorded cases, there are innumerable *yinao* cases that are unreported and solved locally under the political pressure to maintain stability. In the municipality in which my field site is located, there were 550 recorded medical disputes that took place between 2008 and 2011, approximately one medical dispute every two days. Medical conflicts and disputes erupted in local hospitals every month. Rising numbers of health professionals have experienced verbal or physical violence from patients.

Various factors contribute to this increase in medically-related disputes: a rising consciousness of patient rights, the deepening misunderstanding between patients and doctors, inflammatory media reporting, the absence of a formal institution for dealing with medical disputes, and problems related to the health system more generally (Tucker et al. 2015; He and Qian 2016). Yet, the use of *nao* in medical disputes has received little social science scrutiny. This chapter tries to fill this lacuna by studying the outbreak and practice of *yinao*. It explores how both patients and doctors employ the tactics of *nao* to defend their interests, and in the process reconfigure the power relations between patients and doctors. The use of 'power game' rather than 'power dynamic' is to emphasise the performance side of *nao*—how people use the tactics of *nao* and carry them out will influence the result of *nao*. *Yinao* being tolerated, solved or unsolved suggests not only the relationship between patients and doctors, but also the ways in which the state relates to the citizens and practice governance. Thus, this chapter also reflects on the current government measures to contain disputes: how the state frames civilised and legal behaviour, and tries to control *nao*—the uncivilised and backward practice. It highlights the strategies, complexities, and limitations of the practice of *nao* in an era of 'harmonious society', explores the power dynamics between patients, doctors, hospitals, and governments in the process of *nao*.

6.1 The Outbreak of *Yinao*: From Forgiveness to Revenge

During my fieldwork, several cases of doctors being attacked by patients have been widely circulated and discussed nationwide. One of the most influential cases is the 'Harbin' incident described in the beginning of the book. A young man in the city of Harbin in northern China stabbed four members of hospital staff in March 2012. Since this incident, I began to incorporate it into my interviews. I asked my respondents to comment on this incident. The question always evoked emotional responses from local residents. While many people showed their sympathy towards the deceased physician, stating that it was wrong to kill, they also expressed a high degree of understanding towards the extreme behaviour of the patient. 'There must be something wrong with the doctors or the hospital, or else how could the patient come to attack you [doctors]!' many of my interviewees speculated. Indeed, for many interviewees, their first reaction was to suspect the doctors and hospital involved of wrongdoing. My respondents recalled their own unhappy encounters with doctors and hospitals or recounted stories of others' experiences that they had heard about: instances where patients were overcharged, rejected from a hospital for not having sufficient money, mistreated by health professionals, or ignored, literally, to death. Typical was the way this elderly couple that I interviewed expressed their views:

> Grandpa Xu: I reckon the doctor might have done something bad, caused great resentment. You [the health professional who was killed] were a doctor, how could he [the patient] kill you [without a reason]? …
>
> Grandma Xu: In the past, it was less typical. He [the patient] could forgive you [the doctor]. Honestly, in the past, how did you [the doctor] behave towards patients? Your primary concern was to save him, your professional responsibility was to save the patient. Thus, the patient's family could forgive you. Now, even for a minor illness, your main focus is to make money, therefore if something goes wrong, they [the patient's family] will certainly argue with you until they take back more money from you.
>
> Grandpa Xu: The people [patients and their relatives] are just too resentful. His [the doctor's] attitude is really bad…Some [doctors] are too arrogant, they [patients' relatives] killed you then, anyway, one life redeems another life… (Interview P32)

Grandpa and Grandma Xu's comments were informed by memories of an earlier era. During the Maoist period, the socialist system provided almost universal, albeit very basic, healthcare to Chinese citizens. Doctors were encouraged to selflessly 'serve the people' and put saving lives first. Patients recognised that doctors had dedication, which enabled them to be more 'forgiving' when medical accidents occurred. However, in the post-reform era, patients often depict doctors as insensitive towards human suffering, and as putting profit before patient care. Patients become increasingly resentful: they get little information about their treatment, are frequently ignored by health professionals, and sometimes are even pressured to give gift or have expensive drugs. As an interviewee vividly described, 'we patients are like the meat on the chopping board, everyone wants to cut a piece. The doctors say how much [to pay], we [patients] have to pay that amount, we have no choice' (Interview P37). It depicts a picture of 'vulnerable and disadvantaged patients' vs. 'powerful and authoritative doctors'. Doctors' higher rank in the distributive structure was transformed into power to control and profit from patients. The commercialised healthcare sector opens patients up to an unparalleled regime of exploitation. In response, patients cannot hold lenient attitudes towards doctors and hospitals. When medical accidents occur or misfortune strikes, angry patients and families often target doctors as well as other health professionals, including nurses and administrators, for revenge. In people's reasoning, good intention and good deed are responded with forgiveness, bad intention and action are reacted with violent revenge, and a lost life is replied by taking another life (*yiming di yiming*).

Patient's violence is structured by a moral vision of health care. Hospitals and doctors in the post-reform era seriously violate this vision. In local people's accounts, there is a clear 'us-versus-them' dichotomy, in which doctors are seen as patients' main adversaries. If mothering of medical professions shows people's suspicion and hostility, then the demonization of doctors can justify the attacks. Grandpa Xu's words epitomised many locals' explanations of the violence: patients or their families 'intentionally ignored the law, because by using the law [the doctor escaped punishment or only received a prison sentence], you [the doctor] would continue harming others [after being released from prison]…they just killed you, that's all'. (Interview P32) Killing the 'bad doctor' is understood as a pre-emptive act, a way to prevent future medical malpractice. According to this logic, not only the demonised doctor does not merit a patient's trust, but it is even acceptable for the doctor to experience violent forms of retribution, including murder.

6.2   The Power Game of *Nao*: Violence, Protest and Inequality

6.2.1   Nao *in Daily Medical Setting*

In China, medical institutions at the community level are poorly-equipped.[3] The number of patients overwhelms the upper level medical institutions. The increasing health insurance coverage under the new healthcare reform also enables more patients to seek hospital care, leading to growing numbers of patients in medical institutions at all levels (see Figs. 6.1 and 6.2),[4] but the number of doctors has not increased accordingly. There are 1.5 doctors per thousand of the population in China, many of whom are poorly qualified; the density of doctors with five years of training including an internship is only 0.33 per thousand people, compared with an average of 3.1 per thousand in the OECD area (Herd et al. 2010). Since the market reforms, health care in many hospitals have been streamlined to increase efficiency and economic productivity. Under the new healthcare reform, many hospital staff face a doubled workload. Doctors must further speed up their

---

[3]Under the new healthcare reform, medical institutions at the community level are built up by the state with the hope to take the gatekeeper role, but the effects of these institutions are still limited.

[4]My research of more than 10 local hospitals at the county and township level finds rapid increases of patient number in all these hospitals since the new healthcare reform. The People's Hospital, the biggest hospital in Riverside County, had 500 inpatient beds, but the actual inpatient number ranged from 800 to over 1000 per day in 2011. In 2010, the hospital's annual outpatient number was over 490,000, more than 1300 outpatient visits per day. The TCM Hospital had around 450 beds, but the daily inpatient number usually surpassed 1000. Public hospitals add extra beds in wards and corridors. The overcrowded arrangements have many problems: exhausted health professionals, patient complaints, possible medical mistakes and accidents, etc.

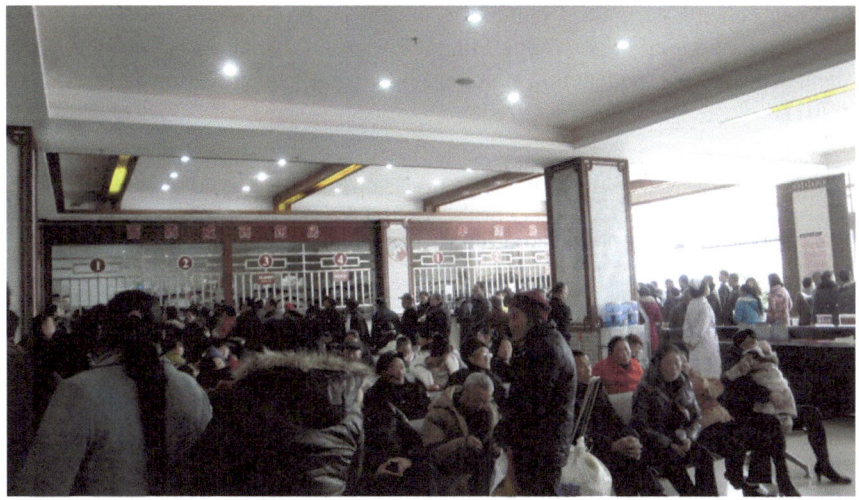

Fig. 6.1 Waiting patients in the TCM hospital

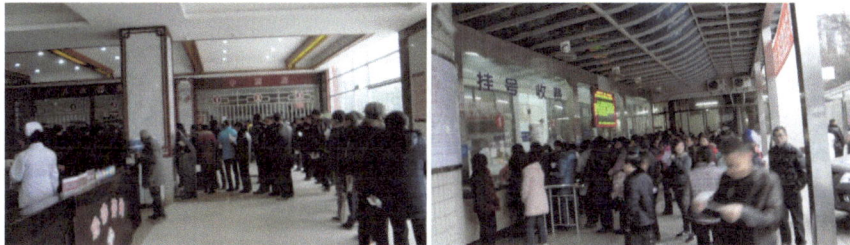

Fig. 6.2 Long queues in front of the registration and cashier widows (Left: the TCM hospital, Right: the People's hospital)

diagnoses and treatment, increasing the number of patients or procedures performed per day. In the local county hospitals, outpatient doctors at the forefront see dozens or even hundreds of patients a day. Pressured by the productivity requirement, doctors have only a few minutes to spend with each patient, which contrasts with each patient's lengthy wait for registration, diagnosis, medication, and tests. Inpatient doctors are also overworked, with long operating lists. Health professionals in the county hospitals and above are pushed to their very limits. Emotionally drained and exhausted, they have neither the time nor energy to pay close heed to individual patient's concerns. These overburdened health professionals sometimes neglect patients' requests. It is their survival strategy to rest whenever they can and sometimes withdraw slightly from their responsibility by ignoring patients' questions and requests, which means that, sometimes, patients who really need help are ignored.

When patients are indeed ignored by health professionals, *nao* is one of their strategies for arguing back. Auntie Liu, a local resident, told me her change from a 'silent and obedient' patient into a 'strong and violent' patient during a hospital visit in 2011:

> Auntie Liu: Now if you don't act violently, he [the health professional] won't pay attention to you…Last winter, I went to the TCM Hospital, he [the doctor] asked me to go into hospital…Later, I waited a long time [in the inpatient department], nobody came to give me a drip. I had handed the prescription to the nurse a long time ago. I asked them about it, and they said they were preparing it for me. Before I went upstairs [to the impatient department], they said they had booked a bed for me, but when I went upstairs, nothing at all, not even a chair to sit on, and nobody gave me a drip. We went to *nao* with them. After the argument, they came to apologise and treated me immediately. If you don't *nao* with them, they just ignore you.

> Community Guard: …Now they are only scared of tough people, if you ask them toughly, they will react to you. If you really think about them, consider how busy they are and wait, then even half a day later they will not have come to you…

> Auntie Liu: Yes, it's like that. At the beginning I stood there waiting quietly, I thought the staff were busy, I should wait, but I waited until all these nurses began to rest and chat to each other, they still didn't pay any attention to me. I spoke to them, and a nurse even said 'You should find a chair for yourself to sit down'. This angered me. I said: 'I'm an inpatient, you ask me to find a chair, where can I find one? Inpatient care should have a bed. If you don't have a bed [for me], at least you should find me a seat'. She said I should find it by myself…How could I find a seat? All these places are full of patients [and their relatives], only if health professionals went to ask, they would spare one. If I went to ask myself, they [the other patients] who were sitting on them wouldn't spare one [seat] for me, only your hospital staff could do that. If I did not *nao*, they would not react. After my argument, the head [of the department] came, and asked her [the nurse] to find a seat for me… (Interview P37)

In the busy hospital environment, patients are frequently unheard, misheard, or heard but ignored. Patients feel helpless, diminished and resentful, and so choose to *nao* to resist the unfavourable circumstances. Auntie Liu's experience of being ignored and mistreated in the hospital led her to give up obedience to act violently, which finally forced the hospital staff to react. Similar experiences were shared by many locals, who agreed that, in many situations, they had to act strongly, complain violently, or report misconduct to a higher authority in order to have their issue solved. The patients, who had paid their medical fees but were left waiting endlessly, began to use *nao* to interrupt the temporal flow of time and space of the hospital until their issue was solved.

In the market, people increasingly become atomised individuals, who need to secure their own welfare, face conflicts, and defend their interests by themselves. Cooper (2011) attributes the rising number of medical disputes to the general decline in health insurance coverage in China during the past three decades, which lead to the restratification and reprivatisation of risk. The reduction in insurance security forces people to negotiate good care and defend their interests by themselves, which produces a new kind of Chinese biopolitical subject—'the individual risk-bearer and contractor in personal services' (2011: 325). Recently, most Chinese patients have taken out health insurance, but, as Chap. 4 shows, the new health insurance schemes do not guarantee anything beyond a minimum level of health-care coverage. Patients are still required to take responsibility for overseeing their own care and the quality of their care. Besides, the government has failed to respond effectively to medical negligence, accidents and scandals. There are few independent investigations, no public apology, and insufficient official attention. Dissatisfied patients cannot obtain an efficient response if they recourse to the official channels. People are concerned that no-one will listen to them, and so resort to measures like *nao* to attract attention. *Nao* is an individual patient's technique for attracting proper attention, enabling them to be heard and obtain response in an overcrowded hospital environment.

6.2.2 The Practice of Yinao: A Weapon of the Weak?

In Riverside County, several cases of patients committed suicide while in the hospital happened just before and during my fieldwork. The medical dispute that took place in one county hospital in 2011 was especially controversial. It was widely discussed by the locals and repeatedly mentioned by the health professionals I interviewed. The patient had been diagnosed with terminal cancer and was hos-pitalised. Overwhelmed by pain, she jumped off the hospital building one night and died. After the incident, the patient's relatives gathered in the hospital, placed the coffin at the hospital entrance hall, and asked for compensation. The family also employed gangs to *nao* in the hospital. Quarrels broke out between the patient's family and the hospital, resulting in the injury of several members of the hospital staff, including the hospital director. Drawing from archival and online sources, I found many cases of patient suicide that led to violent disputes between hospitals and patients' families. These cases aroused intense discussions about hospital responsibility. When the overcrowded public hospital attributed some daily care responsibility to the patient's family, the family expressed that the hospital should take full responsibility if accident happened during the patient's hospitalisation. Further complicating this matter, existing laws did not specify the distribution of responsibility in cases of suicide in medical facilities. When these disputes went to court, the adjudications varied from case to case. Many families thus relied on themselves to *nao* in order to seek just compensation.

In the case happened in Riverside County, I was not able to hear directly from the patient's family, but I found a long complaint posted on a local internet forum that had been written by the patient's husband soon after the suicide. From the post, I learnt that the patient was left unattended by hospital staff even though they had been informed about the patient's unstable emotional state and suicidal tendencies. Additionally, the corpse was transferred to another mortuary outside the hospital before the family had been informed. In order to 'seek justice' (*tao gongdao*), the family used the internet as a channel to air their complaints. The post was filled with grievances. In the forum discussion, others expressed sympathy towards the family and criticised the hospital violently.

Taking this suicide case as an example, *yinao* is manifested in various scenarios. When a patient dies in a medical setting, the family and extended kin quickly gather together. They wear white gowns, sit or camp in or outside the hospital, set up mourning halls, refuse to move the corpse, display funeral wreathes, burn spirit money, broadcast funeral music, and cry out loudly in the hospital. Sometimes patient's families march around the city, holding banners and placards with emotional words in black and white, such as 'return the life of my parent'. Crying, group gatherings, the employment of traumatic language, and the performance of death rituals are all strategies of *nao*.

The practice of *nao* in medical dispute is infused with local social and cultural meanings. Crying out loud, acting emotionally, displaying funeral equipment, and broadcasting funeral music are common practices in conventional mourning. When a patient dies, the family is justified to engage in these mourning rituals even at the hospital or clinic. Sometimes angry families verbally or physically attack health professionals. At the moment of *nao*, social etiquettes (between patients and health professionals) were temporarily discarded. The patient had just passed away; the relatives overtaken by emotion are entitled to act out of normal social customs. Besides, most of the practices of *nao*, albeit controversial, do not directly violate the law. The hospital and government have to tolerate public demonstration of post-traumatic emotions as long as it does not constitute something that threatens the government. Moreover, the public tends to sympathise with the weak, in this case, the mourning family. The long list of grievances the public has about profit-driven hospitals and 'irresponsible' health professionals also increases their tolerance towards *nao*, which is thought to target those in power.

At the same time, the visible, public, and persistent *nao* is disastrous for health professionals and hospitals. While the position of the patient's relatives as victims affords them moral capital in countering health professionals and hospitals, health professionals who hold less moral capital have limited resources. They generally do not respond to verbal attacks until the situation escalates. In addition, the crying and the display of funeral equipment and corpses meet with Chinese people's fear and avoidance of things related to death. These funeral performances at the hospital are thought to bring '*mei*' (bad luck) to the people who encounter them. These intentional actions by the patient's family are meant to drive patients away, causing the hospital and doctors bad luck in their business. Also, these striking and noisy displays put hospital and doctors in an awkward, humiliating position, and threaten their 'face' (*mianzi*)—the reputations of individual doctors as well as that of the clinic or hospital. Many medical institutions and doctors cannot survive these troubles. In order to save their business and their 'face', hospital administrators and doctors are pressured to meet the family's requests.

Nao has traditionally been used by people in various settings. As the Chinese proverb says, disadvantaged people have three measures to defend their interests: 'first cry, second *nao*, and third threaten to hang oneself' (*yiku ernao sanshangdiao*). People subtly manipulate shouting, crying, and bodily movements to publicly decry mistreatment. In the wider society, people increasingly use extreme measures like *nao* to solve their issues which otherwise would be ignored (Pei 2010; Jing 2010).[5] *Nao* is frequently adopted by people from the lower social strata, who subjectively feel that they have less power and fewer channels to have their voice heard, who are pushed to the extreme and have no other way to defend their interests. Through *nao*, the comparatively weak party who has little to lose reverses the power relations with the other party who needs to preserve their existing interests and reputation. In the health sector, it is the disadvantaged who face a greater possibility of suffering as a result of negligence or bad attitudes (see Chap. 3, pages 68 and 69). The accumulative pent-up anger born of innumerable small indignities, resentment, social and medical neglect break out in the form of violence, leading to a political act of considered resistance by the social margins. Although *nao* may not be the perfect solution, it is a 'weapon of the weak' (Scott 2008), deployed by the marginal groups to counter the unequal power relations between patients and doctors, and creates new sites for contestation over rights.

6.2.3   The Pressure of Preserving Stability

Moreover, the ritualised gathering together of the patient's family, kin, and in some cases, hired gangs has symbolic power. In an era of 'harmonious society'—the political agenda promoted by the Hu-Wen leadership since 2004 to reduce social conflicts—the government feels increasingly insecure in the presence of large group gatherings and demonstrations. For this reason, the government frequently pressurises hospitals to solve disputes as soon as possible and meet patients' demands. Ironically, the government effort to build a harmonious society, to some extent, empowers patients.

In the suicide case I mentioned earlier, the hospital later initiated efforts to negotiate with the family, but no agreement had yet been reached when I conducted research in the county hospital in 2012. 'The amount asked by the family was too much' and the family's attacks on hospital staff effectively suspended the negotiation. The hospital director was furious about being attacked and revealed the bind

---

[5]Pei (2010: 29) suggests that ordinary resisters in China are likely to employ simple and direct forms of defiance; their weapon of choice is street demonstrations, blocking major railways and highways, strikes, and even violent attacks on government building. Jing (2010) also writes about the violent contestations and actions, as well as the use of funeral stuffs in Chinese protests. He points out that the transfer of funeral symbolism to social protests is an important feature of China's political culture. In some recent protests, people also employ funeral symbols to demonstrate their demands, such as the white cloth scroll with black and red petition words on top taken by people in the famous Wukan protest in 2011.

he found himself in, with the family demanding compensation, on the one hand, the government demanding that the hospital maintain stability, on the other:

> At the mediation scene, there were the personnel from health bureau and government office, even two members of the police. I bent down to talk with him [the deceased's husband]. Suddenly he took a tea cup from the table and hit me with it on my head. It hit the corner of my eye, caused the rise of the intraocular pressure, the brain blood pressure increased too, it may have potential risk for my brain…What can I do? I had to be there, to *weiwen* [preserve stability]. The hospital head shouldn't be at the mediation scene. Without the hospital head at the site, the conflict could be eased a little, but the government leader didn't understand this. He only wanted to reduce his pressure [in preserving stability]. There isn't any cooperation [between the hospital and the government]. (Interview D47)

As the hospital director explained, the patient's family would wait for an 'influential' person to show up, then act strongly and even violently to show their determination. The hospital director was aware of the importance of avoiding direct confrontation. 'Instead of forcing the hospital head to go [to meet with the family], it should be the staff specialised in solving disputes who conduct the negotiations', the director commented. However, the local government's pressure to maintain stability forced him to meet with the family, which incited the conflict, leading to the attack even in the presence of police and government personnel. The hospital director further complained about the government's irresponsibility:

> When there is a conflict, the police come to tour the hospital then leave…The court just *moxini* [literally, mix the mud], and even if we win the lawsuit, we still lose. We win the lawsuit but lose the money…Now the state promotes the 'harmonious society', it pursues harmony without the premise of the legal system, this is stupid. It's the government's irresponsibility…The effort to conceal conflict cannot really solve the problem…I feel that our society is headed towards a crisis. The crisis is waiting to happen. That's why our government is so nervous, focusing on maintaining stability which outweighs all other concerns, even pursues stability without principle. They are scared that they cannot control the situation if the fire starts and spreads.

According to my respondents, when medical disputes erupted, the police usually arrived, watched, and then left without doing anything. The police's main concern was to preserve social order at the site. As a result, they were often reluctant to interfere for fear of further escalating the conflict. Given police inaction, the conflict dragged on. When the local government was pressured by the existence of protest group of the patient's family and their loud supporters, it, in turn, pressed the hospital to solve the dispute at any cost. The hospital then became the sole target of medical dispute and the only negotiator with the patient's family. The hospital director pointed out the problem of the court that *moxini*—mediated differences at the sacrifice of principle. The director explained that even if the hospital won the lawsuit, they still needed to pay the patient's family in order to 'buy peace'. The government pursued harmony without the premise of the legal system, acted to peace conflicts but failed to address the root of the conflict. When stability trumps all other goals, a bigger crisis ensues.

6.2.4   The Inequality of Nao

Nao is not only employed by the disadvantaged group, but also consciously used by those who have influence and power to argue for more compensation. During a focus group interview in the local community, the residents told me two stories:

Resident A: In my village, there was an old lady, she was treated in hospital and was about to be discharged. Before leaving hospital, she accidentally fell on the toilet floor [and died]. Her daughter was working at a police station, she asked a group of people [from the police station] to go with her and they surrounded the hospital, demanding compensation. The hospital director came to negotiate with her many times, explaining that her mother's operation had been successful, and she fell by herself [but it did not work]…After several days' *nao*, the hospital director learnt that the old lady's daughter was from the police office, and then paid her 80,000 Yuan in compensation. They were from my village, the old lady died…They surrounded the hospital, did not allow anybody to go inside, even the ambulance with a patient was not allowed to enter…

Resident B: Yes, they said you needed to have power, have influence [to get compensation] …If it was ordinary people, they [the hospital] would not respond to you.

Resident A: They were a gang of people [surrounding the hospital]…They would not leave until you [the hospital] give money.

Resident B: Oh, last time, my nephew, his wife went to give birth in hospital, she was pregnant with twins. At first, they didn't know [they should give a red-packet]. If they had known, they would have given a red-packet earlier, then the twins could have been saved. In the end, the twins died in the womb. (JT: Why?) Because the doctor did not treat her for a long time, did not come to her, because they [the family] did not pay [extra] money… How was it solved at last? My nephew did not want to go to court, he said a lawsuit would take a long time…Finally, it was negotiated privately, the hospital compensated them 20,000 Yuan. It was twins, only 20,000 Yuan, too little…It happened only two or three years ago. They did not know they should give a red-packet, thus the doctor did not operate on her [in time]… (Interview P36)

The contrasts between these two cases are obvious: one with power used violent measures to *nao*, and thus obtained 80,000 Yuan compensation, while the other did not have equivalent influence to *nao* and was reluctant to bring a lawsuit, so negotiated privately for only 20,000 Yuan compensation. It is impossible to evaluate the worth of a life in pure monetary terms. What matters is the local people's comparison between those who 'have power and influence' and the ordinary people. The powerful ones were able to obtain the compensation they desired within a short period by manipulating their power and influence, while the ordinary people had little choice but to accept the private negotiation and limited compensation. Mediated by the uneven distribution of power and resources, *nao*—the weapon of the weak can be transformed into the weapon for manipulation and exploitation by the powerful ones. It thereby reinforces the inequality and advantages those who are already advantaged.

Besides, when hospitals are forced to compromise with those who engage in *nao*, this reinforces the sense that more violence begets more compensation. Over time, this encourages people to use violence and society to follow 'the Rule of the Jungle', as shown by the increasing involvement of organised gangs in medical disputes.

Health professionals and administrators notice that organised gangs (employed by the patient's family to perform *nao* on their behalf) have developed a mature model to argue for compensation: first, they do not allow medical appraisal and autopsy; then, they organise groups to *nao* in hospital and disturb the hospital's order; afterwards, they burn spirit money and display banners around the hospital; last but not least, they use other tools like the internet to influence public opinion, and threaten to invoke 'mass incidents' (*qunti shijian*) (Qiu and Yang 2012). These *yinao* gangs clearly understand the pressure that hospitals and the government face with regard to maintaining stability, and consciously manipulate the protocol of a 'harmonious society' to achieve their demands. During medical disputes, many families strive to attain just compensation, but it is clear that some families work together with *yinao* gangs, trying to take advantage of medical disputes to demand a larger compensation package. Sayings like 'want to become rich? Have surgery; after the surgery, sue the doctor' (*yaoxiang fu, zuo shoushu, zuowan shoushu gao daifu*) indicate that doctors reap profits by performing surgery, and patients also strategically sue doctors following surgery to obtain money in the form of compensation. The doctors' attempt to make money out of surgery in the first place supplies a justification for the patients' subsequent extortion behaviour that frequently involves the *yinao* gangs. After successfully helping a patient's families to obtain a high level of compensation, the *yinao* gangs then claim a large portion of it, thereby reducing the actual benefit to the patient's family while at the same time causing the hospital to suffer an unreasonable loss. In this sense, both the patient's relatives and hospital are being hijacked by the *yinao* gangs.

6.2.5   Doctors' Vulnerability, Defensive Measures, and the Reversal of Power

Medical disputes have become a headache for both the medical institutions and professionals. Hospitals pay large sums annually to solve disputes. Health professionals who are accessible, unarmed and unprotected bear great uncertainty in their daily work. Doctors invariably relate their work to 'risks' and complain about the possibility of being sued or attacked by patients. Some even abandon the medical profession or express an unwillingness to let their children study medicine (Wu et al. 2014).[6] In my interviews with health professionals, almost everyone complained endlessly about medical disputes. A young female doctor who had been attacked by a patient told me that she had felt dramatically less secure ever since:

---

[6]Also see various survey results and innumerable media reports (for instance, People's Net 2014) about doctors' unwillingness to let their children study medicine. The rising tensions and conflicts between patients and doctors are one of the contributing factors.

When I was an intern in the hospital, an old woman in a critical condition passed away one night when I was on duty. Next morning, I had finished work and was chatting with another doctor in the corridor before going home. A middle-aged man came to us and asked 'Who was the doctor on duty last night?' The man looked like an ordinary person in the hospital. I responded, 'It was me', without a second thought. At that moment, the man brought out a walking stick from behind his back and tried to strike me with it. I was immobile with shock. The male doctor next to me warded off the blow with his arm, which was immediately broken. Later, the hospital paid compensation to the patient's family, and also had to fund the treatment of my colleague's broken arm. Prior to this incident, the door to my office was always open so that patients could see me whenever they needed to but, after this attack, I always close my office door. If a patient knocks on it, I always ask who it is before opening it. In the past, my computer was opposite the door, near the window. After the accident, I can't work on my computer sitting with my back to the door. I moved my computer so that I can see at once if someone walks in. My trust in others has decreased dramatically since then. (Interview D39)

These attacks occur without warning, undermining the doctors' sense of security and trust towards others. Although this attack was prevented by another doctor, who was hurt instead, the young doctor remains traumatised by this incident. Insecurity prevails among health professionals, who employ many self-defensive measures: refusing seriously-ill patients, exaggerating patients' conditions at the beginning to avoid trouble in the future, avoiding administering shots and drips to uncertain patients, and so forth. Medical practice is being increasingly constrained by the boundaries of 'safe practice', limiting doctors' efforts to save patients.

The laws regulate that, in medical disputes and lawsuits, medical institutions shall bear the burden of proving their innocence.[7] Health professionals therefore devote an enormous amount of time and energy to keeping meticulous records, which are pivotal evidence in medical disputes and lawsuits. 'Our doctors devote more than 30% of their time to taking records, recording all kinds of mistakes and errors, and make even more efforts to find mistakes' (Interview D52), one local hospital director complained. Health professionals have also increased the tests for patients in order to collect evidence for possible disputes and litigation. The same director justified this practice as follows:

There are many unpredictable factors during treatment. Infectious diseases, such as HIV/AIDS and Hepatitis, are more widespread nowadays. We must provide a comprehensive physical examination of patients prior to treatment. If not, there is risk that our

---

[7]In 2002, 'Some Provisions of the Supreme People's Court on Evidence in Civil Procedures' released by the Supreme People's Court (http://www.court.gov.cn/bsfw/sszn/xgft/201004/t20100426_4533.htm, retrieved 14 January, 2013) and the 'Ordinance on the Handling of Medical Malpractice' released by the State Council (http://www.gov.cn/banshi/2005-08/02/content_19167.htm, retrieved 14 January, 2013) both regulate that the medical institution shall take the responsibility to prove there is no medical fault and no causation between medical practice and harmful consequence in a tort case, in contrary to other civil lawsuits that require the party who litigates to provide evidence. Patients without professional medical knowledge are regarded as the disadvantaged party who are difficult to get medical evidences, thus the burden of proof rests on the medical institutions and health professionals.

health professionals may become infected. More importantly, patients may blame the hospital for their infections. In this case, hospitals must prove that the infection occurred before they went into hospital. All this wastes a lot of time for us.

The safety consideration together with economic motivation has made physical examinations and tests popular in Chinese hospitals. Tests are expensive and largely uncovered by medical insurance. It is a significant source of profit for hospitals, but adds a greater burden to patients, correspondingly provoking more complaints from them. Later, in 2009, the new Tort Law changed the former rule of requiring medical institutions and professionals to provide evidence in the case of medical accidents. It tried to 'balance' evidence from both patients and health care providers. Yet, the uncertain medical environment and economic motivation continue to encourage doctors to order extra tests (He 2014).

Conflicts and uncertainties not only make health professionals undertake much 'unnecessary' work, but also challenge their morale. When interviewing a group of young doctors, one of them commented:

Although only a few people *nao*, 'one rotten apple spoils the whole barrel'.[8] If I [a doctor] treated 1,000 patients, and 999 of them were nice to me...but as long as there was one person who engaged in *nao* and spoke badly of me, I would [be cautious]...Scared of this kind of patient, I have to do a lot of things to prevent disputes, a lot of unnecessary work. Now, we feel that our work isn't stable at all. Something might go wrong if we lose focus for a second...Oh, now our *yishi* [mentality] of being a doctor has changed. Going back 20 years ago, doctors then thought about curing patients' illness to their best ability. Although sometimes they might have wanted to make a little money, they still put patients first...but now it's different. Now, the first thing we think about is how to protect ourselves, not how to treat patients...Our thinking has changed. The influence is not good for patients either. (Interview D28)

The occasional outbreak of *nao* can tarnish trust irreparably. The 'few bad cases' are enough to make physicians scared of being condemned or sued for malpractice, and thus they treat the majority of their patients with caution. Yet, under the name of 'self-protection', the measures for making a profit are also justified. This young doctor felt worried because doctors now think more about self-protection than treating patients. He felt that his morale was challenged in his daily medical practice compared with his ideal when pursuing a medical profession and with doctors 20 years ago who put patients first. Saddened by the patients' mistrust and suspicion and shocked by patients' attacks, doctors have become moral agnostics and some feel more justified about doing what is best for themselves instead of what is best for the 'suspicious' patient. A public doctor in her 50s expressed her frustration as follows:

For me, the doctor, you [the patient] don't trust me anyway, no matter what I do, you don't trust me, thus I take some drug kickbacks, even if I did not take a cent, you [the patient] still don't understand me, you don't think I have benefitted you in any way... (Interview D64)

---

[8]The original words this doctor use is *'yike haozishi dahuai yiguo tang'* (a rat's dropping spoils a whole cauldron of soup).

The doctor justified her grey income by mentioning the patients' mistrust in the first place. The more disputes, suspicion and attacks on the part of patients, doctors are more justified in putting their own interests first, which however causes further resentment and frustration on the part of innocent patients.

When the assault and killing of health professionals happen repeatedly, health professionals increasingly become 'the weak' who cannot protect themselves in the face of violence. They employ a 'scalpel vs. dagger' metaphor, protesting that they use a scalpel to save patients only to be 'repaid' with a dagger. Health professionals accuse patients who chose *nao* instead of legal channels of being greedy for more economic compensation. They compared *yinao* with extortion behaviour in the wider society where someone who lends a helping hand is extorted by the very person he or she helped.[9] The latter situation makes people too afraid to help. *Yinao* also makes health professionals reluctant to save dangerous patients, treat all patients with caution, and place their own protection prior to saving lives. Outraged by the 'misleading' media reports that put all blame on hospitals and health professionals, the health professionals whom I interviewed generally expressed a sense of anger and powerlessness. As one hospital staff member put it, 'Now the social atmosphere and medical environment are like this [antagonistic towards health professionals], if the state doesn't create a policy to address these conflicts, we health professionals have no rights, no power, and no way to negotiate with patients at all' (Interview D45). Lacking government and police protection, some hospitals even employ thugs to counter the *yinao* groups. Hospitals become 'battlegrounds of discontent' (LaFraniere 2010) where conflicts sometimes deteriorate into scuffles between the hospital (comprised of hospital professionals and security guards) and patients' family, friends and hired thugs. Without enforcement agencies, patients and health professionals are forced to take disputes into their own hands, but responding to violence with violence triggers further resentment and conflict between patients and health professionals.

Doctors regard themselves as the scapegoats of the health system and blame the government for its minimal involvement in conflict mediation and the protection of health professionals. In retaliation, health professionals have begun publicly to express their grievances and called for increased government intervention. They, too, employed *nao* by taking to the streets, protesting in front of government buildings, and demanding 'respect and dignity' (*huanwozunyan*), 'justice', and 'punishment of the murder' (*yanchengxiongshou*)—referring to patients who have killed doctors.[10] These tactics finally forced the government to respond.

---

[9]Such as the *pengci* people who pretended to be hit by a passing car and demanded compensation from the driver for injuries not actually received, or the Good Samaritans that help others have been extorted by the very person being helped (see Yan 2009).

[10]See reports such as Sina 2009.

6.3　Governing Disputes: Criminalising *Nao*, Civilising Patients and Juridifying Conflicts

Patients' grievance and health professionals' angry finally target the 'irresponsible' local authorities, from the inactive police forces to the ineffective courts. It poses legitimacy challenge to the authority and force the government to react. Since 2012, the Chinese central and local governments have implemented a series of new regulations and decrees to contain *yinao*. The dispute governance involves multiple measures and techniques, including violent containment, legal channelling and system reforms.

6.3.1　Criminalisation of Nao and 'Civilising' Patients

Before 2012, most hospitals in Riverside County used the decree issued in the late 1980s banning the *yinao*. The *Joint Notice on the Maintenance of Public Order in Hospitals* was issued by the Ministry of Health and the Ministry of Public Security on 30th October 1986, due to 'a series of sabotage and looting of hospitals, attacks and insults of health professionals (that) happened repeatedly in recent months, and seriously disrupted regular hospital work' (MOH and MOPS 1980). The decree included a list of rules. Apart from one clause that mentioned the mutual responsibility of health professionals and patients, all of the other seven clauses targeted patients' 'uncivilised' behaviour.[11] In 2001, the Ministry of Health and the Ministry of Public Security released a new decree—*Maintenance of Public Order in Medical Institutions to ensure Clinical Treatment Carry out Orderly* (MOH and MOPS 2001). The 2001 decree was a revised version of the 1986 decree and suggested the new efforts made by governments to curb medical disputes after years of neglect. In four of the eight clauses of the new decree, patients and health professionals' mutual rights and responsibilities were mentioned.[12] On the other hand, Clause Five

---

[11]These clauses are: patients need to pay medical fees according to regulation; nobody is allowed to check, ask, change or destroy clinic record without the permission of the hospital; patients are not allowed to occupy a hospital bed (after being discharged from the hospital) and refuse to leave; the corpse is not allowed to be put in places other than the morgue of the hospital, any feudal funeral activity is not allowed in the hospital; forbidding to use 'medical accident' as an excuse to *nao* in the hospital without reason; forbidding to make trouble, damage or sabotage in the hospital, forbidding to attack or condemn health professionals, and so on.

[12]The four clauses are: patients' legal rights in medical institution are protected by the law while patients and their families should also obey medical institution's regulation; the society should respect health professionals whose works are protected by the law, while health professionals should serve people wholeheartedly, improve service attitude and quality, pay attention to medical ethics, and improve medical skill; health professionals and patients should maintain good relationship with mutual-understanding and mutual-trust, when medical dispute happens, medical institution should share information with patients and their families, while patients and their families should solve medical disputes through the legal channel; medical institution should

specified eight kinds of misdemeanour committed by patients who violate public security management and even the law. Clause Eight regulated the 'proper' way to handle a corpse when a death occurs. By the 2000s, medical disputes and instances of violence were ever more prominent in the public discourse, particularly with the advent of the internet. However, only after a series of shocking stabbings and killings of health professionals in 2011 and early 2012, a new decree—*Notice on the Maintenance of Public Order in Medical Institutions* was finally issued by the Ministry of Health and the Ministry of Public Security in April 2012 (MOH and MOPS 2012). In three of the seven clauses of the 2012 decree, patients' rights and health professionals' responsibilities are specified. Compared with the 1986 and 2001 notices, the new decree further stresses patients' rights as well as medical institutions and professionals' responsibilities. On the other hand, Clause Seven of the new decree lists a series of behaviour that violates public security management or the law: (1) burning spirit money, setting up a funeral parlour, displaying funeral wreathes, displaying corpses, or gathering trouble-makers together in a medical institution; (2) making trouble in medical institution; (3) illegally taking dangerous, inflammable or explosive items and forbidden tools into medical institution; (4) insulting, threatening, intimidating, and intentionally hurting health professionals, or illegally restricting their personal freedom; (5) the sabotaging, theft, or robbery of public and private property in medical institution; (6) the reselling of medical institutions' registration number (ticket) for profit; (7) other behaviour that disturbs the medical institutions' regular order. These 'misbehavers', as defined in the 2012 decree, show that a new comprehensive effort is being made by the authorities to control disputes.

Immediately prior to the release of the 2012 decree by the central government, the local municipality of Riverside County had already issued a local decree on 30th December 2011—*Notice on the Control of 'Yinao' and other Illegal Activities according to the Law to Maintain the Regular Order of Medical Institutions*. The content of the local notice was solely targeted at patients' 'misbehaviour' and 'illegal behaviour', which are a synthesis of all of the misbehaviour listed by earlier national decrees. Besides, the local decree also defines six categories of medical accident that do *not* constitute medical malpractice, a recount of the regulation in the *Ordinance on Handling Medical Malpractice*. Due to the local governments' pressures to preserve stability, many local governments had issued their local decrees to contain *yinao* prior to the issuance of the national regulation in 2012. In Riverside County, the poster containing the local decree was widely circulated around the county and township hospitals to village clinics and community health centres. The large poster was displayed in every eye-catching place in medical institutions: near the hospital entrance, registration window, stairs, elevator, etc.

---

improve its transparency on fees and charges, is forbidden to charge arbitrarily, should give emergency treatment to serious patients, while patients should pay the medical bill according to regulation.

At the bottom of the black and white poster, there were five red seals of the municipal Court, Procuratorate, Police Bureau, Health Bureau, and Government Legal Affair Office, respectively, adding an aura of authority to the decree. The notice was also widely-broadcast by local TV and radio stations. The high 'visibility' of the state power is warning potential violators of the serious punishment.

These decrees supply legitimacy for the enforcement agencies to contain the *yinao*. In May 2012, the Ministry of Health made an announcement to guide the implementation of the above 2012 national decree. It suggested that all hospitals above Grade 2 should set up an internal police office (*jingwushi*) (MOH 2012). In 2013, the NHFPC and the Ministry of Public Security issued a safety guide to hospitals, suggesting that they should strengthen their protective equipment and security personnel.[13] In Riverside, local hospitals have generally expanded their security personnel.[14] Under pressure to preserve stability, many local hospitals also set up an extra 'comprehensive management and stability preserving office' (*zongzhi weiwen bangongshi*) next to their security office. In December 2013, 11 central government departments released a joint *Action Plan to Fight Medically-related Illegal and Criminal Actions to Preserve Health Care Order* (Xinhua Net 2013). This special task force targeted the *yinao* as 'illegal and criminal actions' and gave police forces standing to act. Since 2012, patients and their relatives have begun to be forcefully detained or punished for disrupting the hospital order and any acts of violence.[15] In April 2014, two patients who had killed doctors were given the death penalty (Xinhua Net 2014), the most serious sentence to date. Meanwhile, the media and official discourses began to link *yinao* with criminal gangs, although the involvement of gangs in medical disputes is uncommon in small counties like Riverside. The decrees and official reports frequently describe the *yinao* with words like 'lawbreakers and criminals' (*weifa fanzui fenzi*), 'illegal and criminal actions'. In early 2018, soon after the central government's release of a new *Notice on Launching a Special Struggle against Criminal Gangs*,[16] many local

---

[13]In 2013, after a new series of violent attacks and killings of hospital doctors, the NHFPC and the Ministry of Public Security released a new document—'Guidance on Strengthening of Hospital's Safety Preventive System' (see NHFPC and MOPS 2013), aiming at building 'safe hospitals' (*pingan yiyuan*). The guide includes suggestions such as hospitals should assign one security guard per 20 beds, and security guards should account for no less than 3% of the total medical staff.

[14]For instance, despite the People's Hospital is located just opposite to the police office, the hospital director's office has still been stationed by two security guards since he was attacked in a medical dispute in 2011. In the TCM Hospital, extra security guards have been recruited, counted to 15 formal guards in early 2012, and a police station plaque was installed outside the guard office at the entrance of the hospital to add more symbolic authority to the office. The county hospitals installed CCTV camera in every corner of hospital buildings. Even private clinics have installed home-camera to record evidence in order to prevent serious loss in cases of dispute.

[15]There are many media reports about patients and their families who acted violently being detained (see, for example, Ifeng 2012a; Sina 2013, 2016).

[16]Central People's Government, PRC (2018).

governments began to list *yinao* as one of their target of struggle. It officially consolidated the criminal status of *yinao* gangs. Yet, these new measures effectively criminalise anyone who engages in violent *nao* and the collective contestation that may 'disturb social order'.

In addition, the official decrees and the media form a dominant discourse that frames *nao* as an uncivilised, backward, and irrational form of behaviour carried out by people with low *suzhi* (social merit and quality), while suggesting that educated, civilised, and modern citizens use legal means to protect their interests. Having carried out a careful, close reading of local people's discourses, I find a complex and ambiguous attitude towards *nao*. Although many sympathised with patients who *nao*, they clearly showed their attitude by describing *nao* as a rude, backward practice and a tactic of the poor and peasants who lack *suzhi*. The public, on the one hand, complained about the difficulties of taking out lawsuits, while on the other emphasised the importance of learning about the law to fend off backwardness, modernise minds, and better protect one's interests. Even those who employ *nao* to defend their rights may not regard it as an 'honourable' choice. *Nao* is thus heavily marginalised. However, the situation is not that people of 'low *suzhi*' actively choose *nao*. Rather, it is that their relative powerlessness places them in a structural position where *nao* is their only option.

6.3.2   The Insufficiency of Current Dispute Resolutions and the Limitations of Nao

Figure 6.3 illustrates the four channels used to solve medical disputes in Riverside County. The first, private negotiation, is where patients frequently practice *nao* to argue for greater compensation from the hospital. It is direct and less bureaucratic. The second, administrative mediation, is carried out by the County Medical Dispute Mediation Centre, which consists of officials from different government departments. They are suspected of having a connection with the local hospitals and are frequently mistrusted by patients' relatives. The third, accident appraisal and mediation, have the most complex procedures and involve a long process. The fourth, lawsuits, appears simple, but are costly and time consuming. They are also suspected by patients of favouring hospitals and health professionals that have a connection with the court. The result of the lawsuit is unpredictable and uncontrollable by patients. The official institutional channels, the legal means and administrative forms of mediation, are considered expensive, complicated, unreliable, and unjust. Accordingly, many prefer to take matters into their own hands, through *nao*. Unlike the official institutional procedures, the practice of *nao* is a more familiar, straightforward, and less costly way to air a medical grievance. *Nao* always enables patient's relatives to achieve something, no matter whether it is a large amount of compensation or a small sum for appeasement. *Nao* thus could be understood as 'alternative politics' (Sztompka 2000: 164) from below to replace the

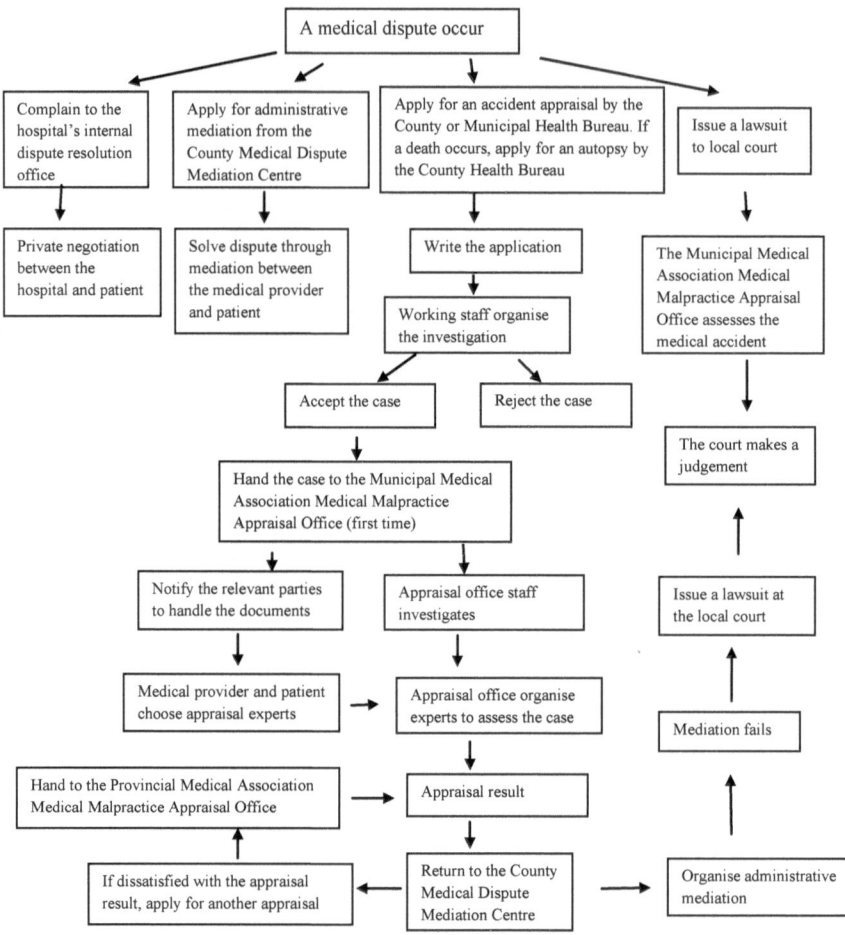

Fig. 6.3 Local medical dispute resolution procedure

official politics, which is distrusted by and less attractive to people. It is politics at the margin of the formal political structure to enforce people's own vision of justice.[17]

The state displays limited tolerance to the alternative politics of *nao* and acts to control and diminish it when it endangers the stability that official policies aims to sustain. The government's efforts to contain *nao* effectively threaten marginalised groups' very means to defend themselves. It is those very disadvantaged people who have little choice but to *nao* who become the target of deterrence and control. The patients who really have power and resources can still use their influence to

---

[17]This dispute resolution procedure image is drawn by the author based upon the image used in local hospitals.

argue for their interests, have more chance to overcome the government's rules, use *nao* to the extreme, even hijacking health professionals, hospitals, and local governments with the 'harmonious society' protocol.[18] The containment of *nao* in the Chinese medical context thus further deepens inequality, reproducing the sub-citizenship (of the disadvantaged group) and super-citizenship (the rich and powerful, who are less likely to be punished). Yet, without effective alternatives to solve their problem, patients continue to ignore the normative order, employing the 'rude, backward, uncivilised' practice of *nao* to defend their interests. As Chinese netizens discussed, when *nao* was forbidden in the hospital, people could still go to *nao* at the doctor's home or on the street, which would be even worse (Deng 2012).[19]

Moreover, it is a mistake to think that the violence facilitates genuine participation and control by patients. Although, *nao* allows the relatively weaker party to reverse the power relations, it is only a momentary reversal. Turner (1986: 26) suggests that in Western history, 'the critical factor in the emergence of citizenship is violence, that is, the overt and conscious struggle of social groups to achieve social participation'. However, the result of employing violent *nao* in the Chinese medical sector is often uncertain and arbitrary—hardly a guarantee that the basic rights of citizenship are restored. The increasing violence on the part of patients consists of individual efforts to argue for immediate economic compensation. When medical malpractice or accidents occur, patients tend to attribute blame to individual doctors and/or hospitals. Individual patients and their relatives employ *nao* against the medical institutions and professionals, in the process seeking help from the government to realise their demands, but do not argue for their rights vis-à-vis the state. Patients' relatives want *gongdao* (justice) and seek just compensation. In the unequal socio-economic order of post-reform China, patients' sense of deprivation and injustice further encourages the practice of *nao* to resist the unequal health system they encounter and the disadvantaged economic situation in which they live. *Nao* in medical disputes should be regarded not as an action for citizenship rights, but as individual agentive efforts to achieve social-economic justice, which sometimes works and sometimes fails.

6.3.3 Juridifying Conflicts and System Reforms

While violently containing *nao*, the authorities also promote legal channels to solve disputes, as characterised by the release of the Tort Law in 2009. Chapter 7 of the

---

[18]A very influential case occurred in 2012 (Ifeng 2012b), when a patient, from a very influential family in local society, died in a private hospital in Shaanxi, the hospital staff (over 40 health professionals) were pressurised to kneel down in the patient's mourning hall to make an apology. Besides, the hospital had to compensate the family 3 million Yuan.

[19]Such a case happened in 2016 when a patient in Guangzhou followed a doctor to his home and attacked the doctor who died subsequently (see http://www.chinanews.com/sh/2016/05-06/7861463.shtml, retrieved 14 March, 2018).

Tort Law regulates on the 'Liability for Medical Malpractice'. It specifies the conditions under which hospitals and health professionals should take responsibility and compensate patients; the conditions under which patients and their relatives can ask compensation from relevant responsible party; and health professionals' rights to be protected, etc. It supplies legal bases for medical dispute resolution and the division of responsibility in medical malpractice, but the juridification of medical disputes also effectively individualises medical accidents, making the pursuit of compensation the responsibility of individual patients and holding individual healthcare providers responsible for compensation. Cooper points out that the introduction of a comprehensive statute on tort law displaced responsibility for managing medical accidents from the administrative structures of the state to the legal channels of civil litigation: hospitals and doctors are made formally liable for medical accidents and other acts of negligence in the course of care (2011: 319); patients are forced to litigate against medical negligence under tort law, becoming, in the process, 'one who must become individually responsible for his or her exposure to risk and refrain from the collective act of protest represented by the mass group incident' (ibid.: 320). In the process, both patients and healthcare providers are required to become responsible juridical subjects. Meanwhile, other legal regulations are being improved. The resolution of medical disputes has been drafted in the Basic Health and Health Promotion Law.[20] A new 'Ordinances on the Prevention and Handing of Medical Disputes' (*yiliao jiufen yufang he chuli tiaoli*)[21] is also under review by the state council in 2018, to replace the outdate regulations in the 2002 Ordinance and to resolve the conflicts on dispute resolution in various regulations. It is worth to see how these will impact the future direction of medical dispute resolution.

Furthermore, efforts are made to build an impartial third party mediator between patients and medical practitioners. In the market, both patients and doctors are urged to take responsibility and risks themselves. Patients have to secure just compensation by themselves. Health professionals and hospitals are also required to prove they are not at fault or use the law to defend themselves. For a long time, there is no public institution that plays a mediating role between the two parties, so patients and medical practitioners confront each other directly. Recently, many localities are experimenting with a People's Mediation Committee of Medical Dispute (*yihuan jiufen renmin tiaojie weiyuanhui*), a named 'independent third party' to resolve dispute, the effect of which is proclaimed to be good.[22] Besides, medical liability insurance and medical accident insurance are encouraged by the

---

[20]A basic health and health promotion law is drafted and under review (see http://health.people. com.cn/n1/2017/1223/c14739-29724759.html, retrieved 31 March, 2018).

[21]'A new "Ordinances on the Prevention and Resolution of Medical Disputes" is forthcoming' (*xinban yiliao jiufen yufang he chuli tiaoli jijiang chutai*) (see http://www.chinanews.com/jk/2015/ 11-26/7641809.shtml, retrieved 13 March, 2018).

[22]For instance, the People's Mediation Committee of Medical Dispute has been listed in Guangdong province's *Regulation on the Prevention and Resolution of Medical Disputes* issued by the provincial government in 2013. The mediation committee is encouraged in the province to

government and experimented in various local organizations, aiming to transfer medical risks and compensations to the insurance system.[23]

The combination of legal channels, mediation and insurance sets up a system to transfer conflicts within the hospital. Since 2016, not only patients and their families are forbidden from the practice of *nao*, medical institutions and practitioners are also guided by the authorities to refuse negotiation with the patient privately and are forbidden from making compensation before a medical appraisal of responsibilities carried out by a legal party,[24] an effort to channel dispute resolution from the hospital to institutions outside the hospital. The authorities also made suggestions to systematically improve the health care quality in order to prevent medical accidents in the first place. These changes however need a long time as the new health care reform progresses.

6.3.4 Conflicts Within Dispute Governance

The slight adjustment of government emphasis from pacifying disputes to legalising disputes recently are in the party state's efforts (under the leadership of Xi Jinping) to correct problems involved in earlier governance that put 'stability as an upmost priority'. Rule by law is reemphasized by the authority to improve its legitimacy, albeit stability is still important. The change suggests the party-state's effort to reform itself to be a better governor, but on the condition of not compromising its fundamental polity. The rules and laws issued by the state constitute a moral and normative order impact on individual behaviours. The channelling of dispute by judicial means, third party mediator or an insurance system shapes people's practice that they are encouraged to solve their own problems including disputes, being exhorted to act civilly and use the formal channel to defend their interests.

In medical dispute governance, rather than a simple shift from coercive practices to the legal means, it is more complex and mixed with multiple modes of technologies from legal measures to coercive practices. The multiple techniques, sometimes conflicting ones, adopted by the authorities to solve dispute still show the authoritarian characters of governance. The state promotes legal channels through which to solve disputes, it also delivers a blow to the rule of law in the name of stability, although some corrections are made later. The dispute containment efforts, from the special task force in the central government to the

---

solve medical dispute and is set up in most municipals (see http://society.people.com.cn/n/2013/0926/c136657-23048180.html, retrieved 16 March, 2018).

[23]'Opinions on strengthening the work of medical liability insurance' (*Guanyu jiaqiang yiliao zeren baoxian gongzuo de yijian*) (see http://www.nhfpc.gov.cn/yzygj/s3589/201407/65d55251804c408581a4e58db41f4bc7.shtml, retrieved 11 March, 2017).

[24]'Notice on further improving the work of medical order maintenance' (*Guanyu jinyibu zuohao weihu yiliao zhixu de tongzhi*) (see http://www.nhfpc.gov.cn/yzygj/s3590/201603/946d95d967474f3c840e9e903f564154.shtml, retrieved 10 March, 2017).

'comprehensive management and stability preserving office' at the bottom, are all temporary institutions outside the existing government and legal system (although constituted by members of the government departments). In the process, local governments are given further impetus and justification to intervene in the local medical sphere and control any 'disharmonious' threat to social stability by resorting to suppressive measures. In the governance of *nao*, both patients and health professionals are easily subjected to the state power once the state steps into intervene in disputes. The strong stance by the authorities to contain *yinao* may evoke people's cynicism about the rules and laws, and even aggravate the sense of injustice among patients. Although the 'professional' *yinao* gang group are decreasing as a result of containment, the acts of *nao* did not come to an end, most *yinao* are now carried out by patient families and relatives in relatively small scale.[25] The combination of authoritarian power, the promotion of rule by law, and the (de)moralisation of individual behaviour in governing disputes will face more tests in the configuration of power among patients (who try to seek better care and argue for proper compensation), health professionals (who seek to make money and protect themselves), commercialised hospitals (that seek to maximise profits and avoid disputes), the local authorities (that attempt to conceal disputes and preserve stability), and the central state (that tries to improve health care, and preserve political legitimacy while reserving social harmony).

In conclusion, various factors contribute to the increase in medically-related disputes: a rising consciousness of patient rights, the deepening misunderstanding between patients and doctors, inflammatory media reporting, the commercialised health care that infringe on people's moral economy, and the absence of a formal institution for dealing with medical disputes. In medical disputes, patients (and their relatives) and doctors (and hospitals) compete in a struggle for power over the control of their interests and safety, and over their moral definitions of justice and rights. When patients are mistreated or die, the moral sentiments of the public who shares many unhappy healthcare experiences are on the side of the patients and their relatives. Patients' relatives who suffer a loss are entitled to act outside the normal social rules, while health professionals and hospitals, having little moral capital, are forced to compromise in front of the patients' relatives. Patients' relatives form a righteous discourse of compensation, which expressively manifests itself in *nao*— the explicit accusation, intrusive noise, and provocative actions that are intended dramatically to disrupt the routine hospital order. The locus of power is shifting from health professionals to patients. However, when health professionals are attacked or killed, they become the weak ones, who cannot protect themselves from violence. They begin to win over public sentiment, gradually accumulating moral capital through their compromises and tolerance, which justifies them in fighting back. They accuse patients of engaging in violent *nao*, propose government

---

[25]'Undercover journalists to disclose inside stories: professional yinao gang extort hospital as well as patients' family' (*Jizhe wodi jie heimu: zhiye yinao e wan yiyuan qiao jiashu*). *Sangxiang City Express* (see http://news.sohu.com/20140701/n401595199.shtml, retrieved 12 December, 2016).

regulation changes and legal action, and finally force the government to release new regulations and subsequent punishments for patients.

The configuration of power between disputing patients and health professionals is shaped by the power of the government. Over the years, the government retains its intervention in hospital affairs and transfers the political pressure of preserving stability to the hospitals. It frequently presses the hospitals to solve disputes and meet the patients' demands. The government's aim of building a harmonious society thus, to some extent, empowers 'weak' patients, who otherwise have little power to counter the hospitals and government bureaus. However, it also encourages *nao*, for many have been led to believe that greater violence leads to greater compensation. Yet, when *nao* endangers the stability that the official politics attempt to sustain, it becomes the target of containment. Government measures try to criminalise *nao*, civilise patients and juridify conflicts. The normative regulations and official discourses delegitimise and stigmatise *nao*, subtly reshaping individuals' conduct and punishing people in the case of transgressions. The incorporation of medical malpractice into the Tort Law and other legal channel seek to juridify conflicts. The juridification places the responsibility for seeking proper compensation on the shoulders of individual patients and holds hospitals and health professionals responsible for compensation. Some other experiments (third party mediation and insurance) are also made to transfer conflicts from the hospital to an outside system. Yet, without an effective, trusted and mature means, people continue to ignore the dominant discourses of civility and rule by law, using *nao* to defend their very interests, although its effect becomes more uncertain.

References

Central People's Government, PRC. 2013. *Why Only 10% Patients Trust in Doctors—Members of CPPCC Pay Attention on Doctor-Patient Conflict* (Weihe jin 10% huanzhe xinren yisheng – daibiao weiyuan guanzhu yihuan maodun). Retrieved 26 Aug 2013. http://www.gov.cn/2013lh/content_2349189.htm.

Central People's Government, PRC. 2018. *Notice on Launching a Special Struggle against Criminal Gangs (Guanyu kaizhan saohei chue zhuanxiang douzheng de tongzhi)*. Retrieved 21 Mar 2018. http://www.gov.cn/zhengce/2018-01/24/content_5260130.htm.

Cooper, Melinda. 2011. Experimental Republic: Medical Accidents (Productive and Unproductive) in Postsocialist China. *East Asian Science, Technology and Society: An International Journal* 5 (3): 313–327.

Deng, Haijian. 2012. *Ending "Yinao", Independent Institute Will Be More Effective than Penalty* (Zhongjie 'yinao', duli jigou bi xingfa geng youxiao). *China Youth (Zhongguo Qinnian Bao)*. Retrieved 7 Jan 2013. http://zqb.cyol.com/html/2012-05/03/nw.D110000zgqnb_20120503_1-02.htm.

He, Alex Jingwei. 2014. The Doctor–Patient Relationship, Defensive Medicine and Overprescription in Chinese Public Hospitals: Evidence from a Cross-Sectional Survey in Shenzhen City. *Social Science and Medicine* 123: 64–71.

He, Alex Jingwei, and Jiwei Qian. 2016. Explaining Medical Disputes in Chinese Public Hospitals: The Doctor-Patient Relationship and its Implications for Health Policy Reforms. *Health Economics, Policy and Law* 11 (4): 359–378.

Herd, Richard, Yu-Wei Hu, and Vincent Koen. 2010. Improving China's Health Care System. OECD Economics Department Working Paper No. 751. Retrieved 11 July 2014. http://www.oecd.org/officialdocuments/publicdisplaydocumentpdf/?doclanguage=en&cote=eco/wkp(2010)7.

Ifeng. 2012a. *Four Yinao People in Henan Xinmi were Sentenced after Besieging Hospital Several Times* (Henan Xinmi 4 ming 'yinao' duoci weidu yiyuan bei panxing). Retrieved 11 May 2012. http://news.ifeng.com/society/1/detail_2012_05/11/14467410_0.shtml.

Ifeng. 2012b. *Shaanxi: Patient Died, over 40 Doctors were Pressured to Kneel Down* (Shannxi: huanzhe siwang, quanyuan yisheng 40 yuren bei bi xiagui). Retrieved 10 May 2012. http://news.ifeng.com/society/1/detail_2012_05/02/14261109_0.shtml.

Jing, Jun. 2010. Environmental Protests in Rural China. In *Chinese Society: Change, Conflict and Resistance*, ed. E. J. Perry and M. Selden, 197–214. London: Routledge.

LaFraniere, Sharon. 2010. Chinese Hospitals are Battlegrounds of Discontent. *New York Times.* Retrieved 28 July 2014. http://www.nytimes.com/2010/08/12/world/asia/12hospital.html.

Ministry of Health and Ministry of Public Security, PRC. 1980. *Joint Notice on the Maintenance of Public Order in Hospitals* (Guanyu weihu yiyuan zhixu de lianhe tonggao). Retrieved 15 Nov 2012. http://www.law-lib.com/law/law_view.asp?id=47792.

Ministry of Health and Ministry of Public Security, PRC. 2001. *Maintenance of Public Order in Medical Institutions to ensure Clinical Treatment Carry out Orderly* (Weishengbu, gonganbu tonggao-weihu yiliaojigou zhengchang de yiliao zhixu, baozheng gexiang zhenliao gongzuo youxu jinxing). Retrieved 13 July 2013. http://www.moh.gov.cn/zhuzhan/wsbmgz/201304/a787769f9a5b4f68b82c02104a197ce2.shtml.

Ministry of Health, PRC. 2012. *Emergency Notice from the General Office of the Ministry of Health about the Implementation of "Notice on the Maintenance of Public Order in Medical Institutions from the Ministry of Health and the Ministry of Public Security"* (Weishengbu bangongting guanyu guanchezhixing < weishengbu gonganbu guanyu weihu yiliao jigou zhixu de tonggao > de jinji tongzhi). Retrieved 21 Dec 2012. http://www.moh.gov.cn/sofpro/cms/previewjspfile/zwgkzt/cms_0000000000000000131_tpl.jsp?requestCode=54607andCategoryID=2746.

Ministry of Health and Ministry of Public Security, PRC. 2012. *Notice on the maintenance of public order in medical institutions* (Guanyu weihu yiliaojigou zhixu de tonggao). Retrieved 28 Dec 2012. http://www.gov.cn/gzdt/2012-05/01/content_2127446.htm.

National Health and Family Planning Commission and Ministry of Public Security, PRC. 2013. *Guidance on Strengthening of Hospital's Safety Preventive System* (Guanyu jiaqiang yiyuan anquan fangfan xitong jianshe zhidao yijian). Retrieved on 25 Oct 2013. http://www.nhfpc.gov.cn/yzygj/s3589/201310/1c98e954a86642b5bdc8b3f33d79f89c.shtml.

Pei, Minxin. 2010. Rights and Resistance: The Changing Contexts of the Dissident Movement. In *Chinese Society: Change, Conflict and Resistance*, ed. E. J. Perry and M. Selden, 23–46. London: Routledge.

People's Net. 2011. *Every Year over 10,000 Doctors were Attacked, the Fragile Doctor-patient Relationship cannot Stand the Heavy Blow of Attacks, When Will the Violence Stop?* (Meinian yiwan yisheng bei ouda, cuiruo yihuan jinbuqi zhongya, baoli shang yisheng heshixiu). Retrieved 6 June 2013. http://health.people.com.cn/GB/16209592.html.

People's Net. 2013. *National Health and Family Planning Commission: Further Improve Village Doctor's Pension Policy* (Guojiaweijiwei: jiang jinyibu wanshan xiangcun yisheng yanglao zhengce). Retrieved 10 Apr 2014. http://politics.people.com.cn/n/2013/1130/c1001-23702409.html.

People's Net. 2014. Nearly 60 Percent Doctors do not Want Their Children to Study Medicine, Medical Environment is the Major Contributing Factor (Jin liucheng yisheng lizu zinv xueyi, yiliao huanjing shi shouyin). Retrieved 12 Aug 2014. http://edu.people.com.cn/n/2014/0731/c1006-25374312.html.

Qiu, Ruixian, and Yang Yang. 2012. Could the Third Party Mediation End Doctor-patient Disputes (Disanfang nengfou zhongjie yihuan jiufen). *Guanzhou Daily (Guangzhou Ribao).* Retrieved 1 Apr 2012. http://gzdaily.dayoo.com/html/2012-01/19/content_1592777.htm.

Scott, James C. 2008. *Weapons of the Weak: Everyday Forms of Peasant Resistance.* New Haven, CT: Yale University Press.

Sina. 2009. Doctor and Patient Conflict in Fujian Nanping: Dozens Doctors Held Sit-in in Front of the Government Building. Retrieved 30 June 2009. http://news.sina.com.cn/c/sd/2009-06-29/092318114728.shtml.

Sina. 2013. *Broke Windows, Attack Nurses, Burn Spirit Money, Display Funeral Wreathes, Two Yinao were Arrested in Baoji* (Za Boli, da hushi, shao zhiqian, bai huaquan, baoji liang yinao bei ju). Retrieved 7 Jan 2013. http://sx.sina.com.cn/news/s/2013-01-07/071541891.html.

Sina. 2016. *Two Hundred Policemen in Hebei Hengshui were Called in for One Yinao case and Nine People were Led Away* (Hebei Hengshui chudong 200 jingli zhizhi yiqi yinao, 9 ren bei daily). Retrieved 13 Mar 2018. http://news.sina.com.cn/c/nd/2016-06-22/doc-ifxtfrrc4142334.shtml.

Sztompka, Piotr. 2000. *Trust: A Sociological Theory*. Cambridge, UK: Cambridge University Press.

Tu, Jiong. 2014. Yinao: Protest and Violence in China's Medical Sector. *Berkeley Journal of Sociology*. http://berkeleyjournal.org/2014/12/yinao-protest-and-violence-in-chinas-medical-sector/.

Tucker, Joseph D., Yu. Cheng, Bonnie Wong, et al. 2015. Patient–Physician Mistrust and Violence Against Physicians in Guangdong Province, China: A Qualitative Study. *British Medical Journal Open* 5 (10): e008221.

Turner, Bryan. 1986. *Citizenship and Capitalism: The Debate over Reformism*. London: Allen and Unwin.

Wang, Zhongming, and Jianhua Li. 2012. The Reason of Medical Disputes and Countering Measures (Yiliaojiufen fasheng de yuanyin ji yingduicuoshi). *Chinese Community Doctor (Zhongguo Shequ Yishi)* 12: 409–410.

Wu, Dan, Yun Wang, Kwok Fai Lam, and Therese Hesketh. 2014. Health System Reforms, Violence Against Doctors and Job Satisfaction in the Medical Profession: A Cross-Sectional Survey in Zhejiang Province, Eastern China. *British Medical Journal Open* 4 (12): e006431.

Xinhua Net. 2013. *11 Departments will jointly Carry out a Special Task to Fight Medically-related Illegal and Criminal Actions* (Woguo 11 ge bumen jiang lianhe kaizhan daji sheyi weifa fanzui zhuanxiang xingdong). Retrieved 25 Mar 2014. http://news.xinhuanet.com/2013-12/20/c_125893851.htm.

Xinhua Net. 2014. *Wang Yingsheng, Wang Yunsheng, the Criminals of Two Cases of Killing Doctors have been Executed with Death Penalty* (Liangqi sha yi an zuifan Wang Yingsheng, Wang yunsheng yi bei zhixing sixing). Retrieved 25 Apr 2014. http://news.xinhuanet.com/legal/2014-04/24/c_126430231.htm.

Xu, Xin, and Lu Rongrong. 2008. Violence and Mistrust: Research on Violence in Medical Treatment in Transforming China (2000–2006) (Baoli yu buxinren – zhuanxin zhongguo de yiliao baoli yanjiu: 2000-2006). *Law and Social Development (Fazhi Yu Shehui Fazhan)* 1: 82–101.

Yan, Yunxiang. 2009. The Good Samaritan's New Trouble: A Study of the Changing Moral Landscape in Contemporary China. *Social Anthropology* 17 (1): 9–24.

Zhang, Xinqing, and Margaret Sleeboom-Faulkner. 2011. Tensions between Medical Professionals and Patients in Mainland China. *Cambridge Quarterly of Healthcare Ethics* 20 (3): 458–465.

Chapter 7
Practice of the Self: 'Barefoot Doctors' in Post-reform China

Previous chapters have shown that Chinese doctors are frequently blamed by patients for misconduct and moral degeneration. Yet health professionals also regard themselves as 'victims' of the health care crisis. Their professional authority is challenged, they are attacked by patients, and they face dilemmas between making money and being a 'good' doctor in the current system. Most doctors I met were bitterly resentful. They frequently experience the clash between what they should do (according to the regulations and laws) and what they can actually do, and are burdened by various and sometimes contradictory demands from hospitals and patients. In the post-reform era, doctors themselves, especially the older doctors, sense a change in morality and are frequently puzzled by the change. This chapter depicts the experience of a group of relatively disadvantaged doctors—the former 'barefoot' doctors.

China's barefoot doctor system is known for having provided inexpensive and accessible medical care to its large rural population in the 1970s.[1] Barefoot doctors, chosen from local farmers, received basic medical training and served in the rural areas afterwards with a focus on the preventive and preliminary health care. The barefoot doctor system together with the Cooperative Medical Scheme in the rural areas became a model for the developing world, which reflected an approach to health care that was 'egalitarian, grassroots-based, decentralised, de-professionalised, low-tech, economically feasible, and culturally appropriate' (Wang 2010). However, the system came to an end with the advent of market

---

Part of this chapter was published in *China Perspectives* 2016/4 (http://www.cefc.com.hk/issue/china-perspectives-20164/) (Tu 2016). This article is reproduced with permission. Thanks for the reviewers' critical comments.

---

[1]The program started from 1965 and became internationally influential in the 1970s. The system was acknowledged by the WHO for securing people's basic health care rights and was a major inspiration to the primary health care movement, leading up to the Alma-Ata conference in 1978 (see Cui 2008).

© Springer Nature Singapore Pte Ltd. 2019
J. Tu, *Health Care Transformation in Contemporary China*,
https://doi.org/10.1007/978-981-13-0788-1_7

reforms in the 1980s and many barefoot doctors either became private doctors or gave up medical practice. In 1985 even the name 'barefoot doctor' was officially abolished, replaced by the name 'village doctor'.[2] By the late 1980s, rural health services had lost 3.7 million employees (Duckett 2007). More than three decades have passed since this change, barefoot doctors seem to have been forgotten. However, the legacy of the barefoot doctor system is still felt in the troubles of ageing former barefoot doctors that now find themselves having no pension. It is estimated that approximately 1.5 million people (Xinhua Net 2003) worked as barefoot doctors in the collective era and today there are still around 1 million[3] former barefoot doctors nationwide. In Riverside County, there were 1868 recorded barefoot doctors by 1977, and even now there are over 1000 remaining former barefoot doctors requesting pensions.[4] In my field, these former barefoot doctors appeared to be one of the most resentful groups in the ongoing healthcare reform. These doctors have practiced medicine since the Mao era and experienced dramatic market change. This chapter thus illustrates how these former barefoot doctors respond to reforms happening around them, take part in changes, and reconcile conflicts and dilemmas in their daily medical practice.

This chapter refers to the Foucauldian concept of 'practice of the self'. Foucault posits that in Western society there is a shift in governance from coercive practices to the practice of the self, which is 'an exercise of self upon self by which one tries to work out, to transform one's self and to attain a certain mode of being' (Foucault 1987: 113). In the 'practice of the self,' self as an ethical project requires one to work on oneself. These practices make possible a way of 'setting up and developing relationships with the self, for self-reflection, self-knowledge, self-examination, for the deciphering of the self by oneself, for the transformation one seeks to accomplish with oneself as object' (Foucault 1985: 29). Through the 'practice of the self' that involves the continue negotiation process of individual with oneself and individual with the wider environment, individuals constitute themselves as subjects of moral conduct. In the neoliberal governance, individuals are encouraged by the authority to become independent, enterprising, and self-reliant. An individual

---

[2]In the post-reform era, although many former barefoot doctors become village doctor, other people (such as new practitioners graduated from local medical school) also join the village doctor group. Thus village doctors are not a homogeneous group.

[3]The data of 1 million came from various predictions and checks through interviews and internet search. However, there is no official data about the actual number of former 'barefoot doctors' who are still alive.

[4]The numbers of barefoot doctors increased rapidly between the middle 1960s and the Cultural Revolution (1966–1976). By 1977, the number of barefoot came to a peak. The number in 1977 was recorded in *Riverside County Medical Chorography* (1988) and *Riverside County Chorography* (1990). The current number of former barefoot doctors comes from predictions by local village doctors and health officials. Besides these ageing former barefoot doctors, there were also thousands of former paramedical workers, who served in the rural areas during the collective era, demanding proper compensation, but their voices are not as loud as the voices of these former barefoot doctors. I could not collect enough materials about this group, which is thus outside the scope of this chapter.

constitutes him- or herself as a self-governing and self-engineering subject. The 'practice of the self' thus produces new subjects of power that expose individuals to new regimes of governance. Yet, the 'practice of the self' is also relatively independent of the practices of the 'government of others or of the state', is 'not only instruments in the pursuit of political, social and economic goals but also means of resistance to other forms of government' (Dean 2010: 21). Applying this concept to the Chinese health sector, market transformations over the last three decades have reshaped individual responsibility and standards of behaviour. The changing context profoundly reshapes the old village doctors as inadequate and in need of self-transformation. The state urges them to become self-enterprising and self-responsible to take charge of their own life, work, and retirement pension. However, different from Foucault's 'practice of the self', these doctors did not and could not successfully use 'the practice of the self' to resist other forms of government. This chapter explores how these former barefoot doctors manoeuvre to work on themselves. It outlines these doctors being rejected of their past, their sense of loss and puzzlement in the market era, their reflective negotiations with multiple moral frameworks in daily work, their self-making and self-legitimation in order to shape themselves as ethical and worthy subjects, and their struggles for state recognition and material subsistence.

In early 2012, my acquaintance introduced me to a village doctor—Doctor Lian from Revival Town, who was in his 60s. I visited Doctor Lian, interviewed him and two more village doctors he introduced to me. The next morning, I got a phone call from another village doctor in the same town, who had heard of my visit and wanted me to visit him as well. 'I have a lot to say', he stated on the phone. I went to Revival Town again, met Doctor Li, a 76-year-old former barefoot doctor. A few days later, another doctor from Revival Town called me, and informed me that a group of them would be gathering for a meeting in the township hospital and would like to meet me afterwards to 'express their thoughts'. I subsequently met Doctor Zhao and around 10 more village doctors who were in their 50s, 60s, and 70s. All these doctors were former 'barefoot doctors' who continued medical practice after their collective medical teams were dismantled. After these encounters, I visited 16 village clinics and 12 private clinics around the county, meeting dozens of current and former village doctors.

7.1 Barefoot Doctors in Transition: Self-doubt and Self-transformation

7.1.1 The Disappearing Collective Clinics

In the early 1980s, the collective production system in rural China was replaced by the household production system. Rural collective clinics supported by the collective production system were unable to sustain themselves. Meanwhile, the state re-legalised private medical practice that had been forbidden previously.[5] Doctor Wei, Doctor Li, Doctor Lian, and another doctor, who worked in the same medical team as barefoot doctors in the 1970s, thus contracted the collective clinic together by paying an annual fee to their village. This tentative collaboration lasted for only a few years. Without external funding, the clinic's business could not sustain the livelihood of four doctors. Subsequently, Doctor Li left the medical team and opened his own clinic in the town. Doctor Lian opened a clinic in his village, worked partly as a village doctor while doing some other businesses to support his family. Doctor Wei and his son kept the collective clinic licence, but moved the clinic to the town, which became a de facto private clinic. The other doctor changed his profession and became a village teacher. Although the collective medical team licence was continued under the name of the four doctors, the clinic had already disappeared in the 1980s.

Doctor Zhao from Revival Town experienced a similar destiny. In the collective era, the medical team of his production brigade had three barefoot doctors. They performed outstandingly and were called a 'model medical team' (*xianjin yiliaozu*). In the post-reform era, one of the doctors joined the township hospital in the 1980s, another old doctor died in the 1990s. Doctor Zhao then operated the old clinic alone in his village. The medical team originally occupied a house in the village centre. In 2008, a poor villager's house collapsed in the earthquake. As a way to help the family, the village committee sold the house occupied by the clinic to the poor family. The committee arranged for the clinic to move to the village school, which had been empty since the school was relocated to the town, but the old school was at the border of the village. Few patients came to visit after students moved out. Besides, the clinic was burglarised not long afterwards. The incident made Doctor Zhao decide to move the clinic back to his own home. In 2012 when I visited Doctor Zhao at his home, I could hardly recognise it as being a clinic, except for the clinic licence on the wall, a medical box and some medicine bottles on the table of the living room (see Fig. 7.1).

In the post-reform era, many collective clinics in the countryside experienced similar destinies, being sold to individuals, being contracted by former barefoot doctors, or silently disappearing. Records documented the privatisation of a large percent of local clinics in this period (Henderson et al. 1994; Duckett 2007). Lost alongside the collective clinic is the material and space manifestation of state care in the life of ordinary villagers, and the symbolic locus of connection between individual

---

[5]Due to the shortage of public healthcare services, in 1980, the Ministry of Health issued a *Report on the Granting of Permission for Solo Private Medical Practice* (*Weishengbu guanyu yunxu geti kaiye xingyi wenti*) (http://law.people.com.cn/showdetail.action?id=2568900, retrieved 17 February, 2010), which recommended legalising private medical practice while regulating it strictly.

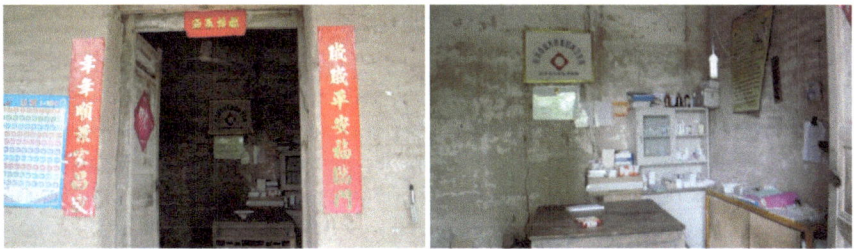

Fig. 7.1 'Barefoot' doctor Zhao's clinic at his home

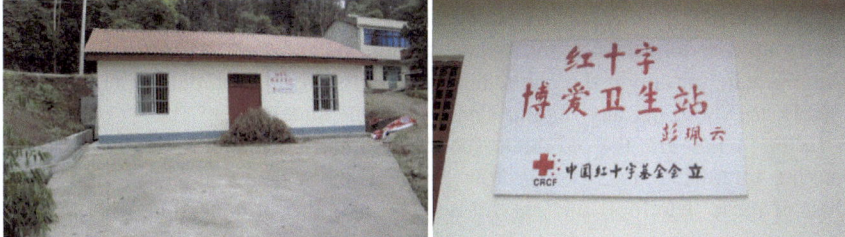

Fig. 7.2 One of the empty 'red-cross' clinics

villagers and the socialist collective. While many old 'barefoot' doctors occupied poor clinics, there were also newly-built village clinics donated by the Chinese Red Cross Foundation to poor areas, which however were emptied and abandoned at the side of rural road due to its poor quality and improper design (see Fig. 7.2).[6] Suspecting corruption associated with the building of these new clinics, the old village doctors, who still occupied poor clinic or practice medicine at their own home, expressed a strong sense of injustice and resentment.

---

[6]Improper design, such as these clinics do not have a toilet, it is not convenient for patients who need to go to toilet after taking drips; improper locations, most of these clinics are located at the side of rural road for official checks. The donation of new clinics to poor areas by Chinese Red Cross Foundation originally aims to relieve poverty and improve fairness. However, in practice, it increases sense of injustice among village doctors. Besides, since the new healthcare reform, the local authority has named two kinds of village clinics. One is advanced new village clinics (*jiaji cunweishengshi*), which have better facilities and are mostly operated by relatively younger village doctors. The other is ordinary village clinics (*putong cunweishengshi*), many of which are in poor conditions and mostly operated by elderly village doctors who cannot renovate their clinics to become an advanced one. The former clinics also get more subsidies than the latter ones.

7.1.2 Self-reinvention and Self-legitimation in Post-reform China

In the post-reform era, most former barefoot doctors changed from being affiliated and supported by the collective commune to entrepreneurial individuals in the market to support themselves. While experiencing reduced state involvement in their livelihood and welfare, village doctors faced new administrative 'exploitation' in their private medical 'business'. In the 1990s, they were asked to pay various fees and taxes by local administrative agencies. Many experienced difficulties in their medical work. Some doctors then changed their private clinics into public-oriented village clinics. The change required them to take public health work without any salary. Instead they could get exemption on some taxes and fees. Only since the new healthcare reform in 2009, village doctors have begun to get some subsidies from the state to support the public health work they carry out, but, till now, village doctors are yet to get any regular salary from the state.

In the market era, the old doctors were frequently depicted by local officials as 'lacking qualifications', having 'low medical skills' and 'outdated knowledge'. Most of these 'barefoot' doctors did not get institutional education and qualification. In the collective era, the training of these barefoot doctors and primary health workers was shortened considerably compared with regular medical training. Usually they started with a six-month initial course concerning rudimentary and preventive medical care, followed by in-service training, which might be achieved by working with a qualified doctor in the countryside, by secondment to a hospital, or by taking courses arranged by a teaching hospital (Kane 1984). In Riverside County, the training of rural health professionals combined the school/hospital education and the traditional master-apprentice training. Most local health professionals had already got some traditional medical training from their families or senior doctors before enrolling into schools or hospital courses. Barefoot doctors were chosen from these half-trained personnel, educated again in local medical school or hospital shortly for preventive and western medical knowledge, and returned to work in their villages afterwards.

In the post-reform era, village doctors were subjected to a new regime of evaluation about their 'qualifications' and the 'modernity' of their knowledge and skills. The local authorities require rural health professionals to take exam to gain new qualifications. Local records show that, through an examination in 1983, 367 medical practitioners became licensed 'village doctor' and 1201 professionals got the certificate of primary health worker (the total numbers of rural health professionals in 1977 were 1868 barefoot doctors and 4880 health workers).[7] Other research similarly shows that barefoot doctors everywhere were taking the certification examinations at the beginning of the market reform (Rosenthal and Greiner 1982). Those barefoot doctors who continued medical practice had to constantly

---

[7]Data comes from *Riverside County Medical Chorography* (1988) and *Riverside County Chorography* (1990).

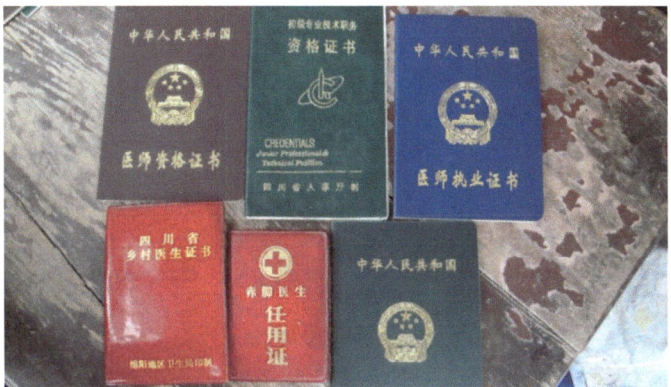

Fig. 7.3 From Barefoot Doctor to licensed physician: a village doctor's certificates

update themselves with new knowledge to meet rising medical requirements. They took further training, worked towards gaining new diplomas and certificates, and passed various assessments in order to become licensed physicians. Doctor Wei showed me his six certificates (see Fig. 7.3): the 'barefoot doctor' certificate from the 70s, the primary professional qualification certificate and the village doctor certificate from the 80s, the village doctor practice certificate, the physician qualification certificate, and the physician practice certificate from the 90s. Some village doctors also got a secondary medical qualification and other certificates. These certificates record and trace a village doctor's professional life from a barefoot doctor to a registered physician, and document an individual doctor's efforts to transform him- or herself into a modern and qualified physician.

However, in general, village doctors' qualifications are still very low. Research shows that up to 70% of medical professionals have no qualifications beyond junior high school in poor rural counties (Eggleston et al. 2008). In Riverside, the former barefoot doctors who continue medical practice in the rural villages mostly specialise in TCM, and some elderly doctors could not pass the certification examinations to become a registered physician. The former barefoot doctors' low qualification, limited western medical knowledge, and the authority's active depiction of them as outdated and unqualified in turn justified local officials' rejection of them. The doctors who could not pass qualification tests were under regular assault from local administrative authorities. Some old doctors were asked to stop medical practice to give way to a younger generation.[8] A few years ago when 76-year-old Doctor Li's clinic was involved in a medical dispute, he was persuaded by local health officials to stop medical practice due to his old age. He rejected the proposal by saying that 'I will stop [medical practice] only if you give

---

[8]The local government regulates that male village doctors over 60 years old and female village doctors over 55 years old will not be given medical practice licence. However, without pension, many elderly village doctors continued medical practices in the rural areas.

me a pension. Now I need to work to earn food to eat'. Besides, he emphasised that he was always welcomed by local patients, who would come to seek help from him even if he stopped medical practice. Old village doctors like Doctor Li rejected their loss of value in the market era. They tried to present themselves as possessing qualities and skills that were needed by their patients. They attempted to prove themselves as being capable and worthy labourers by displaying the certificates they had collected throughout their lifetimes. When the socialist collective—the source and foundation of their social and moral status—disappeared, these old doctors were expected to generate their own legitimacy and value via self-enterprising and self-investment.

7.1.3 Economic Struggle and Moral Responsibility

It is ironic that while these elderly doctors were rejected by local authorities as being not valuable any more, there were few young doctors likely to serve in the rural areas of an interior county and peasants still relied heavily on these old doctors to provide basic health care.[9]

In the rural areas of Riverside County, it is increasingly a case of the 'old' serving the 'old': a group of ageing village doctors were left to serve those elderly 'left-behinds' in the village. Rural areas face the problem of a decreasing and ageing population. The young and middle-aged have migrated to the city or coastal areas to work. Those left behind are mainly children and the elderly, who need health care more than others, but there is a shortage of health professionals in the rural areas. Young doctors do not want to stay in the 'undesirable' village. Middle-aged doctors with heavy burdens to sustain their families are likely to move their clinics to the town or city. Elderly doctors, many of whom are former barefoot doctors, work on meagre incomes in their villages, but the number of these doctors is decreasing. Some villages do not have any doctor once their old doctor passes away. Many of these doctors who continue to practice medicine in the rural areas have to develop several businesses to increase their incomes: opening a grocery store at the side of the clinic, doing farm work, selling commercial insurance, selling fertilizer, etc. In one interview, village doctor Zhao worryingly commented about another village doctor's works:

---

[9]In the post-reform era, many of the former barefoot doctors become the village doctor, however, 'village doctors' in rural areas are actually a diversified group. They included former barefoot doctors who are between 50 and 80 years old now; the village doctors who started medical practice in the post-reform era (some of them are the sons and daughters of the former barefoot doctors, see Huang et al. 2002: 363–371); and former township/commune hospital professionals who took village doctor role after their hospital dissolved in the 1980s and 90s. The writing of 'village doctors' in this section still focuses on the group of former barefoot doctors who continued medical practices in the rural areas after the changes in the 1980s and 90s, although some of their situations are experienced by all village doctors.

What has he done? Farm fish, operate a mill, sell pesticide, treat people, treat pigs [animals], and finally sell insurance. These village doctors, few practice medicine seriously nowadays. Patients are fewer, seeing one or two patients a day can hardly support a family. (Interview D80)

Doctor Zhao was worried that these side-line activities would draw village doctors away from their medical professions, yet he acknowledged the situation of being a village doctor that could not 'support a family'.

Still, many former barefoot doctors uphold their moral responsibility to provide health care for the peasants even with fewer patients in the rural areas. 'If the dozens patients are left in the village without care, this will become a serious social problem', 58-year-old Doctor Yao from a local village stated. The left-behind elderly and children in his village depended heavily on his service. Pointing to the hill opposite his clinic, Doctor Yao told me that on several occasions he had run from his clinic to the top of the hill like a crazy man within several minutes in order to save the unconscious elderly or children who lived on the hill. Decades' work in the rural areas convinced him the importance of village doctors for the left-behind villagers who otherwise would not get immediate help. In another village, Doctor Li, in his 50s, expressed similar thoughts:

We have dealt with peasants for our whole lives, and we have affection towards them. Many old people have chronic illnesses such as asthma, they can't walk to my clinic, some have grandchildren to take care of at home, and some keep livestock in the yard which may be stolen if left unattended. I always go to treat them in their homes. (Interview D23)

These doctors exhibit a sense of responsibility to their fellow villagers and to the community they have always served. Transformed to entrepreneurial private doctors in the market era, the former barefoot doctors generally work very hard to attract patients and to supply good services in order to earn money through patients' private payment. Located in the moral relationship with fellow villagers, they also practice medicine with affection. They leave telephone number to villagers, receive phone calls anytime, and arrange work on villagers' requests. They visit patients at home when they are too sick to come to the clinic, and relatively younger village doctors even pick and drive the serious patients back home on rainy days. Following the earlier practices in the collective era, these doctors continue to serve in rural communities with inexpensive and convenient health care, despite providing only basic care. Their services embody 'an earlier attempt by the state to reach out to peasants by offering affordable care' (Lora-Wainwright 2005: 487), although villagers are well aware that such institutions are not funded by the state.

7.1.4 Moral Reconfiguration in the Market Era: Revolt Against the Past

Generally, these former barefoot doctors have good relationship with local residents. However, social and moral changes in the post-reform countryside continually challenge the former barefoot doctors' long-held values in medical practice. Doctor Zhao, who is in his 60s, recounted one of his troubling experiences:

> A few years ago, a man in my village went to work in Shanxi Province and suffered a stroke while there. The boss, who was also from our village, thought the patient was sick before joining his construction team and refused to pay for the treatment. Without any other choice, another villager [a distant relative of this patient] brought this patient back to the village and handed him to me. When the patient was carried to my place in a wooden cart, he was like a dead man. I gave him several injections, and he gradually recovered consciousness. He had experienced a stroke, couldn't move and needed daily care. His relatives all refused to take him. They said: 'Who handled him, who cured him, who should take care of him'. I had nowhere to send this patient and couldn't see him die, thus began to take care of his daily life: cooking, feeding, and even washing his clothes…My wife wasn't happy with me…I went to ask for help at the Civil Affair Office, the Social Security Management Office, and the Health Office. The health officer even told me: 'You should have refused to treat this serious patient in the first place'. But I am a doctor, I have worked since 1965. Being a doctor for decades, I have to *jiusifushang* [heal the wounded and rescue the dying]. At last, the officer xx in the Social Security Management Office gave me support. He said: 'Asking the villagers to take this patient to me, I will send him back to the person who sent him to you in the very beginning'. When we took the patient back to this person [the distant relative of the patient], he was so angry that he even cursed me. Till now he has never spoken a word to me, and treats me like an enemy. (Interview D80)

Doctor Zhao felt that he took full responsibility for treating and taking care of the unattended patient, even washing his clothes. However, his deeds only led to bitterness, family blame and hatred from another villager. Doctor Zhao sighed in a sad tone: 'Since this case, my consciousness became more indifferent, I am reluctant to treat seriously-ill patients. Society in general has become indifferent; the humanitarian thing between people has been diminished'. This former barefoot doctor had upheld the principle of 'healing the wounded and rescuing the dying' for over four decades, but started to feel confused and doubt his long-held principles. Proud of having good relationships with and being respected by the villagers, he now began to be treated 'like an enemy'. After this troubling experience, he was not willing to treat serious patients anymore. Doctor Zhao's experiences correlate with the wider social and moral changes in rural China: the withdrawal of the state from welfare provision—taking care of the unattended patient in this case; the shift from collective to individual responsibilities that individual villagers have to take care of themselves; the changing family structure and responsibility—no relative in the extended family would like to take care of the patient; and the shirking of responsibility by various government departments. All these changes bring challenges to Doctor Zhao's medical work.

In the collective era, doctors were indoctrinated with the rules and ethics of 'serving the people', 'healing the wounded and rescuing the dying' (*jiusifushang*), and 'sacrificing individual interests to serve the collective'. Yet, the changing social context in the market era challenges doctors' habitus. The event above presented Doctor Zhao with a moral dilemma or 'moral breakdown' (Zigon 2007) (the breakdown of the former moral principles), forcing him to reflect upon an appropriate response to overcome this dilemma. The doctor responded by abandoning his long-held principle of 'saving lives first' and became reluctant to treat serious patients. However, he could not soon reconstruct a new moral guideline, and was left with moral puzzlement. This moral puzzlement is the status of many old doctors, who were pushed to doubt their long-held values and even partly abandon the old values without finding an alternative to guide their everyday practice.

Doctor Zhao also recounted an uneasy encounter with another villager. Thirty years ago, the woman was pregnant after having two daughters already. The enforcement of birth planning policy was at its peak.[10] Barefoot doctors were the main actors in implementing family planning and birth control work. The village party committee found the woman at midnight and asked Doctor Zhao to help carry out an abortion. However, the woman escaped from Doctor Zhao's clinic, where she was kept, before the abortion was carried out. The woman gave birth to a son. Thirty years later, she passed by the doctor's front door with her little grand-daughter. She introduced the little girl (the daughter of her son who she gave birth to thirty years ago) to Doctor Zhao, and asked the little girl to call Doctor Zhao 'grandpa'. Yet, she complained sarcastically: 'Doctor Zhao, you are a good man, do things for the communist party, follow the rules. That time, I was lucky to run away fast, otherwise, you would not have this girl call you grandpa today'. Resentment permeated her simple words. The villager's memory of the past recorded not only the doctor's 'saving' but also his 'killing'. Barefoot doctors' practices in birth control such as enforced abortion and sterilization were especially disturbing for local villagers (Xu 2012: 145), which are in sharp contrast with their early work to aid birth and safeguard children and women's health. In the post-reform era, their historical role was openly questioned by some villagers. Blamed by the woman for his previous abortion practice, Doctor Zhao felt sad and disoriented. He claimed that he just loyally followed the state policy and tried to accomplish the population control task.

Researching moral discourse in a Chinese village, Oxfeld (2010) shows how memories of the past experiences are important in the formation of people's current social relationships. Referring to the Chinese sayings that 'when you drink water, [you] remember the source', she suggests that obligation and debt from the past are not forgotten, and that people remember moral debt and repay it in later social relationships. However, in the rapidly changing and mobile rural communities of Riverside County, Doctor Zhao felt that his past memory of serving the state was remembered by some villagers as hurt and killing, and his help and rescue of fellow villagers were forgotten. His kind deeds were not appreciated, but led to resentment and hatred. The obligation and reciprocity, the redemption and reward that was shaped by the remembrance seems difficult to uphold in a setting where people are increasingly mobile, live apart and do not interact daily. On the wall of Doctor Zhao's house front, he had written several words after a dispute with a patient:

[10]Although the 'one-child policy' formally started in 1980, the birth control efforts had already initiated in the 1970s and came to the peak in the 1980s.

'Tolerance, lenience, communication, understanding, and self-striving' (*renrang, kuanrong, goutong, lijie, zifen*). The doctor, who had worked to safeguard health care in the village for a whole lifetime, now confronted resentment, blame, conflict, even hatred from some fellow villagers. He felt sad and found it hard to understand the situation, and thus wrote these words for self-encouragement.

Doctor Zhao did express moral disapproval of abortion practice nowadays, but he emphasised that he just followed the state rule and took only an assisting role in the abortion practice, which was mainly carried out by gynaecologists under the leadership of local cadres.

> When the [strict] birth planning [period] ended, they [the authorities] attributed the achievement to gynaecologists, midwives, and woman affair cadres, not us [village doctors]. The gynaecologists and midwives get subsidies now, even village woman affair cadres have some salary, but village doctors get nothing, nothing at all!

For Doctor Zhao, the question of his contribution came not only from some villagers, but also from the authorities that did not acknowledge his past contributions and reward his work now when he was old. Over the years, village doctors have yet to get any regular salary or pension. Rejections from patients and governments have made these doctors feel, not only *tongxin* (aching heart, sad), but also *hanxin* (chilling heart, desolate). The feeling of abandonment by the change of time entrenched their very sense of being in the post-collective world.

7.2　Moral Economic Struggle for Subsistence

7.2.1　Ungoverned Professionals—'Work Needs Payment'

Village doctors' persistent moral responsibility towards their fellow villagers does not mean they would continue work like 'barefoot doctors' of the past, they too increasingly ask for justified payment from the state.

The outbreak of SARS in 2003 was the most recent time that the state 'successfully' mobilised the whole country to 'fight' against the disease. Health professionals from village doctors to high level hospital professionals all devoted themselves in the 'fight'. Village Doctor Yao recalled his and his colleague's experiences during that period:

> Every person who came back [home from other areas] had to be registered and followed up by us...As Doctor Ma [in another village] said, the peasants did not follow [our] guide [after coming back] and went to work in the paddy, we even had to take off our shoes to check their body temperatures in the paddy, or climbed up to the hill to monitor their situation...It just so happened that our village had a villager, he came back from Yunnan province, got a cold on the way, his temperature reached 38.9 degree with a constant cough. I called the health office, they asked me to diagnose and monitor him...I had to make contact with this patient every day, it was really scary, [by then] many people had died, we were at the front-line...My records of the SARS period are still here. (Interview D15)

Taking off several notebooks that hung on his clinic wall, Doctor Yao showed me his records. They were normal notebooks used by teachers to prepare lectures, obtained by Doctor Yao from local retail shop. After several years, the notebooks' covers had become yellowish, but Doctor Yao's hand writing on the cover was still clear: 'Promote Chinese medical ethics, help and save human beings, unite all the people, conquer the SARS'. It was a slogan he used to encourage himself to work under the dangerous circumstances, which expressed his sincere wish to help the national emergency. He showed me page by page which villager had come back to the village on which day and what check he had carried out for them. However, after all this hard work, he got nothing, except the dozens Yuan subsidy from local authorities for the telephone bill he used to report epidemic progress to the township health office. It was the same for other village doctors in Riverside County, most of whom were 'only left with a (white) mask as a souvenir'.

In the rural areas, the Maoist 'prevention first' policy and the mobilisation-based public health system were effective in tackling some major public health challenges and rapidly curbing the infectious diseases in the collective era. However, the state investment in public health was greatly reduced since the 1980s. Many village doctors ceased to provide preventive health services for which they were not compensated (Huang 2013). As a result, the 'prevention first' policy virtually came to an end by the late 1980s. In some areas, the infectious diseases that reduced in the Mao era re-emerged. The outbreak of SARS in 2003, the re-emergence of some infectious diseases, and the presence of new epidemiological threats such as HIV/ AIDS exposed the problems of Chinese health care system that neglected public health, primary and preventive care. Meanwhile, chronic diseases have already become the major disease burden as the population are ageing (Yip et al. 2010). The change in population structure and disease pattern puts forth a renewed interest in primary and community care. The state has made efforts to set up a sustainable primary and public health system. Village doctors and their clinics constitute an important part of this new system,[11] but the government can no longer effectively mobilise village doctors.

SARS was the most recent and also the last time local doctors were mobilised to risk their lives in order to fight disease. After SARS, there have been several other public health movements (such as countering H1N1 influenza pandemic, prevention of avian influenza, and TCM promotion work) implemented locally that echo the health movements and social campaigns of the Maoist era. In the new healthcare reform, the local health authorities continue to ask village doctors to fulfil their 'responsibility and duty' (*zeren he yiwu*) in reform programmes. Yet village doctors have begun to refuse to take on 'voluntary' work and started requesting payment for their labour.

---

[11]For instance, in May 2014, the central government released the document '2014 Working Tasks to Deepen Healthcare Reform' (CPG 2014). It suggests transferring 40% of all public health work to village doctors.

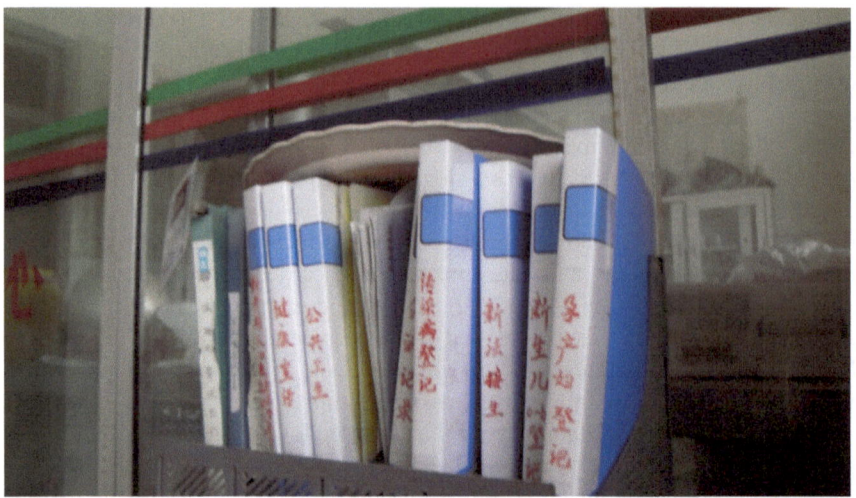

Fig. 7.4 Eight record books a village doctor keep in 2012

Indeed, in the new healthcare reform, the local authority relies heavily on the control and allocation of resources and subsidies from the higher level government in order to mobilise village doctors carrying out public health work. Village doctors began to get some subsidies for the public health work they carried out, but the amount they got was only hundreds or a few thousand Yuan a year, varying according to their performance in fulfilling the allocated tasks. Village doctors are subjected to a set of audits and evaluations, which gives them numeric measurements according to the amount of public health work they have carried out, the number of health checks they have done, how many forms they have filled, the number of records they have written, etc. (see Figs. 7.4 and 7.5). In 2011, the allocated subsidy for every village clinic was 3000 Yuan.[12] Yet, the amount was subjected to deduction by the local health authority according to the evaluation of a village doctor's accomplishment of working targets. Most village doctors I met get only 1000 to just over 2000 Yuan after those deductions.

The audit system ties individual doctor's performance to subsidies, and is designed to produce scientific management and promote fulfilment of responsibilities in health work. Yet, health care work is translated into crude and blunt numbers. Village doctors' actual hard work and humane care are not measured and cannot be measured. The ongoing healthcare reform attempts to shift village doctors' focus from curative work to prevention and public health work. If focusing on achieving these allocated working targets to earn the state subsidy, village doctors

---

[12]The subsidies have increased gradually over the years, but have yet reached a satisfactory level for village doctors.

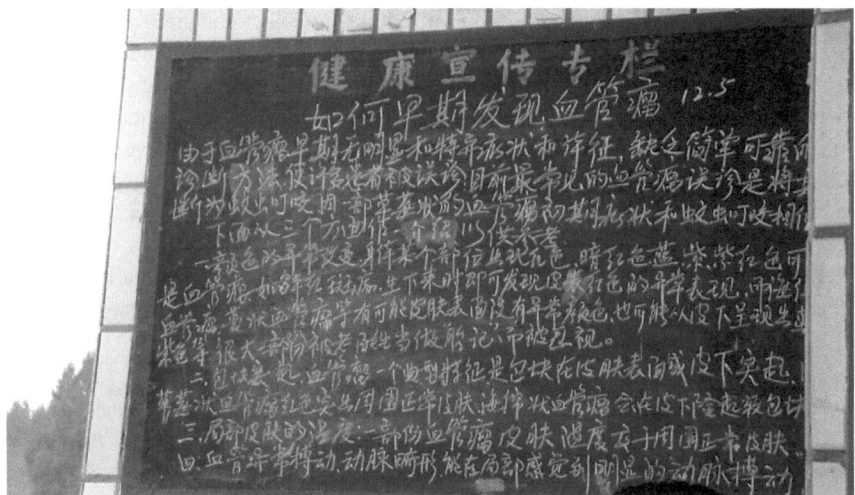

Fig. 7.5 Health Propaganda Billboards outside a village clinic—a requirement in the new healthcare reform

may transfer patients, who they used to treat as individual patients personally, into 'patient numbers' to fulfil a target, ignoring individual needs of concrete care.

Besides, due to the low subsidy and serious deduction by the local administrative authorities, village doctors view these new public health works as 'unprofitable' tasks. Rather than regarding the audit as neoliberal governance, old village doctors in my research frequently relate these evaluations to the socialist past when barefoot doctors were subjected to strict evaluations and were required to take on much voluntary work. The 'audit' technology is regarded by village doctors as socialist practice.[13] Public health work is interpreted by village doctors as requiring them to 'voluntarily and selflessly contribute'. Elderly village doctors add their own history into their interpretation of policies and, in the process, redefine the official meaning of these policy interventions. Village doctors complain about these record writing and non-treatment works. Many show resistance in performing these 'useless' tasks and react with counter-strategies such as faking records. Local doctors complained about the unreasonable deductions of their subsidies, some reported the delay of the subsidies they should have received (both in my interviews and on internet), and many suspected that the local administrative authorities used their audit power to gain from village doctors' subsidies. If all these accusations were true, performance audits then lead to 'non- and anti-neoliberal outcomes' and 'the development of new, efficiency-hindering practices' (Kipnis 2008: 285) rather than neoliberal results.

---

[13]This is similarly found by Kipnis (2008) among Chinese workers who describe the performance audits in the market era as 'socialist' rather than neoliberal governmentality.

Village doctors also employ market rationales to reject carrying out these 'unprofitable' new tasks. Many regard their labour as being underpaid and undervalued in the new audit system. Without sufficient operating funds, village doctors still focus on treatment work to make their own revenue, instead of dedicating time to public health work. '[The government] ask us to work, but doesn't give us [enough] subsistence, it's just like "forcing the horse to run without feeding it", it won't work' (Interview D73), said an old village doctor, who used to be a 'barefoot doctor' and who did not get much over the past decades, and was expecting a change in the new reform. Doctor Yao too, defied the public duties the local health bureau put on him and justified his actions in terms of market logic:

> I only know work needs payment, that's the logic! Oh, the society is economic society, it means responsibility and income should be consistent...but we do the work without [sufficient] repayment, is that reasonable? He [the local health official] only uses the rules to pressurise us, but the rules should be set on a reasonable base. If it isn't reasonable, we won't obey it. (Interview D15)

These village doctors, who have been liberated in the market for decades, adopt the work-reward mentality to argue for their payment from the government,[14] and resist being shaped by the socialist discourse of 'selfless dedication' and by the new audit system. For the village doctors, health care changes from a political and moral mission to a source of economic revenue and a terrain to argue for their compensation. However, old village doctors have few opportunities to earn appreciable sums of money that are enough to support them in the post-reform era. Every year increasing numbers of elderly village doctors become too old to continue practicing medicine. Facing subsistence crises, they begin to demand pensions.

7.2.2   Moral Economic Claim to Pension

In the field, I collected several autobiographies and petition letters from these former barefoot doctors, who eagerly wrote down their life stories. These old doctors resort to their past contributions to argue for compensation. In their letters, they listed the work they had done at length: educating peasants with health knowledge, sowing and collecting herbs, using acupuncture to treat patients; delivering babies, spreading birth planning propaganda, securing maternal and child health, birth surveillance and control, operating on ligation and abortion; carrying out surveillance on epidemics, infectious disease prevention, providing vaccinations, tackling emergent public health incidents, etc. They highlighted their selfless

---

[14]This new market 'work-reward' logic is somewhat different from the 'work point' system adopted in the socialist period. 'Work point' was very crude evaluation. In Riverside County, a barefoot doctor' daily work was counted as 1.2 ordinary villager's daily work points, but they needed to take many works that were not evaluated. The market 'work-reward' logic tends to put everything into evaluation, village doctors have clear ideas about the value of their labour and have specific demand of the amount of monetary rewards.

contributions under difficult working conditions: visiting the peasants whenever they were called, working at night and in all kinds of weather conditions, saving innumerable lives with limited medical resources, etc. Some even traced their contribution back to the time before they became 'barefoot doctors'.

The letters they wrote are full of strong emotional words: 'broken heart', 'disappointed and depressed', 'lonely and desolate', 'driven to despair', etc. The barefoot doctor generation regarded themselves as the most unfortunate. When they were young and able, they followed the socialist guide to serving the people without making money for themselves. Now they are old and will soon lose their working ability, but do not have pension to secure their livelihood. They felt they should be compensated for their past contributions, but found they were ignored by the market reform.

> I've worked more than four decades, even if you denied my achievement, I deserve some recognition for my hard work; if no credit went to hard work, at least I should be rewarded for being exhausted (*meiyou gonglao you kulao, meiyou kulao you pilao*). (Interview D72)

Doctor Wei in his late 60s stated resentfully. His words expressed the collective sentiments shared by many former barefoot doctors, who felt lost and forgotten, and felt they did not get decent credit for what they had done and were doing. By depicting themselves as self-sacrificing contributors, barefoot doctors gained moral legitimacy for themselves, in order to argue for pension in old age. 'We have contributed to the country for decades, we are old, we need to eat', 76-year-old Doctor Li expressed. By using their past hardworking experience and current poor livelihood, village doctors formed a moral economy claim to subsistence. The subsistence crisis was real and urgent. 'We are pushed to the edge of life, the communist party says the old will get care (*laoyousuoyang*), but now we are not cared for (*laole meidei yang*)' (Interview D79), Doctor Zhao resented. Ironies abounded in his words, which echo the perspective and experience typical of the old generation. These old doctors watched news, shared information with one another, and were extremely knowledgeable about state policies. Recent state efforts to reconstruct social safety nets provide them a new terrain to articulate their claims. 'At this year's national congress, premier Wen Jiabao said that even the vagrants would be given food to eat, how could we not?' (Interview D72) Doctor Lian questioned. Premier Wen was popular among the general public. In the media, he always showed his benevolent concerns towards people at the bottom. The central government positions itself as a protector for the people at the bottom. Reciting the premier's words and the party's proposal endowed these elderly doctors more legitimacy to seek their own entitlement for subsistence.

Yet in the local government, 'Those people [officials] just think about making money, they deny our contribution for all those years. We have been completely forgotten', Doctor Li complained resentfully. The words raised village doctors' shared concerns that the local government focused on economic development while ignoring their welfare entitlement. By comparing the central government's good proposal and the local dismal situation, these old doctors implied that the local government failed to take on its duty and did not live up to the ideals of the media representations. These old doctors regarded themselves as having contributed selflessly to the socialism, and thus being deserving of the promised subsistence guarantees. Yet they were refused pensions, which for them symbolised the rejection of their past contribution and a breach of the moral contract between the state and the people. While strongly resentful, they did not show any subversive attitudes towards the central government and the party. Instead in their letter, they praised the good policies and positive changes the party had established in the rural areas in the past few years, and called for 'grace' to come upon them too.

Facing the dismal situation today, village doctors became sentimental of the past:

> In the 70s, peasants got the medicine for free, only 4 pence diagnosing fee, a doctor's daily work accounted for 1.2 villager's working days. If a villager earned 100 work credits a day, we earned 120 credits. On top of that, we had 6 Yuan subsidy every month. Besides, we were treated at the same level as village cadres. We felt respected and had a sense of honour as a doctor. Now we feel insecure and unsure about our future. (Interview D15)

Doctor Yao recounted with great nostalgia. Most old doctors I interviewed could clearly recall their incomes in the collective era, when they got not only higher work points, but also additional cash income. Besides, they had prestigious status, equal to village cadres. 'Even the cadres needed to come to us [when they were sick]', many old doctors said proudly. Historical research also shows that barefoot doctors had relatively better social and economic status in rural communities during the collective era (Yang 2011). People of the collective generation from all walks of life tend to use the past to criticise the unsatisfactory aspects of the present (Ku 2003; Tong 2006; Hurst and O'Brien 2002). Lee (2000) research of laid-off workers in north-eastern China suggests, in workers' narratives of Maoism, retrieving accurate chronologies of the past was less important than the shared vision of history they constructed, which provided them common values and class sentiments to mobilise solidarity for action, and served as an alternative to their present predicament. It is similar for these old village doctors, who used their experience in the Mao era to express their dissatisfaction at present and call for changes. Yet, their memories of the past are not just idealisations, but also a genuine yearning for an era, when they were at the peaks of their careers, and their labour and values were appreciated. In the rural community of the collective era, barefoot doctors had real privileges, both symbolically and materially. However, in the post-reform era, they have gradually lost their labour values and correspondingly their economic values, and in the process they have also lost their symbolical and social status in an era when status is increasingly determined by economic conditions.

The old doctors had great expectations regarding the new healthcare reform's ability to solve their pension problem, but, as the reform progressed, they found nothing changed and subsequently they felt more and more disappointed. Their extreme disappointment has lasted for years. Since 2000, village teachers, veterinarians, and other professional groups, who took public posts in the rural areas during the collective era, have received pension one by one. However, the village doctor's pension problem was still not solved.[15] Village doctors felt they were being left behind by the development and became increasingly upset. 'The doctors who treat pigs [animals] are much better off now than we who treat human beings', I heard this words repeatedly from almost every elderly village doctor I encountered. It highlighted the difference between other pension receiving groups and village doctors' own dismal circumstances. If the neglect of village doctors in the beginning of the market reform could be justified as necessary sacrifice for economic development, later as the state became 'richer and stronger' and more people benefited from the market reform, these old doctors could not stand anymore, but regarded their situation as the failure of the (local levels of) government to provide minimum protection to realise the state's promise of subsistence.

7.2.3 Action for Pension

Since 2000s, local village doctors began to put their pension claims into action. They wrote autobiographies of their career lives, sent complaint letters to authorities, sought out media attention, visited government offices, and organised petitions. Meeting up with me was also one of their strategies to express complaints, with the hope that my research could help solve their problems, but, hearing the lost generation's lament, I could not do much more than lend a sympathetic ear. Their petition letters and autobiographies were targeted to an imagined high level official, with the hope that the upright official would solve their issue after reading their materials. However, in reality, they could not find such a high level official to hand the petition letter. At last, they could only write down the name of the county health bureau chief, the highest official they could possibly reach out to. However, their letters did not get them any response.

In 2008, local village doctors attempted to organise a collective petition. Doctor Lian and Doctor Zhao were two of the organisers. They recounted to me in detail how they contacted village doctors in the whole county, even village doctors in neighbouring counties, but only dozens of village doctors came. They gathered in a square in the county capital and planned to March to the county health bureau to pressurise the bureau leaders to solve their pension issues, but their gathering was learnt by local authorities. A government official came to the square, bringing a document about prohibition of collective actions. The official warned them that those organising petitions or protests would be detained. Faced with this dramatic turn, the group village doctors I met became emotional:

---

[15]As I show in this article later, many factors contributed to the fact that the former barefoot doctors are treated differently from other groups, such as the former barefoot doctors' inability to organize themselves to act collectively, the large number of former barefoot doctors that made solving their pension issue difficult financially (compared with the relatively smaller number of village teachers and veterans).

Doctor Lian: We village doctors, we doctors [who have worked] since the 70s reported our situation to the authority, but our personal safety couldn't be secured. [We were] not allowed to petition, gathering was regarded as trouble making.

Doctor A: They [the local officials] said our action would disturb social stability.

Doctor Zhao: Two years ago, the county released a document which stated that the one who organised the petition or protest would be arrested; it had the official seals from five departments.

Doctor B: The radio station has broadcast it.

Doctor C: It has been broadcast on the TV too…

Doctor Zhao: If we organise a petition, it is an illegal action. They will detain people [involved]. It makes us difficult to act.

Doctor A: Or else, we would have already gone to [petition in] the provincial capital. (Interview D79)

The village doctors were quickly discouraged by the containment measure from local authorities in a period of 'tightening' social control before the Beijing Olympics in 2008. Scared of being accused of 'disrupting social order', village doctors quit their petition attempts and dissolved themselves from future collective action, but their resentment did not go away. After the attempt in 2008, local village doctors continually took part in some small actions. They supported any act that was in accordance with their own interests, piggybacked their pension concern to other issues relevant to their daily medical practices. When village doctors in a neighbouring town protested against the charge of an unnamed 'development fee' by their township health office in 2010, village doctors in Revival Town also signed their names in support of the protest. Over these years, village doctors continually consulted their issues to any 'knowledgeable' person they could reach, handed their complaint and petition letters to the authorities, met up in each other's clinics, and contacted one another through telephone and the internet. The younger village doctors, who shared the same worries with the former barefoot doctors about salary and pension (albeit not that imminently), took their complaints to the internet, posted videos about the village doctor's miserable life,[16] and created village doctor's chat groups to discuss work-related issues, including the pension problem. However, generally village doctors' actions were limited to these fragmented acts. After years of struggle, these village doctors have yet to see any concrete results. Some old doctors passed away without getting any compensation.

---

[16]See one of the video about village doctor's miserable life: 'Xiangcun yisheng de xinsheng' (The voices of village doctors), available at http://v.youku.com/v_show/id_XMzkyOTYyNzcy.html, retrieved 27 October, 2014.

7.3 Governance of the 'Left-behind' Doctors

7.3.1 Government Responses

Former barefoot doctors' pensions are a long lasting issue. The central government unequivocally recognises these elderly doctors' pension needs, but is unable to shoulder the pension responsibility for the large numbers of former barefoot doctors. It thus redistributes pension responsibility to individual provinces and local municipal authorities. While provinces and municipalities in more developed regions may have better financial ability to tackle the pension issue,[17] resource-strapped and poorer agricultural localities such as Riverside County face difficulties handling such an immense financial burden. In Riverside County, there were 1868 recorded barefoot doctors by 1977, even now there are still over 1000 former barefoot doctors requesting pension compensation, not to mention the thousands of paramedical workers who served in the rural areas during the collective era. Without a clear national mandate on pension resolution and lacking public funding from the higher level government, the local authority is not willing to and not able to shoulder the pension responsibility.

In the past, the local authority did not even admit village doctors' livelihood difficulty. It suggested that village doctors, who had land to supplement their medical practice, would not have subsistence problem. The authority also emphasised that the family should take responsibility for supporting the elderly relatives. Yet, it ignored the situation that these elderly doctors might become too old and feeble to continue medical practice and farm work, and the children of these doctors from the rural areas of this less developed county may be financially unable to support their aged parents. The 'barefoot' doctors are like other 'lost' groups (such as laid-off workers) who once depended heavily upon the collective for livelihood. In the market, these groups become 'potential sources of surplus value (as capital and labour)' (Anagnost 2004). Yet, when their labour and knowledge became 'outdated' without immediate values to contribute, they become the 'forgotten' ones and are asked to find their own solution. In the market era, individuals are encouraged by the authority to become independent, enterprising, and self-reliant. The old doctors' 'waiting' (*deng*)—waiting for a solution of their pension issue, 'demanding' (*yao*)—demanding compensation for their past contribution, and 'relying' (*kao*)—wanting to rely on the government for subsistence in old age, are exactly the 'backward' mentalities the government criticises.

In recent years, the state has started to recognise the importance of village doctors' services in current health system. Elderly village doctors' pension issue also came to the attention of the government. In 2011, the state council released a

---

[17]For instance, the coastal Guangdong Province began to give livelihood subsidy to these former 'barefoot doctors' and midwives who served in the rural areas during the collective era (see China Daily 2013). In Jiangsu Province, elderly village doctors were given public employee pension insurance (see People's Net 2013).

'Guideline to Further Strengthen the Building of Village Doctor Team'.[18] It advices all levels of government to actively solve village doctors' pension issue, guiding village doctors to join the national rural pension scheme and adopting various measures (e.g. subsidy) to secure elderly village doctors' livelihood, but the implementation is up to the local government according to its financial ability. In 2013, the National Health and Family Planning Commission issued a document indicating that it will 'further improve village doctors' pension policy, increase village doctors' income, and secure the function of rural healthcare network' (NHFPC 2013). In 2014, the central government again released a document—'2014 Working Tasks to Deepen Healthcare Reform' (People's Net 2014), stating 'policies about village doctors' pension should be implemented, [local governments should] adopt various measures to properly solve elderly village doctors' pension and difficult livelihood, and set up a retirement mechanism for village doctors'. Following these state guidelines, provincial and municipal levels of government nationwide also issued similar guidelines. Yet, all these guidelines have not specified how to fund village doctors' pension. The responsibility is then transferred from the central to the local government, from the provincial to the municipal and then county government.

Accompanying these changes, the local authority at least began to recognise village doctor's pension needs. During an interview of an official from the county health bureau in early 2012, he admitted:

> There are many conflicts in our work, such as the barefoot doctors. They earned their own salary in the 80s and 90s, now they are old, cannot earn enough money, life becomes difficult, but the country hasn't given them a pence. (Interview D8)

The official granted symbolic and verbal recognition of the former barefoot doctors' pension needs, but felt helpless to solve the problem without funding from the higher level government. Since 2012 when the national rural pension scheme began to be implemented in Riverside County, the local authority has encouraged village doctors to buy their own pension insurance like other villagers. However, not having received compensation for their past 'contributions', village doctors do not agree with this proposal. They are still waiting for the 'lucky chance' (jiyuan) to come, which will solve their pension issue. They have waited for the lucky chance for years. They thought the chance would come after the SARS epidemic in 2003, during the Hu-Wen leadership since 2004, after the earthquake disaster in 2008, during the new healthcare reform since 2009, and in Xi Jinping's new leadership since 2012. However, when I finished my fieldwork in Riverside County, they were still waiting for the 'lucky chance' without immediate hope. In 2017 when Doctor Lian—the first barefoot doctor I encountered in Revival Town was diagnosed with cancer and was in financial difficulty, he wrote a petition letter again to the local health authority, a response was received this time which stated: 'village doctors'

---

[18]Central People's Government, PRC. 'Guideline to Further Strengthen the Building of Village Doctor Team' (Guanyu jinyibu jiaqiang xiangcun yisheng duiwu jianshe de zhidao yijian). Retrieved on 11 November, 2017 (http://www.gov.cn/zwgk/2011-07/14/content_1906244.htm).

identity is peasant in nature, they should join the national rural pension scheme, based on the principle of voluntary participation'. In another words, village doctors (unlike public hospital doctors) are not entitled to the pension for public institution employees, and should not expect the government to subside them in pension. They should be responsible for their own pension.

7.3.2 Moral Economic Struggle, Practice of the Self, and Governance of the 'Left-behind' Doctors

Elderly village doctors constitute one of the most vulnerable groups in the new socio-economic order of post-reform China. The barefoot doctors, who had been motivated to work hard and contribute to the health of the mass peasants since the collective era, had improved health care in the rural areas. Yet in the post-reform era, they were quickly forgotten in the state's aims of economic development, the scientific development of medicine, and the modernisation of the health system. Barefoot doctors changed to village doctors, had to continue medical practice without any salary or a pension. They lack institutional training and qualifications, are viewed by the authorities as being inadequate and in need of self-investment and self-transformation. They are urged by the government to become self-sufficient, to improve their *suzhi* (social merit and quality), and to modernise their medical knowledge. Indeed, these former barefoot doctors actively fostered their own transformation by gaining further training and qualifications, working hard to earn their own salary, experiencing what Colin Gordon (1991: 44) calls the 'entrepreneurialization of the self'. Yet it is not easy or feasible for every doctor to rapidly adapt to the market. Old, vulnerable, and less productive, many of them become uncompetitive in the market. The state's frame of the self-responsible, neoliberal subject is inherent with conflicts for these old doctors, who become too old and frail to be productive and self-reliant.

The dominance of the market in the post-reform era has resulted in a questioning of the socialist values held by the older generation. Prior to the market reform, the 'good' doctors were those who 'selflessly' served the people and 'heroically' saved the patients,[19] who were both 'red and expert', having good medical skills and upholding correct political ideology. However, in post-reform rural China, old village doctors' heroic lifesaving actions began to take them hatred from villagers, their medical practices in the collective era (such as abortion practice) began to be questioned by villagers, and their contributions in the past were ignored by the authority. 'Red' political purity was replaced by the ability to generate profits. The changing social and economic landscape has thrown these elderly doctors into dismay and puzzlement. Many are left to ponder the meaning of their youth years,

---

[19]No matter was doctors in the Maoist era really act 'selflessly' and 'heroically', the good doctor in official discourse was frequently depicted as acting 'selflessly' and 'heroically'.

and to reform themselves to become rational, enterprising and self-reliant economic beings. The former barefoot doctors reflexively react to the changing social world and embrace a new market ideology but, for many elderly doctors who were endowed with a collective habitus, the formation of a rational 'economic habitus' (Bourdieu 2000) is not easy. Many express varying degrees of nostalgia towards the Maoist era, when their values and worthiness were appreciated. Yet, village doctors are not really calling for a return to the past, nor are they rejecting the market reform. What they are against is the overt rejection of their basic needs by the local government, and the extreme inequality produced in the market. They also employ the market logic to argue that they 'deserve' sufficient payment for their services in the rural areas. They try to prove themselves as a body of value by displaying their certificates. They resist the requirements put on them by local health authorities to take on 'voluntary' public health work and demand sufficient payment. For them, when the authority did not hold its moral responsibility in safeguarding their livelihood, they would not obey its governance and rules in health care work.

The former barefoot doctors become increasingly disappointed when they are confronted with subsistence needs, sense their loss of status, and perceive the difference between themselves and other professional groups. These doctors iterate their past contribution, draw on their current difficult livelihood and old age, and employ the moral rhetoric of both the socialist ideals of securing people's livelihood and the work-reward logic of the market era to argue for pensions. They refer to the 'need'—the need to eat (*yao chifan*) and the need to survive (*yao shengcun*)—to show the moral imperative of pensions. They recount their contribution and hardship in the Maoist countryside to demonstrate their 'deserving' of pensions when they are old. They display their medical practice now to show that they have already made the best efforts to be self-responsible, but face losing their working ability soon. For these old doctors, pension is both a real subsistent need and their 'deserved' entitlement for their past contribution and current work in the rural areas. Pension is also the socialist contract between the government and the generation who have worked since the collective era. It symbolises the state's recognition of their devoted services. When local health officials attribute financial constraints for their inability to provide pensions, these old doctors voice their feelings of disappointment, betrayal, and frustration. Their plight is exacerbated by their perceived local corruption. While receiving information from the state media about various good policies, which, however, do not reach them, these elderly doctors are further convinced that the local administrators are corrupt. They rally around policy slogans promulgated by the central government for securing people's livelihood, and criticise the fact that the local government fails to provide the promised subsistence to them.

Yet, these former barefoot doctors generally have few effective measures to defend themselves. They seek to address their issues by pressuring the local government or reporting to higher levels of authority. They regard the central party-state as a repository of justice and are looking for an upright high official to solve their issue. They praise the party's good policies in the past decades and look for the 'grace' coming upon them too. Their actions are not a matter of contesting rights vis-à-vis the state, but take the form of state recognition for their status, identity, and correspondingly the compensation they deserve. However, their acts reproduce the dominant ideology and their subordinate position. The current system continually disappoints them. The letters they submitted to higher levels of government did not get them any response, their office visits were frequently ignored or avoided by officials, and their petition efforts were easily aborted. They lodge collective actions only when they become extremely disappointed and desperate as they are ageing. However, their localised and disorganised actions have limited influence. Operating individual clinics in the vast rural areas, village doctors lack horizontal linkages and cooperation among themselves. Village doctor are divided groups with diversified interests and demands, which makes them unable to form a unified action group: the former barefoot doctors, who continued medical practice in the rural area, are the most resentful ones, but these doctors are aged between 50s and 80s, some of them are too old and feeble to join any collective action; the village doctors, who started medical practice in the post-reform era, are generally younger and do not consider their pension issue as pressing as the older barefoot doctors, although they also are demanding a pension system; and the former township/commune hospital professionals, who took village doctor role after their hospital dissolved in the market era, fight for their pension within their own 'township hospital professional' group and argue their interests differently from the barefoot doctors. Besides, there is no health professional association to represent these doctors' interests. The only Chinese Medical Doctor Association founded in 2002 claims to protect the rights and interests of the practice physicians.[20] However, it is more like an official association in guiding physician's practice than an association to protect physician's interests, especially when physicians argue their entitlements vis-à-vis the government. Moreover, local doctors are under the administrative control of government health bureaus, which constrain their action ability. The idealised memories of the past, dashed expectations, dismal current situations, and futile actions come together making these old doctors extremely resentful. The feeling of being abandoned by reforms entrenches their very sense of being in the post-Mao era. Without a foreseeable and realistic economic solution, these old doctors are still facing a long and ongoing battle for pensions.

The governance of these doctors combines various techniques and measures: the promotion of self-governance, the repressive measures towards their collective actions, and the institutional control and surveillance. Rather than the shift from coercive practices to the practice of the self, as shown by Foucault (1987) in Western society, Chinese governance is more complex and mixed with the practice of the self and coercive practices. The 'practice of the self' operates as a technology of power through which individual doctors are subject to new forms of governance. The emphasis on individual skills, self-transformation, and self-enterprising transfers the responsibility of salary and pension from the state to individual doctors. It

---

[20]See the official web of Chinese Medical Doctor Association at http://www.cmda.gov.cn/ (in Chinese), http://cmdae.org/en/index.php (in English), retrieved March 24, 2013.

also attributes inequalities in the new market order to individual abilities rather than the system issue, but even the government efforts to shape these doctors into becoming new market individuals sometimes are practiced with coercive elements that remind these old doctors of the socialist past (such as the audit system that pressurise them to take certain tasks). The new governance is thus a hybrid of old socialist practices and new market rationalities and mechanisms.

However, the result of these governance is that these former barefoot doctors are characterised as being 'backwards' and having 'low quality', and are forgotten in China's efforts to strive for economic development and modernity. These former barefoot doctors failed to use 'the practice of the self' to resist other forms of government (as stated in Foucault's concept of the 'practice of the self'). They are excluded from the proper policy design and public health system. They are anonymous individuals, working at the bottom of the health system without formal title and full-time, salaried status. Yet, the services of these old doctors remain crucial for peasants (especially those in remote areas). In the new healthcare reform, the authorities start to recognise the importance of village doctors' services and give village doctors subsidies in an effort to set up a sustainable primary and community health care system, but the current system still puts them in an inferior position without equal status with other public health professionals. The issues surrounding the former barefoot doctors and current village doctors are related to China's chronic rural-urban divide that both doctors and patients are segregated between rural and urban areas with different entitlements. The change of the status of village doctors needs systematical reform of the rural-urban divide that persists in the Chinese society. After all, having a generation of doctors like barefoot doctors who are willing to stay and serve in the local communities is critical to China's healthcare reforms. With the imminent retirement of these former barefoot doctors, rural China will face a serious shortage of health professionals. The unmet pension needs and unrecognised status of these old village doctors will seriously discourage younger generations from serving in the rural areas. In the ongoing healthcare reform, China should reflect its policies towards these old doctors and village doctors in general, and readjust its policies from temporary subsidy to long-term pension, from symbolic recognition to systemic inclusion.

References

Anagnost, Ann. 2004. The Corporeal Politics of Quality (suzhi). *Public Culture* 16 (2): 189–208.
Bourdieu, Pierre. 2000. Making the Economic Habitus Algerian Workers Revisited. *Ethnography* 1 (1): 17–41.
Central People's Government, PRC. 2014. *2014 Working Tasks to Deepen Healthcare Reform* [Shenhua yiyao weisheng tizhi gaige 2014 nian zhongdian gongzuo renwu]. Retrieved 31 May, 2014. (http://www.gov.cn/zhengce/content/2014-05/28/content_8832.htm.

China Daily. 2013. *Retired Barefoot Doctors in Guangdong can Get Subsidy Up to 900 Yuan per Month* [Guangdong wei ligang chijiaoyisheng fafang buzhu, zuigao meiren meiyue 900 yuan]. Retrieved 10 Apr, 2014 (http://www.chinadaily.com.cn/hqgj/jryw/2013–01-16/content_ 8049578.html).

Cui, Weiyuan. 2008. China's Village Doctors Take Great Strides. *Bulletin of the World Health Organisation* 86 (12): 914–915. Retrieved 13 July, 2014 (http://www.who.int/bulletin/ volumes/86/12/08-021208/en/).

Dean, Mitchell. 2010. *Governmentality: Power and Rule in Modern Society*, 2nd ed. London: Sage Publications.

Duckett, Jane. 2007. Local Governance, Health Finance, and Changing Patterns of Inequality in Access to Health Services. In *Paying for Progress in China: Public Finance, Human Welfare, and Changing Patterns of Inequality*, ed. V. Shue and C.P. Wong, 46–68. London: Routledge.

Eggleston, Karen, Li Ling, Meng Qingyue, Magnus Lindelow, and Adam Wagstaff. 2008. Health Service Delivery in China: A Literature Review. *Health Economics* 17 (2): 149–165.

Foucault, Michel. 1985. *The Use of Pleasure: The History of Sexuality*. New York: Vintage.

Foucault, Michel. 1987. The Ethic of Care for the Self as a Practice of Freedom: An Interview with Michel Foucault on January 20, 1984 in The Final Foucault: Studies on Michel Foucault's Last Works. *Philosophy and Social Criticism* 12 (2–3): 112–131.

Gordon, Colin. 1991. Governmentality Rationality: An Introduction. In *The Foucault Effect: Studies in Governmentality*, ed. G. Burchell, C. Gordon, and P. Miller, 1–52. Chicago: University of Chicago Press.

Henderson, Gail, John Akin, Li Zhiming, Jin Shuigao, Ma. Haijiang, and Ge Keyou. 1994. Equity and the Utilization of Health Services Report of an Eight-Province Survey in China. *Social Science and Medicine* 39 (5): 687–699.

Huang, Yanzhong. 2013. *Governing Health in Contemporary China*. New York: Routledge.

Huang, Ying, and Zhang Kaining. 2002. The impact of village doctors' hereditary phenomenon on the quality of rural health services (xiangcun yisheng shixi xianxiang dui nongcun jiceng weisheng fuwu zhiliang yingxiang tanxi). In *From Barefoot Doctors to Village Doctors (Cong Chijiao Yisheng Dao Xiangcun Yisheng)*, ed. Zhang Kaining, Wen Yiqun, and Liang Ping. Kunming: Yunnan Renmin chubanshe. (in Chinese).

Hurst, William, and Kevin J. O'Brien. 2002. China's Contentious Pensioners. *The China Quarterly* 170: 345–360.

Kane, Penny. 1984. An Assessment of China's Health Care. *The Australian Journal of Chinese Affairs* 11: 1–24.

Kipnis, Andrew. 2008. Audit Cultures: Neoliberal Governmentality, Socialist Legacy, or Technologies of Governing? *American Ethnologist* 35 (2): 275–289.

Ku, Hok Bun. 2003. *Moral Politics in a South Chinese Village: Responsibility, Reciprocity, and Resistance*. Lanham, MD: Rowman and Littlefield.

Lee, Ching Kwan. 2000. The Revenge of History: Collective Memories and Labor Protests in North-Eastern China. *Ethnography* 1 (2): 217–237.

Lora-Wainwright, Anna. 2005. Using Local Resources: Barefoot Doctors and Bone Manipulation in Rural Langzhong, Sichuan Province, PRC. *Asian Medicine* 1 (2): 470–489.

National Health and Family Planning Commission, PRC. 2013. *Further Improve Village Doctors' Pension Policy, Increase Village Doctors' Income* [Jinyibu wanshan xiangcun yisheng yanglao zhengce, tigao xiangcun yisheng daiyu de tongzhi]. Retrieved 15 June, 2014 (http://www. nhfpc.gov.cn/jws/s3581/201308/ca329d50ec4e4e56af4fb7a5c519d245.shtml).

Oxfeld, Ellen. 2010. *Drink Water, but Remember the Source: Moral Discourse in a Chinese Village*. Berkeley: University of California Press.

People's Net. 2013. *National Health and Family Planning Commission: Further Improve Village Doctor's Pension Policy* [Guojiaweijiwei: jiang jinyibu wanshan xiangcun yisheng yanglao zhengce]. Retrieved 10 Apr, 2014 (http://politics.people.com.cn/n/2013/1130/c1001- 23702409.html).

People's Net. 2014. *2014 Working Tasks to Deepen Healthcare Reform*. Retrieved 31 May, 2014 (http://politics.people.com.cn/n/2014/0528/c1001-25075751-2.html).

Rosenthal, Marilynn M., and Jay R. Greiner. 1982. The Barefoot Doctors of China: from Political Creation to Professionalization. *Human Organization* 41 (4): 330–341.

Tong, Xin. 2006. Continued Socialist Cultural Tradition: An Analysis of Collective Action of Workers at a State-owned Enterprise. *Sociological Studies* 1: 59–76.

Tu, Jiong. 2016. The Lost Generation: "Barefoot Doctors" in Post-reform China. *China Perspectives* 4: 7–17.

Wang, Shaoguang. 2010. China's Double Movement in Health Care. *Socialist Register* 46: 240–261.

Xinhua Net. 2003. *The Sources and Contributions of Village Doctor* [Xiangcun yisheng de laiyuan he zuoyong]. Retrieved 4 May, 2014 (http://news.xinhuanet.com/zhengfu/2003-08/18/content_1030667.htm).

Xu, Sanchun. 2012. *The Medical System of Chinese Country since Qing Dynasty: from Caozelingyi to Barefoot Doctor* [Qing yilai de xiangcun yiliao zhidu]. Doctoral Dissertation, Nankai University (in Chinese).

Yang, Nianqun. 2011. Memories of the Barefoot Doctor System. In *Governance of Life in Chinese Moral Experience: The Quest for an Adequate Life*, ed. E. Zhang, A. Kleinman, and W. Tu, 131–145. London: Routledge.

Yip, Winnie Chi-Man, William C. Hsiao, Qingyue Meng, Wen Chen, and Xiaoming Sun. 2010. Realignment of Incentives for Health-care Providers in China. *The Lancet* 375 (9720): 1120–1130.

Zigon, Jarrett. 2007. Moral Breakdown and the Ethical Demand. A Theoretical Framework for an Anthropology of Moralities. *Anthropological Theory* 7 (2): 131–150.

Chapter 8
Conclusion: Moral Experience in a Socialist Neoliberal Polity

The Chinese health sector is a sphere of assemblage.[1] It assembles diversified visions of health care: the social welfare view of health care as a public good supplied by the state, a Confucian vision of health care based on the family-structure of health care provision (see Fan 2008), and the market vision of health care that promotes individual responsibility and promises access to the best care for all even though it cannot realistically be secured. Health care is seen as a business embedded in the market, a political project of the state to improve its legitimacy, and a system in the vision of modernity and scientific development. It is also a 'global assemblage' (Ong and Collier 2004) of thoughts, technologies and products from different localities: the introduction of western medicine and technology, nationally and globally-produced medical products and equipment, capital expansion in the health sector, the adoption of health systems from other countries —the Soviet model since the early PRC, the neoliberal reform (mainly learnt from the US in the 1980s and 1990s), and the recent 'new socialist' reform that refers to welfare states in Europe. Chinese health sector has become a site of contestation among these different visions, ideologies, and practices. It is where the state power, market forces, medical institutions, health professionals, and patients converge and negotiate in everyday life. The various issues and phenomena in health sector are not only individual, but also related to the wider organizational, procedural, and institutional contexts individuals situate. Health care supplies a site to explore how the state thinks about individuals, the way in which they act upon citizens' needs and welfare, and the relationship between power and subjectivity. Drawing on Foucault's concept of governmentality and its critical use in the Chinese context by other researchers, the book investigates the diverse governing activities in the Chinese health sector, the way in which governance frames people's identity and subjectivity, how these government activities produce dilemma for various actors in the health sector, and how these governing practices were conceived, constituted,

---

[1]I got inspiration from reading Saxer (2013) research of Tibetan Medicine. He describes that the Tibetan medicine industry as an assemblage both spatially and temporally.

© Springer Nature Singapore Pte Ltd. 2019
J. Tu, *Health Care Transformation in Contemporary China*,
https://doi.org/10.1007/978-981-13-0788-1_8

negotiated and resisted by the people. Chinese health policy and governance are marked by an extreme form of hybridity, and the medical experience of both health professionals and patients are filled with conflicts.

8.1 Making Governable Subjects: Hybrid Moral Experience in a Socialist Neoliberal Polity

Market reforms in the Chinese health sector and the recent reverse of the market reforms have generated hybrid experiences for Chinese people. Both patients and health professionals experience hidden anxieties during medical encounters. Patients are concerned that they may not get the right diagnosis, pay more than they should, be over prescribed or mistreated by health professionals, and even be rejected by hospitals unless they pay upfront. In the market, patients become the target of profit-calculation, and increasingly feel victimised by commercialised hospitals and profit-driven professionals. Doctors worry that they may not diagnose precisely, not meet the patients' requirements, be mistrusted, criticised, and even attacked by patients. Doctors' professional authority is constantly challenged by more informed patients and increasingly intervened by administrative agencies. Doctors see themselves as victims of not only their patients (who attack them) but also a failed health system. The doctor-patient relationship becomes a commercial one, a bureaucratic one, and a conflicting one. The relations and power dynamics between doctors and patients are being reconfigured in the multiple and changing governance.

8.1.1 Self-responsible Patients and Differential Citizenship

For the general public, their health has improved together with the improvement in their overall material life. However, until recent years, the dismantlement of the barefoot doctor system and the CMS in the rural areas and the reduction in insurance coverage in the urban areas have made accessing health care difficult for many. The market reform has transformed individual patients into clients and consumers, who are urged to become self-responsible citizens and care for themselves and their relatives. Market logics increasingly inform and organise people's life. Health care is determined according to patients' financial status. Patients become more active and calculating consumers in seeking health care and bargaining medical prices. The market reform forces people to face risks and uncertainty by themselves. With reduced social security and incomplete protection by the state, many people have a heightened sense of vulnerability.

Patients do not act as ideal neoliberal subjects who are autonomous, rational and self-regulating. Their views of health care are mixed with the ideals of collective welfare, traditional philanthropic provision, and commercial products in the market. Their resentment and sense of injustice has risen when encountering opaque medical charges, irresponsible health professionals, and hospitals that put money first. The empirical medical economy subjects patients to 'exploitation' and infringes their moral economy. Patients brand the capitalist outlook of hospitals and profit-driven doctors as a moral problem, and are increasingly 'unable to forgive' hospitals and doctors in medical disputes. Sensing the loss of health care benefits and rising health care inequality, many question their place and very rights in the post-reform society. The socialist past has been constantly reconstructed by patients to criticise the current dissatisfactory aspects. People also question the neoliberal trend of health care change by referring to the party-state's very promise to satisfy people's needs. Health care is understood by them as a need-based right or entitlement rather than simply another service to be bought only by those who can afford it, but people also want to purchase better, qualified health care in the market if their financial status allows it. In recent years, the state began to reverse the market trajectory of the healthcare reform. People began to have medical insurance and improved health care access, but the same group still frequently faces negligence, misconduct, and rampant corruption from the local administrative agencies, hospitals, and health professionals. The recent new healthcare reform is guided by ideas of both individual responsibility and state welfare. Patients' vision of health care is mixed with a moral economy of needs, deservingness in the neoliberal market, and a budding sense of rights. The troubling issue for the new healthcare reform is how to create a proper balance between satisfying the basic needs and meeting the rising expectations arising from the country's change from socialist equality to the comprehensive 'equality of opportunities' in the market, and to the recent 'equality of redistribution'.[2]

Health care operates as a technology of power through which individuals reshape themselves. The aspects of individual responsibility, consumer patients, and rule-abiding patients constitute a form of biopower, through which the state not only disciplines individual life and regulates the population, but also redirects health care responsibly towards individual households. Health policies produce power/knowledge, defining 'qualified', 'unqualified', and 'partially-qualified' patients, sanctioning certain treatments while rejecting others, including and excluding certain populations. Insurance schemes function as the 'biopolitical technologies' of the state that exercise influence over the conduct of individuals and the population. They force the beneficiary 'voluntarily' to comply with the rules in order to gain benefits. The citizenship attainment process paradoxically individualises responsibility that patients must present themselves as qualified, responsible, 'deserving' citizens in order to demand inclusion and so receive benefits. Health care entitlements easily become earned privileges through individual efforts.

[2]I got ideas about the 'socialist equality', the 'equality of opportunities', and the 'equality of redistribution' from reading 'A Conversation with Wang Hui' (Battaglia 2013).

In China's health sector, there is a 'differential citizenship' (Wu 2010; Whyte 2010), framed by the combination of market forces, socialist legacies, and state policies: the *hukou* system, the rural-urban division, the different health insurance schemes, and the individual social economic capital in the unfolding of market reforms. Although the official rhetoric is to secure people's health care needs and rights, in practice health care is frequently based on neither needs nor rights. The commercialised health sector places priority on maximising profit rather than meeting human needs. Differential citizenship is embedded in the political economy of the market era that requires productivity and self-reliance when the state retreats from welfare provision. Moreover, the structural arrangements and health policies frame a set of conceptual categories and norms about social worth and qualifications, which lead to the unequal distribution of health care access and insurance benefits. It is the combination of the socialist legacies of control (such as household registration) and the neoliberal market forces (in creating self-responsible patients, and the deservedness of patients) that constitute a form of governance to fit the market economy with 'Chinese characteristics', under which differential citizenship is inevitable. The new healthcare reform in recent years tries to supply universal basic health care, but patients are still required to take responsibility for their own quality care, to make informed decisions about their medical treatment, and to obey the state rules to become qualified for insurance benefits. Moreover, claims over citizenship can even be held hostage by officially-sanctioned programmes, such as birth planning, and by hospitals and professionals who seek to promote their own interests. The excessive administrative interference and abuse of power easily encroach on the promised social and economic rights. The official regulation of health care rights is insufficient to enable people to secure health care entitlement (actually accessing the required health care), which is based on their purchasing ability, willingness to submit to a set of established rules, and qualification evaluation. Health care entitlement is still 'bestowed' on the people rather than constituting an inalienable right.

While health care becomes increasingly differentiated, people have become sufficiently well-informed to resist separate standards of care. Patients negotiate medical prices and better care, map their own suffering to argue for health care needs, and try to qualify themselves for insurance reimbursement. There are many creative measures that are adopted by patients to circumvent structural obstacles to health care access: for instance, seeking media reports or officials' attention, using the relationship to become 'qualified' patients, and seeking reliable health care through informal transactions of money and gift. However, patients' ability to make good choices and negotiate in the medical market varies according to their socio-economic conditions. The powerful, resourceful ones are more able to obtain 'entitlement' to welfare and subsidies, while the poor and well-less connected have less agentive ability to argue for their health care access. The unequal individual ability to negotiate structural barriers poses another symbolic 'violence' to the disadvantaged (generating a sense of futileness, injustice, and vulnerability). Besides, patients may have insufficient knowledge to make accurate plans. Their successful negotiations with doctors are frequently limited to minor treatment, chronic illness and outpatient care. In more urgent, complex situations, patients largely depend on doctors to make decisions for them, and their bargain has a limited effect in reducing their financial burden in the case of major illness. Moreover, patients' efforts, such as informal transactions, to overcome the structural barriers are sometimes extorted by health professionals to reap more profits. Perceiving injustice, some patients hit back by taking advantage of health policy and making false insurance claims. They find ways to turn their victim status into a demand for compensation (in the case of malpractice), and even act violently in order to argue for more compensation. Many show a willingness to engage in norm transgressions for self-gain whenever the opportunity arises. Patients thus simultaneous exploit and are exploited by the commercialised health system (among others).

Albeit resenting unequal health care, patients may not necessarily question the system through which they obtain health care. The public resentment about health care targets the chaotic policy implementation, local corruption, and 'immoral' behaviour of the health professionals whom the patients encounter daily, rather than the health system or the healthcare reform itself. Thus no matter how resentful they may feel, patients do not protest against the authorities, apart from individual cases of attacking medical professionals, blocking hospitals, and resisting maltreatment. Patients negotiate health care with the health professionals, medical institutions, and local authorities (such as government insurance bureau), but seldom argue health care rights vis-à-vis the state. Their arguments are normally need-based concerns about socio-economic justice and to realise the medical entitlement they obtained only recently. People's everyday actions remain in the frames set by the state. In the market, patients become consumers without necessarily becoming citizens with inalienable rights. Many still regard the new welfare as being 'granted' by the state. They strive to be included in the unequal health care agenda, rather than act against the unequal system itself.

This research does realise that China, with its large geographical areas and about a fifth of the world's population, could hardly provide a universal identical healthcare system for all. What this book argues is the recognition of health care as an inalienable basic right for all and a distribution of health care based mainly on the common experience of the 'frailty and precariousness' of human beings (Turner 2008: 244) and the fundamental needs of the human body, rather than an economic rationale and political priority. Only when health care benefits change from 'qualification' to inalienable rights and the 'eligible' people become the 'entitled' will the stratified citizenship become more equal citizenship.

8.1.2   The Self-enterprise, Discipline and Resistance of Health Professionals

In the market reform, health professionals are generally required to advance their own life and maximise their 'entrepreneurial comportment' (Rose 1996: 340). Public doctors are pressured by hospitals to achieve work efficiency and make a financial contribution. They are subject to a series of performance audits based on economic rationales. Private doctors open their own clinics by overcoming administrative obstacles and work extremely hard to attract 'customers'. The former 'barefoot' doctors reinvent themselves by undertaking further training and attempt to demonstrate that they are capable, valuable labour in the market. Hospital administrators too are required to become entrepreneurs in order to manage their hospitals to maximise profits. Even government officials apply an economic rationale to the management of individuals, institutions, and government agents. The entrepreneurial model of conduct dominates local governments and medical organisations, and so, correspondingly, the officials, hospital administrators and professionals within them.

The conflicts experienced by Chinese doctors are associated with the multiple, often contradictory demands put on them. The government requires public hospitals and health professionals to practice medicine as public welfare while reducing investment and asking them to be responsible for their own income. The state regulates on doctors' treatment and lifesaving responsibilities but, in actual medical practice, it is challenging for doctors to meet these requirements. They may even be fined by their hospital if they offer the 'wrong' treatment that fails to generate profits or causes economic loss for the hospital. Doctors struggle with the contradictions between socialist morality, the official ethic codes, and the daily pressures and opportunities presented in the market. Being a 'good' doctor in the post-reform era is about 'technologies of the self' to balance the competing and sometimes contradictory requirements of daily practice, to improve one's medical skills, and to adapt to the changing circumstance. While public doctors cannot save all poor patients under their hospital's 'economically rational' rules, they express their sympathy and kindness through their individual actions. Even though doctors accept red-packets and over-prescribe to gain more, they also save money for uninsured patients and return these red-packets to poor families. For many doctors, health care is not just a locus for profit-generation but also a set of professional duties and a site for identity and meaning-making. Doctors' rhetoric of income combines the idea of being outstanding in the market, the socialist value of egalitarianism, and a moral economy of justice. They complain about the growing income difference between ordinary health professionals and hospital administrators. Many exhibit anxiety about falling behind in a competitive market. Health professionals are both exploited by and exploiting the existing system. They resent the corruption within the health sector, yet actively exploit the market opportunities and morally ambiguous means for self-gain. They take advantage of the state investment and gain from insurance funds, but also feel somewhat embarrassed about their 'grey' incomes. Yet, without sufficient income via the formal channel, many do not hesitate to manoeuvre the system to obtain more. 'Stealing' from the state is justified by hospitals and doctors provided that it does not directly compromise the patients' interests.

The changing health sector in the past few decades has forced many doctors to confront a situation in which their commitment is 'challenged, undermined, even lost' (Kleinman 2005: x). Prior to the market reforms, the 'good' doctors were those who selflessly served the people and heroically saved patients, who were both 'red and expert', equipped with good medical skills and the correct political ideology. In post-reform China, public doctors' link to the pre-existing moral and political order, through which they gained their identity and fulfilment, was broken. The heroic rescue of patients would cause problems for doctors if the patients failed to pay their medical fees. 'Red' political purity was replaced by the ability to generate profits. A doctor's value resided in their ability to mobilise resources, produce profits, and pursue the institution's economic goal. The changing external environment casts some doctors into a moral uncertainty that continually questions their previously-held values. Many middle-aged and elderly doctors are left to reform their 'thoughts' and turn themselves into rational, enterprising and self-reliant economic beings. Yet it is not easy for every doctor to rapidly adapt to the market condition. Elderly doctors who are unable to adapt rapidly (such as the former 'barefoot' doctors) are even criticised for their lack of education, skills and qualifications. Many seem to be left behind in the rapidly-developing Chinese society, caught up in a dramatic change which they cannot control.

In the governance of Chinese health professionals, there has been a combination of suppressive measures of discipline and the promotion of self-governance. In the collective era, doctors were strictly controlled under the *danwei* system. They were governed by a combination of authoritarian power in the form of punishment, ideological indoctrination and moral mobilisation. In the post-reform era, the health system seems to gives doctors greater autonomy over their daily medical practice (to arrange their own work), but their institutions and local health authorities remain closely administrate them. They are not allowed to change job freely and face administrative interventions in their medical practice. In addition, they are subjects to new technologies of control through a set of performance audits promoted by their hospital. Their treatment decisions come under increasing scrutiny of profit-focused administrators. Health professionals are being shaped to become 'rational' economy beings, and are forced to increase their capability, productivity and docility to promote production and accumulation. Besides, under the new healthcare reform, public doctors encounter extra audit and budgetary scrutiny by insurance bureaus and the local authorities that seek to control medical funding and regulate in treatment, medication, and budgets. Moreover, the administrative authorities directly issue various decrees, behaviour codes, and laws to police the conduct of professionals. Government agencies and the public media attribute problems in the health sector (such as gift-taking, letting patients die incidents, medical corruption, and medical accidents) to the moral failure of individual health professionals. The intense focus on the actions of professionals at the frontline, to some extent, draws attention away from the system's issue and role of the government that is committed to affordable, accessible medical services while reducing its involvement. This 'moral displacement' (Hansen 2013: 52) individualises systemic issue and enables the party-state to portray itself as the moral centre in implementing good governance and as the source of the solution to local problems (see Hsu 2001; Hansen 2013; Thornton 2007). It provides further justification for the state to control professionals. The authorities have issued a variety of rules and codes on professional behaviour and obligations, but health professionals' daily medical practice is frequently at odds with the external system of norms and rules. Some of these containment measures evoke fresh resentments among health professionals. Furthermore, moral displacement leads to patients' increasing resentment towards health professionals, and correspondingly rising conflicts between the two.

The individualisation of health care problems is violently rejected by health professionals. However, health professionals generally cannot access many effective measures with which to publicly defend themselves. Working inside the bureaucratic system and trained in the state institutions, they are more constrained by the normative power of the state and are yet to act as autonomous, independent agents. Even if they were to organise joint action, it would be easily suppressed by the public security management. Constrained by the disciplinary discourses of civility and *suzhi*, doctors generally refrain from violent actions, which are not in accord with the image of civilised, educated doctors. They generally seek out official institutions to solve their issues. In the case of elderly village doctors, they struggle to receive their pension, and want the state to recognise their decades of contribution, and correspondingly the benefits and compensation they deserve. Yet their individual contestations can rarely be collectively organised, their complaints and petitions to the authority do not give them any response, and their pension entitlement remain unrecognised. Health professionals are intensely governed in general. Many feel a strong sense of powerlessness and cynicism, when faced with the conflicting demands of administrative agencies and attacks by patients, while being unable to change the situation in any way.

8.1.3 An Assemblage of Governmental Rationalities and Technologies

In the market era, the state retreated from investment and introduced a market mechanism into the health sector. At the same time, it continues to govern the health sector through a planning and administrative rationality that has been predominant since the collective era (by allocating resources, pricing, regulating medical institutions and professional mobility, and deciding patients' entitlement), although the measures employed are more to 'steer' and 'guide' (Sigley 2006). The state governs both directly and at a distance, combining the market norms, bio-political intervention, socialist planning, and sovereign power, and now increasingly relies on individuals' aspirations, choices, and capacity (as both con-sumers and entrepreneurs in the market). Governance in the health sector works through multiple actors within and outside the state bureaucracies. The party-state continues to play a decisive role in the governance of populations and individuals. Local levels of government even use their administrative power directly to extract profits from the health sector. Health policies promote tactical intervention and constitute knowledge and systems of discipline that attempt to classify, shape and order individuals and populations. Health insurances form the regulatory, normal-ising apparatus, bringing out new sets of hierarchies and controls to reinforce governance. People are governed by others as well as by themselves. Entrepreneurial, self-responsible, self-reliant citizens are produced by the new modes of governance, and also constitute part of the governance structure and process.

Health care functions as a biopower, maximising the energy and capacity of individuals and institutions while prohibiting certain acts, ensuring that certain members of the population are nurtured and have entitlement while others are marginalised and neglected. In the market era, both doctors and patients are required to be self-responsible and self-enterprising, solve their conflicts and deal with risks themselves, while at the same time obeying the rules and acting docilely within the system. Individual responsibility still contains a premise of a collective end (reducing the family and state burden). Patient autonomy and individual freedom to choose in the market also gives hospitals and doctors an 'excuse' to reject patients who are unable to pay in the market. Rather than the old sovereign power to 'take life or let live', China has transformed itself into an authoritarian, neoliberal regime, where biopower works to 'make live or let die'. The market reforms have improved many people's material life and so, to some extent, have fostered life, but also ignore certain lives and let the unproductive and disadvan-taged die. Recently, the state has fostered life by continuing to improving the health care conditions and other welfare programmes, yet it has issued many regulations and normative rules related to the entitlement to care, which underlies the value of the self-responsibility of individuals to satisfy the criteria in order to obtain enti-tlement. Patients continue to be segmented by structures such as the household registration system that prevent some from receiving care. The state rules certain citizens 'qualified' to access health care, who thus have more chance to 'live', and others 'unqualified' for health care coverage, who thus have more risks to 'die'. Besides, the government tends to make state projects (such as birth control) at a priority, often at the expense of individual rights. The biopower to foster life is frequently compromised in the face of the more dominant political and adminis-trative power (that concerns stability, population control, and economic efficiency) which functions to punish, contain or eliminate. The rights and interests of health professionals are also insufficiently protected. They are not protected from harm or attack from patients. When they grow old and unproductive, some are regarded as inadequate, are required by the government to improve their quality, and do not receive adequate pensions.

How and to what extent individuals can negotiate the processes through which they are governed? In the health sector, the authorities form a regime of truth, regulating on how to prescribe medicine, what are medical accidents, what constitutes medical malpractice, what is unreasonable *nao* in medical disputes, and so on. Individual's behaviour is interpreted, evaluated, regulated and restricted through the 'regime of truth'. However, increasingly, people feel dissatisfied, question the normative 'truth', and are unwilling to obey rules that they consider unreasonable and unjust. When patients felt exploited and manipulated, health professionals felt oppressed and alienated by the reform policies, the link was lost between (official) ideology and (individual) consciousness, 'the normative power of modern government lost its ideological grip' (Shore and Wright 1997: 24). The state itself is riddled with ambiguities and contradictions with regard to its policies, governance and political rationales, and thus is vulnerable to pressure, instability and resistance. The forms of governance represented by these policies were then met with questions, challenges and resistance. Both patients and health professionals interpret and manipulate the available resources and customs to counter the dissatisfactory health policies. They skirt around sharp corners to launch their 'resistance' by 'taking advantage of the policies', 'violating the regulations', 'informal networks and gifts', and so on. The normative regulations and official discourses shape a moral environment to encourage people to act civilly and use the law to defend their interests but, without an alternative, people practically employ the disruptive measure to defend their interests, such as patients' violent outbreaks of *nao* in the case of medical disputes. Patients and doctors, among others, strive for their entitlements and rights, and fight against perceived injustice, malpractice and corruption through their personal stratagems, even by employing morally ambiguous measures. During these processes, they construct their own moral discourses and rules that lie outside the official ones.

However, in the non-liberal context of China, the space for people to act, participate and resist is limited. Both patients and health professionals' actions could hardly go beyond the established organisational structure that the state shapes, confines and manages. Patients' actions aim to express their resentment towards the medical providers, to put pressure to the local authorities, and place their cases higher on the local government's agenda. They strive to be included in the social programme, but not for their inalienable rights. They articulate rights against doctors and hospitals, but do not argue rights vis-à-vis the state. For health professionals, their arguments about their income and pension are based on subsistent needs, deservingness, and justice, which seem to follow the moral economy path of livelihood rather than the liberal tradition of rights. People could hardly distance themselves from the government even though their thinking and behaviour are frequently incongruent with a state-framed subject position and they could adopt a critical attitude. People continue to resort to various levels of government that affirm the top-down authority hierarchy. When their issues cannot be solved privately, they seek help from the local government agencies; when the lower level government cannot solve their problem, they go to the higher level government which is believed to be more just. This is the order of both the administrative hierarchy of political power and the moral order in people's political imagination but, when the authorities cannot right the local wrongs, they take their rights into their own hands. Yet, their extra-legal struggles are fragmented, localised with unpredictable results and can easily be suppressed by the authorities. Individuals are responsible for defending their interests and rights themselves in the market era, while the state retains control and is ready to intervene at any moment under the political agendas, such as a 'harmonious society'. The government responses to people's actions range from tolerance, suppression, a delay in solving some problems, and making material concessions to some immediate issues. People are easily alienated in an inaccessible, un-transparent policy-making and implementation process. Overall, Chinese people remain intensely governed, and the rights of individual patients and doctors are still insufficiently protected. They contribute to the reconstruction of the powers and structures that govern them and by which they govern themselves through their active participation and contentious actions.

8.2 Healthcare Reform and the Moral Economy of the State

Health care is the site of contestation, struggle, rebuilding, and legitimation of governance. Individual and the population's health in the official discourses are linked to national strengthening, political legitimacy, and China's international image. The ongoing healthcare reforms provide a window for exploring the political rationale and moral economy of the state.

The Chinese health system, that used to be an exemplar of socialist altruism, an agency of social integration, and a vision of socialist superiority and a 'good' society, has gradually lost its value in the post-reform era. The dismantlement of the erstwhile socialist system of universal, albeit basic, health care, and the adoption of the new market-oriented health system has launched an aggravated assault on the moral weight of health care and the moral value that people attached to it. The market-oriented healthcare reform raised moral and existential issues for the individuals within the system, and endangered the moral image of the authority. In the post-reform era, the socialist ideology cannot effectively exert its influence, the state cannot find an alternative core value to replace it and, at the same time, the Chinese leaders are not elected by a recognised procedure. Thus, the party-state lacks both ideology and procedure legitimacy, relying mainly, or even solely, on the performance for legitimacy (Zhao 2012). The state increasingly relies on economic performance, represented by GDP growth. It pursues GDP growth, regardless of the social costs that this might involve. The economic improvement is accompanied by growing inequality, rampant corruption, a deteriorating environment, and rising public resentment. The leadership tries to find new sources of legitimacy by providing public services and continually improving people's livelihood. The idea that good governance rests upon guaranteeing the livelihood of ordinary people has been a hallmark of Chinese political philosophy from the traditional society to the Maoist era (Perry 2008). Improving livelihoods is the moral obligation of the party-state towards the people. In return, the party-state receives the people's indebtedness and support. The Chinese government in recent years has taken steps to transform itself into a 'service-oriented government' (*fuwuxing zhengfu*) (Yu 2008: 52). It adjusts its policies to react to public sentiment: the abolishment of the agricultural tax, the improvement of migrant workers' conditions, the rebuilding of the social safety net, and so on. Healthcare reform is one of the state's responses to laying a legitimate foundation for governing, and is part of the state's efforts to project it as caring for people's interests. The party's rhetoric frequently refers to the historical improvement in people's life through its policies, and proclaims that it will continue do so through the substantial support of health care and other welfare programmes.

The governing legitimacy also lies in the party-state's continual commitment to lead China to modernity and global prominence. Modernisation was the most powerful ideology in China (Tu 2001) and continually shapes Chinese society today. In the process of chasing modernity, the government subjects itself to the normative power of modernism and developmentalism. Kohrman (2005: 24–25), in his research on disability in China, writes: 'not only are state institutions and the people working within them extraordinarily influential in producing distinctive iterations of biopower, the institutions themselves are highly subject to biopower's increasingly international framework'; the normative framework evaluates modernity and civility in terms of how the state cares for the disabled, the Chinese party-state was thus compelled to shore up their authority by generating a new bio-bureaucracy to care for the disabled. The dominant discourse of modernity and development with a gradation hierarchy from developed to developing and from advanced to backward countries continually influences the Chinese government, who regards western science and technology as part of the solution to the Chinese problem, as China is seeking to frame itself as a modern, moral state on the international stage. In the health sector, the modernising normative gazes compelled the party-state to reform the health sector along the lines of neoliberal change in the 1980s and 90s by emphasising biomedicine, advanced medical technology, and imported drugs, and focusing on treatment while gradually ignoring preventive care. Concerned about its global image and social stability, the party-state in recent years has begun to return to the public welfare nature of health care. As the new healthcare reform progresses, the state continually updates its reform plan to address the newly-emerging issues. In the wider society, 'the moderately prosperous society' (*xiaokang shehui*) promulgated by Deng Xiaoping promises people an improved material life (see Wong 1998). 'The three represents' (*sange daibiao*) concept of Jiang Zemin puts the party and its cadres in the place to 'represent' the advanced productive forces, the advanced culture, and people's fundamental interests (People's Net 2006).[3] Hu Jintao proposed the 'scientific development concept' (*kexue fazhanguan*) that aims to promote a 'people first' and 'comprehensive, coordinated and sustainable development', and the concept of 'harmonious society' (*hexie shehui*) that aims to build 'a harmonious socialist society' and promote 'fairness and justice' (China Net 2007). The recent 'China Dream' slogan promulgated by the new leader, Xi Jinping, as the 'realisation of national prosperity, national rejuvenation and people's happiness' (Xinhua Net 2013) is also a self-engineering project that helps the state to overcome the national limit and improve both itself and the lives of its people. These slogans demonstrate the CCP's efforts to keep engineering itself to adapt to new situations and renew its ideology. As Pieke writes, the key to the party's ability to renew its charisma is not simply a capability to change its policies according to the shifting social concerns, but also 'its skill in redefining its mission to change China, creating a moving target that is always many years away' (2009: 192).[4] The moving target from 'the moderately prosperous society' to 'the China dream' gives people a sense of optimism and new hope, which is predicated on the rule of the party who is the sole agent in making the country stable and improving people's lives. The legitimacy of the party-state has transformed from one based on ideology to a mixture of economic performance, the improvement of living standards, moral righteousness, social welfare provisions, modernisation, and political stability. In the process, the party-state itself is subject to the normative power of modern discourses and moral rhetoric, and strives hard to engineer itself to become a modern state and a coherent moral agent on the international stage. It is an ongoing ideological and moral project which will never end in the party-state's renewal and reinvention of itself.

The changing health sector epitomises the continuous state efforts to update and modernise society and itself. The party-state employs various values and rationales to reinvent its ideologies and to justify its policies in the health sector. It promotes traditional family values to encourage families to care for their members at a time of state retreat from welfare provision, adopts traditional values to tackle the ideology and moral vacuum that besiege Chinese society, and reinvents Confucian ideas of social harmony to promote a 'harmonious society' in the face of the growing social conflicts. The traditional moral obligation of the state to satisfy people's needs for legitimacy continues to have significant currency. Market rationales are also promoted by the state to ask individual patients to arrange their own care, and to require health professionals and hospitals to compete in the market and secure their own incomes. Socialist equality is still regularly deployed in the official discourses.

---

[3]The 'three represents' also legitimate the introduction of capitalism and market mechanism to the government itself, legitimate the accepting of entrepreneurs into the party, and produced many entrepreneur party-members. It is very market-oriented, enables the alliance of economic and political elites.

[4]Researching on communist party cadres' training in contemporary China, Pieke (2009) notes that the party-state has developed specific disciplinary, educational and surveillance techniques which are part of a larger strategy of governmentality that takes the party-state and its leaders themselves as its object. This book gets many inspirations from his work.

Socialist values are also promoted by the state to require people to take responsibility, be public-spirited, work hard and avoid becoming a burden on the state. The health sector in the post-reform era thus shows the paradoxical nature of China's socialist modernity. The state uses market values and neoliberal technologies to serve the state socialism, but not necessarily adopt the neoliberal ideology. These discourses of individual responsibility and market values are still premised on a common good and serve both the state projects and sovereign power, leading to non-neoliberal practice and outcomes. The party-state seeks to be both a moral and business representative, and increasingly uses the latter to serve the former. It promotes the spread of capitalism into new domains to contribute to socialism, articulates a libertarian version of the market with an authoritarian version of one-party rule, and uses all kinds of technologies of power to consolidate the sovereignty. Overall, governance in contemporary China is an innovative mixture of technologies and rationalities that serves the legitimacy of the party-state, who are less concerned (and sometimes unconcerned) about the contradictions, with a 'broader understanding of socialism' (Goodman 1994: 94–101) originated from Deng Xiaoping since he promoted the market reform three decades ago. Society shows the continuity of the socialist ideology, the adaptation of neoliberalism in varied local contexts, and anti-liberal governance. These collisions and convergences of neoliberal economics and authoritarian rule, the suturing together of neoliberal techniques and a strong state socialism fundamentally serve a moral political end—that of making the party-state more able to govern.[5]

8.3 Governance, Conflicts and Limitations

Currently the party-state retains wide public support and continues to generate its legitimacy from sustaining stability, economic growth, material prosperity, and China's global rise (the sense of national pride it inspires in people),[6] but the party-state also faces a challenge to be a moral exemplar. There is a serious gap

---

[5]The author got inspiration from reading Brown (2006), who writes that in America the combination, collisions and convergences of neoliberalism and neoconservatism are the coming together of a market political rationality and a moral-political rationality. The moralism, statism, and authoritarianism of neoconservatism are enabled by neoliberal rationality, even the two are not concordant. The intersection of neoliberal and neoconservative rationalities produced new political form: '(1) the devaluation of political autonomy, (2) the transformation of political problems into individual problems with market solutions, (3) the production of the consumer-citizen as available to a heavy degree of governance and authority, and (4) the legitimation of statism' (2006: 703).

[6]Stability, material prosperity, and the sense of national pride are viable sources of legitimation due to the recent Chinese history of humiliation in the world, the experiences and memories of many elderly and middle-aged people about deprivations, scarcity, instability, wars, and political movements during the Mao era and the time before Mao. Other researcher such as Pei (2014) writes that the party's survival strategy relies on four pillars—robust growth, sophisticated repression, state-sponsored nationalism and co-opting of social elites.

between moral governance and local moral practice. The government technologies and government ideologies seem in out tone sometimes.

Traditionally, Confucianism persuaded the ruler to embody certain moral actions and to set a moral example to people.[7] The communist leaders in the collective era embodied not only the political and administrative power, but also the moral authority to think and serve the people. In the post-reform era, 'the Party-Government is the only institutional initiator and authorizer of moral norms' (Ci 2009: 23). However, it cannot provide an effective moral framework for people on a day-to-day basis. The state withdraws itself from the moral centre and the withering away of the state as the 'organ of moral discipline' has been accepted by the CCP as a necessary component in the pursuit of economic reform (Keane 2001; Thornton 2007: 20). The authorities that administer hospitals and other social organisations lack moral credibility themselves. Over the years, the party-state has always tried to find new moral narratives. As shown above, the moral language of the party-state continually commits itself to providing public services and improving people's livelihoods, the central leaders constantly display their symbolic caring for the people. The official discourse presents the party as the vanguard of Chinese modernity and morality. Indeed, the central government is portrayed and conceived by many as willing to continue its moral commitment to serve the people, but the dismal local reality has led to widespread criticism of the local authorities. The public discourse reveals a bifurcation between the perceptions of central and local government. High levels of satisfaction are generally expressed in respect of the central government, but that satisfaction and trust decline progressively with regard to the lower levels of government (see Pei 2006; Fewsmith 2008; O'Brien 2002; Saich 2011; Li 2004).[8] When the current issues began to trigger wide public criticism, the party centre tended to attribute blame to local corruption, local administrative failure, or the morality of individual officials and professionals, which to some extent preserves the legitimacy of the power centre. Yet, over time, an ever-widening gap has developed between the central proposal and people's experience, which has produced a deepening sense of precariousness. The mismatch between the centre and the local also makes the state unable to operate as a relatively consistent whole. The local government is perceived as corrupt, while the

---

[7]The traditional moral exemplar is different from the moral exemplar in current discourses. As Festa (2006) writes, while the conception of traditional Chinese model derived from a heavenly mandate, the modern moral regulation in the post-reform era is grounded in the secular rationality of the market economy, which is open to multiple appropriations within micro practices of everyday life.

[8]Many factors contribute to this disparity. The up-ward performance based political system makes local officials tend to respond to the upper level government, but show poor performance in the provision of public goods for the people below who lack power in surveillance and decision making. The discrepancy between the central and local images is also due to the conflicting policies promulgated at the centre which produce many 'unfunded mandates' to the local government (Birney 2014). Without being financially backed by the central government, the local government frequently directs their loyalty to the central but discounts its policy (Zhang 2011).

central government is distant and inaccessible. Resentment thus permeates and endangers the moral legitimacy of the power centre.

The problem has been identified by the authorities, and many measures (recent anti-corruption champion, for instance) are taken to tackle emerging problems, but effective solutions have not yet been fully implemented. Health care reform is such an example. Health care transformation in China over the past few decades, albeit dramatic, is still an ongoing process of adjustment, improvisation and rearrangement. The Chinese healthcare reforms are filled with many contingent or temporary remedies for solving the emerging social problems: following the SARS outbreak, the government enhanced the public health infrastructure and disease surveillance; after growing media reports of poor patients being rejected by hospitals, emergency funds and regulations were set up to ensure that hospitals and doctors did not 'ask for money first'; with the increasing medical disputes, the government released various regulations to control conflict and explored systematic measures to solve disputes; facing patients' wide complaints about inhuman care, a new 'human-oriented' (*yirenweiben*) approach[9] to health care was promoted as part of the new healthcare reform amidst the national discourse of 'human-oriented' or 'people-centred governance'. The state periodically makes 'its power visible' (Anagnost 1994: 244) to reassert control and legitimacy. The government's 'harmonious society' proposal in an era of increasing instability, the promotion of healthcare reform and welfare programmes, the tackling of corruption issues amid rising public resentment and the support for 'rule by law' were all efforts made by the party-state to improve the social and political situation. The authority is adaptable and versatile in handling social problems that threaten its legitimacy. The responsive and adaptive policy style can be traced back to Mao, who emphasised learning from experience (Heilmann and Perry 2011), as well as Deng, who guided China's market reform as 'crossing the river by touching the stone'. The state continually revises its track in health care reform. The actual implementation of the healthcare reforms emerge out of a political, economic and social struggle amid China's ongoing exploration of a suitable development route with 'Chinese characteristics', and these reform efforts will never end accompanying China's changing social circumstances.[10]

---

[9]It explicates that the patient should be at the centre of health care and the nature of health care as public goods should be restored.

[10]As an official from the Medical Reform Office of the State Council expressed in an interview: people's dissatisfactions and complaints are the authority's motivation for reform, health care reform cannot accomplish its intended result at one stroke, it needs to be carried out in practice and in many steps. The reform is an endless circle. It will be always on the way, always on-going without an end. (see 'Liang Wannian interview: health care reform is always ongoing without an end', from http://politics.people.com.cn/n1/2018/0305/c1001-29847274.html, retrieved 1 April, 2018).

Contingency has allowed flexibility and relative stability during the rapid social changes,[11] but also leads to many contradictions, arbitrariness and local variations in policy implementation. First, the contingent measures and technologies adopted in China's governance fill the system with paradoxical facts. China, while increasingly pursing neoliberal economic policies, has recently also witnessed a substantial rise in social spending. The reform issue that troubles the government is the balance between social justice and economic development, between maintaining equity and motivating hard work, between ensuring health care for all and enabling those who are willing to pay get better care, and between promoting material prosperity and the fair distribution of wealth. Moreover, some temporary remedies in China's contingent governance may even have a negative impact in the long run. In the health sector, it is already clear that the very policy designed to make health care more accessible is used by health professionals to reap more profits by sacrificing patients' interests; the laws designed to protect patients unexpectedly leads to their interests being further encroached upon; the measures to control medical disputes sometimes result in more conflicts. The policies lead to unintended consequences, different from those for which they were originally designed. This is partly because the function of the health system and organisations follows a familiar set of norms, incentives, and power relations that are embedded within the governance apparatus and market mechanism formed in the past few decades. If health care and other welfare programmes can be regarded as 'gifts' from the central state to the people for redistribution and legitimacy building, the local authorities and public medical institutions then frequently maximise the profits from these redistributive 'gifts' and so people benefit less than expected, which raises questions regarding the broader ineffectiveness and corruption of the regime. The collusion amongst bureaucracy, market forces, and local interest groups obstructs the implementation of the central government policy (also see Zhou 2010). The reform is thus hampered by the lack of mutual interest and confidence between the local and central powers, and by conflicting goals within the various institutions of the state.

Despite the vigorous state attempts to control the problems within the health system and bring about reform, these efforts are limited unless the structural sources of the problems are addressed. These problems are intimately related to the polity that leaves government power unsupervised, and to the 'authoritarian capitalism' that power and market forces work together in kidnapping the whole system and the reform itself. Researchers note that China today has entered a 'trapped transition' (Pei 2006) or fallen into a 'transitional trap' (Sun 2012) whereby the political and economic elites form an alliance, leading to extremely unfair distribution. 'The nature of neoliberalism without political liberalism' (Ong and Zhang 2008: 19) and 'the system that combines the state power and the market' (Sun 2012) create much

---

[11]As Bloom et al. (2001) notes, China, compared with many other ex-command economies, has preserved a more effective health sector during a time of great transition, which was largely due to its management of transition—most changes have taken place under local experimental initiatives and then emulated by other localities.

ambivalence and many problems. The party-state itself is well aware of its limi-
tation and works to adjust without compromise its fundamental 'characteristics'—
the one party rule. Despite the changes in the mode of governance over time, the
party-state is still the primary driving force behind national development and the
goal of the reforms (to preserve its rule). The socialism with Chinese characteristics
is socialism with neoliberal characteristics. Market technologies are used to further
CCP rule, and thus are implemented in modified ways in the local context, without
the complete 'innovation and adaptation' of a legal and institutional framework
meeting the practical needs of a market. Recently, the authorities have made efforts
systematically to solve some social problems (through, for instance, promoting a
better safe-net, welfare programmes, a complaint system, and rule by law).
However, behind these specific changes, it avoids any broad structural reform,
especially any that might influence the existing political system. The ongoing
healthcare reform could hardly overcome the limits inherent in the routine practices
of the system, but continually reinforces these practices with unchallenged power
and an official structure preserved in the socialist neoliberal polity.

The result is that the party-state inaugurates a system that expands its power and
governance, often at the expense of individuals' needs and rights. Zhang (2011: 22)
rightly concludes that China today is paying 'high attention to *minsheng* (the
livelihood of the people)' without a 'fully developed *minquan* (the rights of the
people)'. In the heath sector, the implementation of many reform measures fail to
target patients and doctors, but aim rather to achieve certain goals, projects, and
statistical improvements. Individual rights are easily compromised in favour of
'grand' state projects or 'common goals'. Neoliberal subjectivity is reduced to
self-care, and is oriented towards the common good. It makes citizens more subject
to administrative power and extensive governance through a set of means-testing,
qualification checks, audits, and the moral requirements with regard to
self-responsibility. Neoliberal citizenship thus does not necessarily make the
improvement of citizenship right in China, 'may be antagonistic and detrimental to
it, especially when it appears on the heels of a system of governmentally granted
benefits' (Solinger 1999). Both patients and doctors have less chance to participate
in the policy-making and surveillance of the policy implementation. Besides, the
state still employs old-fashioned totalitarian rule to government. People's acts are
ruthlessly suppressed by the authority when their acts challenge or endanger what is
fundamental to the CCP rule (such as social stability). In addition, in the ongoing
healthcare reforms, interest groups resist the reform policies, making profits at the
price of patients' interests. Patients easily become the targets of fraud, extortion and
the abuse of power. The combination of neoliberal techniques, authoritarian rule,
and moralistic political rationality produces more compliant subjects, but also
increasingly resentful subjects with insufficiently protected rights.

Health care is vulnerable to being deformed by political and economic forces.
The current healthcare reform has been constrained by its own logics and routine
practice. This book argues that reform policy design and intention should also be
accompanied by improvements in the government itself. The health system needs to
be strengthened by structural change: making the state the moral authority as well

as moral exemplar, whose behaviour is under public surveillance, developing a more transparent system, shortening the 'decisional distance' between a decision made and the individual it concerns (Foucault 1988: 168), opening up the space for participation (in decision making and surveillance, among others things), allowing the development of civil organisations to check and balance power and represent people's interests and express their voices, promoting the rule of law, reforming the social structure that segregates citizens, changing the market mechanism that dominates the Chinese health system, restoring the public welfare nature of health care, and most importantly recognising health care as the inalienable right of every citizen based on the fundamental vulnerability of human beings. Many of these proposals need far more social transformation than the current reform measures, and target exactly the characters of the 'effective' Chinese modes of governance, with the one party rule, socialist principle and market mechanism at their heart. Nevertheless, the robust state power under the CCP rule is pushing forward the concrete steps of healthcare reform. The ongoing healthcare reform is heading in the right direction in the sense that it is seeking to restore the public welfare nature of healthcare. Yet, as the reform moves forward, if it cannot significantly improve people's health care experience and handle the entanglement of various interest forces, the reform and government effectiveness may continue to be questioned by the people. On the way towards modernity and the reinvention of its governance by adopting various modes of power, techniques and values, the Chinese state faces tough questions about what kind of combination it can formulate, how it will maintain a suitable balance or mixture to suit China's unique social, economic, political and population conditions, and how to overcome its own institutional and political limits.

Health, illness, and health care are the very arenas in which people struggle daily. China's health care reform concerns the life of the world's largest population. Through an ethnographically-based study from a distinctive geographical and historical context, the book shows the logics and modes of governance in the Chinese health sector, reviews the continuities and changes of multiple values in the health sector, outlines people's moral experience of health care transformation, and explores the government's ability to reinvent itself and its limitations. Hearing directly from the voices of patients and health professionals, this research shows people's articulation of their worries and hopes as they experience the healthcare reforms. Health care contestation can be understood in a broad sense as people's search for a meaningful life. Within that search and exploration, an ethical and moral space emerges that allows one's very sense of being to find a (temporary) dwelling place in the transformational Chinese society. Health care change thus supplies a window for viewing people's search for their moral and political existence in China today. The ongoing reform also provides a window for seeing the political rationales, governance, and ideologies within China's transformation. The understanding of the hybridity of Chinese governance may illuminate the wider discussions of the direction of China's social, political and economic reforms. It may also enrich the international discourses of governmentaltiy as China rises as an alternative model of development in the global stage. China's new healthcare reform is tackling unprecedented challenges as it moves forward. Further research will be required to assess how the 'socialist' state manages to handle its problems and overcome its limitations in the rapidly-changing global age.

References

Anagnost, Ann. 1994. The Politics of Ritual Displacement. In *Asian Visions of Authority: Religion and the Modern States of East and Southeast Asia*, ed. C.F. Keyes, L. Kendall, and H. Hardacre, 221–254. Honolulu: University of Hawaii Press.

Battaglia, Gabriele. 2013. A Conversation with Wang Hui. *Asia Times*. Retrieved 22 September, 2013 (http://www.atimes.com/atimes/China/CHIN-01-030713.html).

Birney, Mayling. 2014. Decentralization and Veiled Corruption under China's "Rule of Mandates". *World Development* 53: 55–67.

Bloom, Gerald, Leiya Han, and Xiang Li. 2001. How Health Workers Earn a Living in China. *Human Resources for Health Development Journal* 5 (1–3): 25–38.

Brown, Wendy. 2006. American Nightmare Neoliberalism, Neoconservatism, and De-Democratization. *Political Theory* 34 (6): 690–714.

Ci, Jiwei. 2009. The Moral Crisis in Post-Mao China: Prolegomenon to a Philosophical Analysis. *Diogenes* 56 (1): 19–25.

China Net. 2007. *Scientific Concept of Development and Harmonious Society*. Retrieved 10 Sept, 2014 (http://www.china.org.cn/english/congress/227029.htm).

Fan, Ruiping. 2008. A Reconstructionist Confucian Approach to Chinese Health Care. In *China: Bioethics, Trust, and the Challenge of the Market*, ed. J.L.P.W. Tao, 117–133. New York: Springer.

Fewsmith, Joseph. 2008. Staying in Power: What does the Chinese Communist Party Have to do? In *China's Changing Political Landscape: Prospects for Democracy*, ed. C. Li, 212–226. Washington, DC: Brookings Institution Press.

Festa, Paul E. 2006. Mahjong Politics in Contemporary China: Civility, Chineseness, and Mass Culture. *Positions: East Asia Cultures Critique* 14 (1): 7–35.

Foucault, Michel. 1988. In *Politics, Philosophy, Culture: Interviews and Other Writings, 1977–1984*, ed. L.D. Kritzman. London: Routledge.

Goodman, David. 1994. *Deng Xiaoping and the Chinese Revolution: A Political Biography*. London: Routledge.

Heilmann, Sebastian, and Elizabeth J. Perry (eds.). 2011. *Mao's Invisible Hand: The Foundations of Adaptive Governance in China*. Cambridge, MA: Harvard University Press.

Hansen, Anders Sybrandt. 2013. Purity and Corruption: Chinese Communist Party Applicants and the Problem of Evil. *Ethnos: Journal of Anthropology* 78 (1): 47–74.

Hsu, Carolyn L. 2001. Political Narratives and the Production of Legitimacy: The Case of Corruption in Post-Mao China. *Qualitative Sociology* 24 (1): 25–54.

Keane, Michael. 2001. Redefining Chinese citizenship. *Economy and Society* 30 (1): 1–17.

Kleinman, Arthur. 2005. Forward. In *Behind the Silence: Chinese Voices on Abortion*, ed. J.B. Nie, viii–x. Lanham, MD: Rowman and Littlefield.

Kohrman, Matthew. 2005. *Bodies of Difference: Experiences of Disability and Institutional Advocacy in the Making of Modern China*. Berkeley: University of California Press.

Li, Lianjiang. 2004. Political Trust in Rural China. *Modern China* 30 (2): 228–258.

O'Brien, Kevin J. 2002. Collective Action in the Chinese Countryside. *The China Journal* 48: 139–154.

Ong, Aihwa, and Li Zhang. 2008. Introduction: Privatizing China: Powers of the Self, Socialism from Afar. In *Privatizing China: Socialism from Afar*, ed. C.F. Keyes, L. Kendall, and H. Hardacre, 1–20. Ithaca, NY: Cornell University Press.

Ong, Aihwa, and Stephen J. Collier (eds.). 2004. *Global Assemblages: Technology, Politics, and Ethics as Anthropological Problems*. Malden, MA: Blackwell.

Pei, Minxin. 2006. *China's Trapped Transition: The Limits of Developmental Autocracy*. Cambridge, MA: Harvard University Press.

Pieke, Fank. 2009. *The Good Communist: Elite Training and State Building in Today's China*. Cambridge, UK: Cambridge University Press.

People's Net. 2006. *The Three Represents* [Sange daibiao]. Retrieved 10 Apr 2014 (http://english. cpc.people.com.cn/66739/4521344.html).

Minxin, Pei. 2014. China's Very Success Could Cost the Regime Dearly. *Financial Times*. Retrieved 12 July, 2014 (http://www.ft.com/cms/s/0/658376dc-dc57-11e3-9016-00144feabdc0.html#axzz39zQXrI7W).

Perry, Elizabeth. 2008. Chinese Conceptions of "Rights": From Mencius to Mao—And Now. *Perspectives on Politics* 6 (1): 37–50.

Rose, Nikolas. 1996. *Inventing Our Selves: Psychology, Power and Personhood*. Cambridge, UK: Cambridge University Press.

Shore, Cris, and Susan Wright. 1997. Policy: A New Field of Anthropology. In *Anthropology of Policy: Critical Perspectives on Governance and Power*, ed. C. Shore and S. Wright, 3–42. New York: Routledge.

Sigley, Gary. 2006. Chinese Governmentalities: Government, Governance and the Socialist Market Economy. *Economy and Society* 35 (4): 487–508.

Saich, Tony. 2011. Chinese Governance Seen through the People's Eyes. *East Asia Forum*. Retrieved 21 Sept 2013 (http://www.eastasiaforum.org/2011/07/24/chinese-governance-seen-through-the-people-s-eyes/).

Saxer, Martin. 2013. *Manufacturing Tibetan Medicine: The Creation of an Industry and the Moral Economy of Tibetanness*. Oxford: Berghahn.

Solinger, Dorothy. 1999. *Contesting Citizenship in Urban China: Peasant Migrants, the State, and the Logic of the Market*. Berkeley: University of California Press.

Sun, Liping. 2012. "Middle Income Trap" or "Transition Trap"? ['Zhongdeng shouru xianjing' haishi 'zhuanxin xianjing']. *Open Times* [*Kaifang Shidai*]. Retrieved 11 Jan 2013 (http://www. opentimes.cn/bencandy.php?fid=332&aid=1588).

Thornton, Patricia M. 2007. *Disciplining the State: Virtue, Violence, and State-Making in Modern China*. Cambridge, MA: Harvard University Press.

Tu, Weiming. 2001. The Ecological Turn in New Confucian Humanism: Implications for China and the World. *Daedalus* 130 (4): 243–264.

Turner, Bryan. 2008. *The Body and Society: Explorations in Social Theory*, 3rd ed. London: Sage.

Whyte, Martin King (ed.). 2010. *One Country, Two Societies: Rural-urban Inequality in Contemporary China*. Cambridge, MA: Harvard University Press.

Wong, John. 1998. Xiao-kang: Deng Xiaoping's Socio-economic Development Target for China. *Journal of Contemporary China* 7 (17): 141–152.

Wu, Fei. 2010. *Suicide and Justice: A Chinese Perspective*. London: Routledge.

Xinhua Net. 2013. *Xi Jinping Explain "China Dream"* [Xi Jinping zongshuji chanshi 'zhongguomeng']. Retrieved 12 Dec, 2013 (http://news.youth.cn/gn/201303/t20130317_2988865.htm).

Yu, Keping. 2008. Ideological Change and Incremental Democracy in Reform-Era China. In *China's Changing Political Landscape: Prospects for Democracy*, ed. C. Li, 44–58. Washington, DC: Brookings Institution Press.

Zhao, Dingxin. 2012. Will Revolution Come Again in Contemporary China [Dangjin zhongguo huibuhui zai fasheng gemin]. *Twenty-First Century (Ershiyi Shiji)* 134: 4–16.

Zhang, Everett Yuehong. 2011. Governmentality in China. In *Governance of Life in Chinese Moral Experience: The Quest for an Adequate Life*, ed. E. Zhang, A. Kleinman, and W. Tu, 1–30. London: Routledge.

Zhou, Xueguang. 2010. The Institutional Logic of Collusion among Local Governments in China. *Modern China* 46 (1): 47–78.

Appendix A
Health Care Transformation in China in the Last Several Decades

1949, the funding of PRC

Late 1950s, the start of the rural CMS

1965, the start of barefoot doctor system

Since 1978, the market reform

    the end of barefoot doctor system

    the privatisation of village clinics and township hospitals

    the commercialisation of public hospitals

    the decline of insurance coverage

1998, the start of worker medical insurance scheme

2003, the outbreak of SARS

    the start of new rural CMS

    the rebuilding of preventive and primary health care

2007, the start of urban resident health care insurance

2009, the new healthcare reform first five year plan: universal basic health care

2014, next five year plan: the deepening of healthcare reform

© Springer Nature Singapore Pte Ltd. 2019
J. Tu, *Health Care Transformation in Contemporary China*,
https://doi.org/10.1007/978-981-13-0788-1

Appendix B
Interview List of Health Professionals and Administrators[1]

Number Dx	Name	Gender: M = Male, F = Female	Age	Professional background	Interview context and length
D1	Doctor Tu	M	Around 50	Public health professional in the local Centre for Disease Control and Prevention	I interviewed Doctor Tu individually for about 2 h at the beginning of the fieldwork, but talked with him informally whenever he accompanied me to interview other health professionals
D2	Doctor Xu	M	Around 40	Private doctor, open a clinic in the city without a licence	Interviewed him individually for about an hour at the beginning of the fieldwork, but visited his clinic and chatted with him regularly during the fieldwork
D3	Teacher Cai	F	Around 50	Teacher in the local Primary Medical School. Before joining the school, she was a nurse in the People's Hospital	Interviewed her individually for about an hour at the beginning of the fieldwork, but chatted with her whenever I met her in the medical school
D4	Herbal Doctor Huang	M	Around 60	Private doctor, open a herbal medicine shop in the city, which is also a private clinic	First interview with him was two years ago during my master's fieldwork. This second interview took place at his clinic for over an hour, during which patients came frequently

(continued)

---

[1]This is the list of formal interviews took place during 2011 and 2012. I had many informal talks with other health professionals, medical school students and teachers, and some interviews outside Riverside County, which are not listed here.

© Springer Nature Singapore Pte Ltd. 2019
J. Tu, *Health Care Transformation in Contemporary China*,
https://doi.org/10.1007/978-981-13-0788-1

(continued)

Number Dx	Name	Gender: M = Male, F = Female	Age	Professional background	Interview context and length
D5	Doctor Yang	M	Around 45	Doctor of the Chinese medical team in Tunisia. In China, he works as a TCM doctor in a public TCM hospital in Jiangxi Province	Interview for about one hour and a half through internet at the beginning of my fieldwork, but also talked with him face-to-face before my fieldwork
D6	Dentist Deng	M	Around 40	Private doctor, open a private dentist clinic in a local town. His father is a TCM doctor, opens a private clinic in the city. His daughter is studying at the local medical school, prepares to be a doctor	First interviewed him in my mater's study. In the Ph.D. research, I interviewed him for over an hour at the beginning of my fieldwork, later visited his clinic many times
D7	Doctor Xu	M	Around 40	Director and chief doctor of the Department of Digestion and Urology, the People's Hospital	Interviewed him for over half hour at his office, ended by an emergency meeting in his department, later chatted with him in many other occasions
D8	Chief of Riverside County Health Bureau	M	Around 50	Head of the Health Bureau, Riverside County	Interview lasted for around 2 h at his office, with many interruptions in the middle by phone calls
D9	Doctor Ren	M	Around 30	Private doctor, had worked in a local private hospital. At the time of interview, he worked as an assistant doctor in a private clinic	Interviewed him while he treated patients, the interview lasts over 2 h with many interruptions by work
D10	Doctor Du	F	Around 40	Village doctor. Had worked in a township hospital in the 90s, later opened a private clinic, now she changed the private clinic into a public-oriented village clinic	First interview was in my master's fieldwork. During the second interview, she called another doctor to join us. Interview lasted for about one hour and a half, with occasional patient visits

(continued)

(continued)

Number Dx	Name	Gender: M = Male, F = Female	Age	Professional background	Interview context and length
D11	Nurse Wang	F	Around 40	Head nurse, vice director of the Northern City Community Health Centre (one of the four community health centres)	Interview lasted for about 2 h, during which she went out to handle work issue for about 15 min
D12	GYM Village Doctor	M	Around 45	Village doctor, open a village clinic	Interview lasted for about 45 min
D13	Intern Wen	F	21	Intern in the People's Hospital, many of her family members work in the local health sector	Interview lasted for about half hour. Many informal chats in other occasions
D14	Doctor Heng and His Wife	A couple	Around 40	Open a private clinic. The husband works as the main doctor, the wife works as an assistant and pharmacist in the clinic	Interview carried out while they treated patients, lasted for over 2 h
D15	Doctor Zhao	M	Around 58	Village doctor, worked in a private clinic in the city and two village clinics at the same time	The first interview lasted for over 2 h, during which he took me to visit his two clinics in two villages. The second interview lasted for about 45 min
D16	Drug retailer	F	Around 55	Drug retailer, open a herb medicine shop with her husband, who used to work in a public medical product company	My family bought herb medicine from their shop regularly. After acquainted with them, I interviewed the wife for about an hour while the husband was at the side. The interview centred on drug sell and medical products
D17	Doctor Deng	M	Around 40	Village doctor, open a village clinic, and had got the licence to transfer his clinic to a private hospital at the time of interview	The interview took place while he treated patients, lasted for about 2 h, accompanied by observation of doctor-patient encounters
D18	Doctor Tu	M	Around 30	Village doctor, open a village clinic	Interview lasted for about one hour and a half with patient visits in the middle

(continued)

(continued)

Number Dx	Name	Gender: M = Male, F = Female	Age	Professional background	Interview context and length
D19	Dentist Lei	M	Around 65	Private dentist, work in a private dentist clinic after retired from the People's Hospital	Interview in a tea house for over one hour and a half without interruption
D20	Doctor Zheng	M	Around 35	Private doctor. During my fieldwork, he closed his clinic and joined a public hospital	Interview outside his clinic before its closure for half hour
D21	Director of QG Township Hospital	M	Around 40	Director of QG Township Hospital	Interview in a tea house for about an hour without interruption
D22	Doctor Luo's wife	F	Around 40	The couple opens a private clinic (in the town) and a village clinic (in the village) in RH town. The wife works as an assistant in the clinic	Interview at the clinic for about half hour
D23	Doctor Li	M	Around 50	Open a private clinic and a village clinic in RH town	Interview at his clinic for about half hour
D24	Doctor Luo2's Clinic	Group interview	The doctor in his 60s, his son in his 30s, and a group of local residents	Doctor Luo2's clinic is a private clinic as well as a village clinic in RH town, his son works in a private hospital in Chengdu (the capital of Sichuan)	Interview lasted for over an hour and a half. During the visit, many people (doctors, patients, and local residents) join the interview and discussion
D25	Hospital administrative staff	M	25	Graduated from medical school a year ago, and joined the medical affair department of the TCM Hospital	Interview at a park in the city for about one hour without stop
D26	Doctor Wu	M	Around 65	Village doctor, open a village clinic for decades	First interview was during my master's fieldwork. This second interview lasted for over one hour at his clinic

(continued)

(continued)

Number Dx	Name	Gender: M = Male, F = Female	Age	Professional background	Interview context and length
D27	Medical Graduate Student Qin	M	Around 27	Medical Graduate Student in Chongqing. When I finished my fieldwork, he already graduated and started to work at the People's Hospital of Riverside	Interview in a tea house for over one hour and a half without interruption
D28	Group interview with four young doctors	Three male, one female	Aged between 25 and 30	Three residential physician and one pharmacist from different departments of the People's Hospital	Interview in a tea house for over 2 h. Afterwards, I had many gatherings with these doctors
D29	Doctor Zhang	M	25	Public doctor, graduated from medical school one year ago, work as resident physician in a county hospital in Xinjiang Province	Interview in a tea house for over an hour. I interviewed him when he came back to Riverside for new year holiday
D30	Medical Student Deng	F	17	Local medical school student, intern in a local private clinic. Her family opens a dentist clinic	One formal interview at her family's clinic for over 45 min, many informal chats
D31	Doctor Xiang	M	45	Private doctor, open a private clinic	Interview for over one hour at his clinic, where I also took observation and chatted with patients
D32	Rocket Village Doctor	M	50	Village doctor, open a village clinic	Interview at his clinic for over 2 h, during which several villagers came for treatment
D33	Doctor Luo3	M	27	Public Doctor, Resident Physician in the TCM Hospital	First interviewed at the emergency department Doctor Luo worked, continued the interview after work at a fast-food store for over 2 h
D34	Director of the Disease Preventi on Office	F	Around 40	Director of the Disease Prevention Office of the Centre for Disease Control and Prevention	Interview at her office for over half hour without interruption

(continued)

(continued)

Number Dx	Name	Gender: M = Male, F = Female	Age	Professional background	Interview context and length
D35	Head of the Centre for Disease Control and Prevention	M	Around 45	Head of the Centre for Disease Control and Prevention	Interview at his office for over an hour without interruption
D36	Huaxi Doctor	M	71	Doctor in the local private Huaxi Hospital, retired doctor from the People's Hospital	Interview at his office for over half hour, during which two patients were visiting for treatment
D37	Head of the Municipal Health Bureau	M	Around 45	Head of the Health Bureau of the Municipality (govern four county level areas including Riverside)	Interview at his office for over an hour with occasional phone call interruption
D38	Director of the JF Road Community Health Centre	M	Around 38	Director of the JF Road Community Health Centre in the Municipality	Interview at the director's office for over an hour and a half, a female doctor in the centre joined in the middle
D39	Doctor Yang	F	29	Used to work as intern and resident physician in one of the biggest hospitals in Beijing, experienced patient attack	Interviewed her at her home for over an hour
D40	Director Assistant of the Municipal Central Hospital	M	Around 33	Director Assistant of the Municipal Central Hospital (the best hospital in the whole municipality)	Interviewed at his office for about one hour, during which he went out for about 10 min to handle work issue
D41	Vice Director of the People's Hospital	M	Around 50	Vice Director of the People's Hospital, Riverside County	Interviewed him at his office for about half hour
D42	Director and Chief doctor of the Department of Infectious Disease	F	Around 60	Public doctor, Director and Chief doctor of the Department of Infectious Disease, the People's Hospital	Interviewed him at his office for about half hour
D43	Director and Chief doctor of the Paediatrics Department	M	Around 40	Public doctor, Director and Chief doctor of the Paediatrics Department, the People's Hospital	Interviewed him at his office for about twenty minutes (while patients waited outside his office), later had informal chats in other occasions

(continued)

(continued)

Number Dx	Name	Gender: M = Male, F = Female	Age	Professional background	Interview context and length
D44	Vice Director of the Oncology Department	M	Around 35	Public doctor, Vice Director of the Oncology Department, the People's Hospital	Interview at his office for about 40 min, stopped by a patient's call
D45	Technician in the People's Hospital	M	Around 55	Work in the electrocardiogram (ECG) diagnosis division, the People's Hospital	Interview at his office for about an hour
D46	Director of the Department of Clinical Laboratory	M	Around 50	Director of the Department of Clinical Laboratory, the People's Hospital	Interview at his office for about half hour
D47	Director of the People's Hospital	M	Around 45	Director of the People's Hospital	Interview at his office for about one hour and a half, occasionally interrupted by calls
D48	Vice party secretary of the People's Hospital	M	Around 40	A psychiatrist, party secretary and vice director of the People's Hospital	Interview at his office for about half hour
D49	Health Professionals in Riverside Women and Children's Hospital	Two female, two male	One in 20s, the others in their 60s	Two doctors, a head nurse and an intern of Riverside Women and Children's Hospital (a private hospital). Except the intern, all are retired public doctors from the People's Hospital	Interview at the doctors' office for about an hour
D50	Doctor of the TX township hospital	F	Around 40	Public Doctor of the TX township hospital	Interview at the doctor's office for about 40 min, joined by other health professionals occasionally
D51	Director of the DY township hospital	M	Around 45	Director of DY township hospital	Interview at his office for about 20 min, later in his car on the way to the city for about 15 min
D52	Director of the TCM Hospital	M	Around 55	Director of the TCM Hospital	Interview at his office for over an hour, occasionally interrupted by other people's office visit
D53	Doctor of the Southern City Community Health Centre	M	Around 50	Public Doctor of the Southern City Community Health Centre	Interview at his office for about half hour
D54	Nurse of the Southern City Community Health Centre	F	Around 45	Nurse of the Southern City Community Health Centre	Interview at her office for about half hour, later continue the conversation during lunch time

(continued)

(continued)

Number Dx	Name	Gender: M = Male, F = Female	Age	Professional background	Interview context and length
D55	Assistant of the Director of the People's Hospital	M	Around 33	Public Doctor, Assistant of the Director of the People's Hospital	Interview at his office for about one hour and a half
D56	Administrative Staff of the Red-cross Hospital	M	Around 50	Administrative Staff of the Red-cross Hospital (a public hospital)	Interview outside his office for about half hour
D57	Doctor of the Red-cross Hospital	M	Around 55	Public Doctor of the Red-cross Hospital	Interview at his office for about half hour, stopped by a patient's visit
D58	Doctor Chen of Eastern City Community Health Centre	M	Around 50	Public Doctor, Director of the Eastern City Community Health Centre	Interview at his office for about an hour, occasionally interrupted by patients' visits
D59	Doctor He	M	70s	Work in the Safe and Rehabilitation Hospital (a private hospital), after retiring from the People's Hospital	Interview at his office for about one hour and a half
D60	Doctor and Head Xu	M	Around 45	Private doctor, head of the Safe and Rehabilitation Hospital (a private hospital)	Interview at his office for about one hour
D61	Director of LS township hospital	M	Around 40	Public Doctor, Director of LS Township Hospital	Interview at his office for about 45 min
D62	Medical sales representative	M	Around 40	Head of medical sales representative in one region of Sichuan	Interview at his home for about one hour and a half
D63	Obstetrician in the Affiliated Hospital of the Family Planning Centre	F	Around 55	Public Doctor of the Affiliated Hospital of the Family Planning Centre	Interview at her office while she treated patients, lasted for about 40 min
D64	Gynaecologist in the Affiliated Hospital of the Family Planning Centre	F	Around 55	Public Doctor of the Affiliated Hospital of the Family Planning Centre	Interview at her office while she treated patients, lasted for about an hour

(continued)

(continued)

Number Dx	Name	Gender: M = Male, F = Female	Age	Professional background	Interview context and length
D65	Director of the Family Planning Centre	F	Around 50	Director of the Family Planning Centre and head of the Affiliated Hospital of the Family Planning Centre	Interview at his office for about 40 min, two other office staffs joined the discussion later
D66	Head of the Food and Drug Administration	M	Around 45	Head of the County Food and Drug Administration	Interview at his office for over 45 min
D67	Staff of the Food and Drug Administration	M	Around 35	Office Staff of the county Food and Drug Administration	Interview at his office for about half hour
D68	Doctor in WS Township Hospital	F	Around 35	Public Doctor in WS Township Hospital	Interviewed her first individually, later another male doctor join, lasted for about 40 min
D69	Doctor Yang	M	28	Resident physician in a public hospital in Tianjin	Interview through Internet for many times, the first time lasted about 40 min
D70	Doctor TL	M	Around 55	Open a drug store in the city, which is also a private clinic. Retired from a railway hospital in Shanxi Province	Interview at his clinic for over half hour
D71	Doctor DQ	M	Around 40	Village doctor, open a village clinic	Interview in his clinic for about an hour, later was joined by several villagers
D72	Doctor Lian, Doctor Wei, Doctor Wei's son	All male	68, around 65, around 35	Group interview with three village Doctors in Revival Town	Interview at Doctor's Wei's clinic, lasted for about 2 h
D73	Doctor Li	M	76	Open a private clinic in Revival Town, an old village doctor, former barefoot doctor	Interview twice individually at his clinic, the first time lasted for over an hour, the second time lasted for about 40 min
D74	Doctor Qin	M	70	Open a private clinic in WS Town, retired TCM doctor and pre-head of the WS township hospital	Interview at his clinic for about an hour, a few local residents joined the conversation in the middle

(continued)

(continued)

Number Dx	Name	Gender: M = Male, F = Female	Age	Professional background	Interview context and length
D75	Doctor Zhang	M	Around 35	Open a private clinic in WS Town	Interviewed him at his clinic for about one hour and a half, during the interview, patients came for treatment and joined the talk occasionally
D76	Doctor in WS township hospital	M	Around 40	Public doctor, work in WS Township hospital	I first met him and talked with him when interviewing another doctor. This interview was at his office for about half hour
D77	Doctor Gu	F	Around 35	She and her father work in a 'village clinic' in the city as doctors (the community was rural area several years ago)	Interview lasted for about 50 min in her clinic
D78	Doctor Li	M	53	Village doctor, open a village clinic in the border between Riverside County and a neighbouring County	Interview at his clinic for about 2 h while he was treating patients
D79	A group of village doctors	All male	Aged between 50 and 70s	Around 15 village doctors from Revival Town, all former barefoot doctors	Interview last for over 2 h, during which, some left and the number reduced to around 5 doctors at the end
D80	Doctor Zhao	M	60s	Village doctor from Revival Town, former barefoot doctor	Interview at his home for about 2 h

Appendix C
Interview List of Patients and Local Residents[2]

Number Px	Name	Gender: M = Male, F = Female	Age	Background information	Interview context and length
P1	Mr. Huang	M	Around 70	His wife's two times hospital experiences and difficulty in getting insurance reimbursement	Interview for over an hour when I accompanying him to hospital and return home
P2	Mr. Li and Mrs. Ren	A couple	Between 35 and 40	Daughter's experience with medical school; family's experiences of seeking health care	Interview for over an hour
P3	Mr. Li and Mrs. Luo	A couple	29 and 28	Given birth to a daughter during my fieldwork, the whole preparation process and hospital visit experiences	Interviewed them and visited them at hospital for many times. The formal interview took place at their home after the birth for over an hour

(continued)

---

[2]This is the list of formal interviews took place during 2011 and 2012. The interview of patients and local residents were frequently in groups of two or over two people. I also had many informal talks and chats with local residents and patients when taking observations in medical institutions, and some informal interviews outside Riverside County (on the train, coach, plane, and other places), which are not listed here.

© Springer Nature Singapore Pte Ltd. 2019
J. Tu, *Health Care Transformation in Contemporary China*,
https://doi.org/10.1007/978-981-13-0788-1

(continued)

Number Px	Name	Gender: M = Male, F = Female	Age	Background information	Interview context and length
P4	Auntie Liu	F	Around 55	She had many hospital experiences during my fieldwork	I accompanied her to see a doctor and interviewed her on the way before and afterwards for about 1 h and a half
P5	Mr. Tu	M	More than 70	Talked about his view of healthcare reform and his experiences of health care. In September 2012, I visited him daily during his one week acupuncture in the TCM hospital	The formal interview took place at his home, lasted for over 1 h
P6	Auntie Lou	F	30s	Auntie Lou got her leg broken during my fieldwork, was hospitalised and got reimbursed from the new rural cooperative medical insurance	The formal interview lasted for over half hour, afterwards I accompanied her to applied unemployment pension and chatted on the way
P7	Mr. Li	M	Around 55	Had chronic skin problem, had many visits to doctor and chemist during my fieldwork	Interviewed him at his home for over half hour, also accompanied him to visit chemists and doctors
P8	Auntie Luo	F	Around 50	Her daughter just graduated from local medical school, was working as a nurse in a township hospital without formal licence	The interview lasted for over an hour, talked about her daughter's medical education and current hospital work

(continued)

(continued)

Number Px	Name	Gender: M = Male, F = Female	Age	Background information	Interview context and length
P9	Mr. Tu and Mrs. Yang	A couple	Around 60	Had bought medicine through infomercial	Interview at their home for over an hour
P10	A family in RH town	A family	Around 65	Group interview with a family—an old couple, their adult son and daughter-in-law	Interview at their home for over 2 h, centred on the wife's several hospitalisation experiences
P11	Uncle Wen, Auntie Wen	A couple	Between 65 and 70	Wife's recent hospitalisation experience after Bone Fracture and the reimbursement experience	Interview at their home for over 1 h and a half
P12	Auntie Lou, Grandma A, Grandma B	F F F	30s 70s 70s	Talk about their own illness and health seeking experience, their experience of taking care of sick family member	Interview in a park for over an hour. I had interviewed Auntie Lou individually earlier
P13	Mrs. Tu, Mrs. Wen, Mrs. Qin	All female	40s 60s Late 70s	Group interview of three people in DQ village. Two of them have been visited twice	Around 1 h
P14	Miss Zhang	F	27	A primary school teacher, had many recent experiences of visiting doctors (due to her daughter's illness)	Interview took place in her family tea house, lasted for about an hour. I also companied her to visit an acupuncture shop and had many informal chats
P15	Group interview	Two female, one male	Aged 40s (F), 70s (F), and 70s (M)	Group interview of three people in DQ village	Interview lasted for about an hour
P16	Group interview in LJG village	Two female, one male	60s (F), 60s (F), 70s (M)	Individual and group interviews with several villagers about their health seeking	First individual interview with a female villager about her recent hospital visit,

(continued)

(continued)

Number Px	Name	Gender: M = Male, F = Female	Age	Background information	Interview context and length
				behaviours, attitudes towards doctors, public/private hospitals, insurance, etc.	lasted for about 20 min, later joined by a couple, lasted for over half hour
P17	Parkinson patient and wife	A couple	50s (F), 60s (M)	The wife talked about the husband's illness, people around joined and gave her suggestions on how to get medical treatment and financial aid	Interview at a local coach station for about half hour, while the couple waiting for the coach
P18	A mother and a daughter	F	40s and 70s	Patients in the private clinic of WS Town where I did interview with the doctor	Interview lasted for about half hour at the clinic while the mother taking drips
P19	Mrs. Li and Mr. Guo	A couple	40s, 40s	General attitudes towards the current health system and health insurance	Interview at their home, lasted for about 45 min
P20	Mrs. Li	F	70s	The old lady talked about health care before liberation, in the collective era and compared with that now	Interview outside her family restaurant, lasted for about an hour
P21	Mrs. Wen Mrs. Qin	F F	60s 70s	Both interviewees were peasants from DQ village	Interview in Mrs. Qin's home, lasted for over 1 h
P22	Villager of KJY village	M	60s	Peasant	In the interviewee's home, lasted for about 50 min
P23	Group interview of three people	All female	70s 68 40s	All are peasants and housewife, have moved to the city in recent years	Interview lasted for about 40 min in a square in the city
P24	Mrs. Zhou Mr. Li Mr. Wang	F M M	Over 70 Over 55 Over 40	Group interview in ELM village, all interviewees are peasants, but Li and Wang have moved to the city to do small business	Interview took place in Mrs. Zhou's home, lasted for over 1 h

(continued)

(continued)

Number Px	Name	Gender: M = Male, F = Female	Age	Background information	Interview context and length
P25	Mrs. Xu Miss. Li Mrs. Tu	F F F	Over 40 25 70	Group interview in ELM village. All interviewees are peasants, Miss. Li is Mrs. Xu's daughter, and Mrs. Tu has bronchitis	Interview took place in Mrs. Xu's courtyard, lasted for about 50 min
P26	Resident 1 Resident 2 Resident 3 Resident 4 some others	F F F F	Over 70 Over 60 Over 65 Over 75	Group interview of residents in a local community. Resident1 is a housewife. Resident2 is a retired teacher, her daughter is a nurse in a local township hospital. Resident 3 and 4 are peasants, moved to the city with their adult children in recent years	Interview in a resident community in the city, lasted for over 1 h and a half. Some other community members also joined the conversation later
P27	Mrs. Huang, Mrs. Wen, A Retired Doctor	F F M	68 65 75	Mrs. Huang is a housewife with rural health insurance. Mrs. Wen is a peasant and housewife, currently have urban resident's health insurance. The retired doctor is also a local resident	Interview in a resident community, lasted for over 1 h and a half. The retired doctor sat at the side and joined the interview occasionally
P28	Mr. Gao, Mrs. Tian, Mrs. Yang	M F F	66 Over 70 Over 70	Gao is a retired officer of a mine company. Tian and Yang both are landless peasant—local peasant who lost land in the urbanisation process	Interview took place in a resident community, lasted for about 40 min, many other residents joined the conversation during the interview

(continued)

(continued)

Number Px	Name	Gender: M = Male, F = Female	Age	Background information	Interview context and length
P29	Auntie Luo1 Auntie Luo2 Auntie Luo3	All female	Over 60 56 51	Group interview of three people. All used to be peasants and moved to the city with her husband in the last decades	Interview took place in a local park, lasted for about 50 min
P30	Teacher Yang	F	Early 50s	Primary school teacher	Interview took place in a local school, lasted for about an hour
P31	Classmate Xu	M	26	Telecommunication engineer	Interview in a water bar, lasted for about an hour
P32	Grandpa and Grandma Xu	A couple	In their 60s	Grandpa Xu is a retired veterinarian, now opening a shop selling veterinary medicine. Grandma Xu is a peasant and housewife	Interview took place in their retail shop, lasted for over 1 h and a half
P33	Mr. Yang	M	27	Engineer in airplane industry	Interview took place in a tea house for about an hour
P34	Uncle Li Auntie Li	A couple	46 45	Uncle Li is a production administrator of a cloth factory, Auntie Li is a production worker in the same cloth factory	Interview took place in my home, lasted for more than 2 h
P35	Mr. and Mrs. Wen	A couple	77 77	Mrs. Wen was a peasant, her father and grandfather, old brother were all doctors; Mr. Wen is a retired worker. The couple's sons and grandchildren also work in the health care sector	Interview in the interviewees' home, lasted for about 1 h and a half
P36	Community Guard A and B,	All male	Over 50 Late 40s Over 50 Over 60	The two guards were peasants, working as community guard.	Interview took place in a residential community,

(continued)

Number Px	Name	Gender: M = Male, F = Female	Age	Background information	Interview context and length
	Resident A, Resident B			The two residents were peasant and have moved to the city and lived in the community in recent years	lasted for over 2 h, later several more residents joined the conversation
P37	Community Guard A and B Auntie Liu Resident A	M M F F	50s 50s 50s 40s	Interview with two community guards, both were laid-off worker before becoming guard. Later the interviewed was joined by two residents	Interview took place in a residential community, lasted for over an hour
P38	Mr. Chen Miss Zhang Mr. Qin Mr. Li	M F M M	27 27 26 27	Group interview. Chen is a civil servant. Zhang is a vocational school teacher. Qin is a sells person of a construction company. Li is an engineer in a construction company	Interview in a water bar, lasted for about 2 h
P39	Mrs. Deng Mrs. Zhou Mrs. Chen	All female	69 79 77	Mrs. Deng is a peasant and housewife. Mrs. Zhou is a retired worker, has good pension and health insurance. Mrs. Chen is a peasant and housewife	Interview took place in Mrs. Zhou's door front, DY town, lasted for over 1 h
P40	Mr. Zhong Mr. Yang Mr. Zhou	All male	79, over 80, over 70	Group interview with three local residents: Zhong is a retired worker, Yang is a retired worker and lawyer, Zhou is a peasant	Interview lasted for over 2 h in a tea house in DY town
P41	Mrs. Zhao Mr. Liang	F M	78 55	Mrs. Zhao—a housewife, Mr. Liang—Mrs. Zhao's son, worker in a local textile company	Interview at Mrs. Zhou's door front, lasted for about an hour

(continued)

(continued)

Number Px	Name	Gender: M = Male, F = Female	Age	Background information	Interview context and length
P42	Mr. Zhong Mr. Yang Mr. Dai	All male	79, Over 80, 71	Group interview with three residents. Mr. Yang and Mr. Zhong are the same from interview P40, Mr. Dai is a veteran and a retired teacher	Interview lasted for over one hours in a tea house in DY town
P43	Mr. Xie	M	70	Retired postman from the local post office in the town, his son died from cancer several years ago	Interview took place in a tea house in DY town, lasted for about 45 min
P44	Mrs. Peng Mrs. Zhou	F F	83 50	Peng is a peasant, opening a retail shop in the town. Zhou is also a peasant, doing odd jobs	Interview in Mrs. Peng's retail shop, lasted for an hour
P45	Mr. Chen Doctor He	M F	81 Late 60s	Mr. Chen used to be a worker, retired as a local cadre. Doctor He was a retired doctor from local township hospital	Interview took place in Mr. Chen's home, lasted for over 2 h
P46	Teacher Chen	M	70s	Retired teacher with good pension and insurance	Interview took place in a local community tea house, lasted for over 1 h, other people in the tea house joined occasionally
P47	Mrs. Tian Mrs. Feng	F F	72 78	Both interviewees moved to the city and lived with their adult children in the community. Mrs. Tian has coronary heart disease. Mrs. Feng has high blood pressure	Interview took place at the entrance of a local community, lasted for about 1 h
P48	Uncle Liu Auntie Xi	M F	67 60	Interview with two local residents. Both were peasants and recently moved to the city because	Interview took place in their local community, lasted for about 45 min

(continued)

(continued)

Number Px	Name	Gender: M = Male, F = Female	Age	Background information	Interview context and length
				their respective adult children live in the city	
P49	Mr. Chen	M	77	Retired worker from railway industry, later did small business in the town, have pension and insurance	Interview him on the street outside his home, where people gather to chat with each other. The interview lasted for about 1 h
P50	Mr. Liu	M	81	Retired expert from a geographical exportation team, graduated from university in 1960 (1956–1960)	Interview him at his home about his own health condition and health care experience, lasted for over 1 h and a half

Appendix D
Other Data Collected and Used

Types of materials collected	Information of these materials	Reasons of collecting the kinds of data
Ethnographic observation and field notes	The field notes are over 700 pages include observations, conversations, my personal experiences, and interviews that transcribed on the day, addressing topics • Different medical institution's surrounding, arrangement and daily works • Health professionals' daily work, income, and evaluation in different medical institutions • Health professional-patient encounter • Hospital emergency rescue • Patient's healthcare seeking and treatment process in different medical institutions • Discussion about health care costs, health care experience, health care responsibility and rights, and problems in China's health sector by patients, patients' families, and local residents • Patients' health insurance arrangement and reimbursement process • Comparison between health care in the past and that now made by patients, local residents and health professionals	The research was planned to centre on three themes: people's perception toward health care change and reform; health professional-patient relationships; health care responsibility, entitlement and rights. These ethnographic observation and field notes address topics related with the three themes, and provide essential background information for this research
Archives, published materials and local government reports	The county gazetteers used • *Riverside County Medical Gazetteer (Riverside Xian Yiyao Zhi)* (1988) • *Riverside County Gazetteer (Riverside Xianzhi)* (1990) • *Riverside County New Medical Gazetteer (Riverside Xian Xinban Yiyaozhi)* (forthcoming)	The county gazetteers record local history and the history of the local health sector, which provide important background information for this research, and enable me to outline the changes of local health sector overtime

(continued)

© Springer Nature Singapore Pte Ltd. 2019
J. Tu, *Health Care Transformation in Contemporary China*,
https://doi.org/10.1007/978-981-13-0788-1

(continued)

Types of materials collected	Information of these materials	Reasons of collecting the kinds of data
	Published local government reports used • Riverside County Health Department. 2007. 'Statistical Overview of Western and Traditional Health Professionals in the County' (quanxian zhongxiyi renyuan tonngji qingkuang) • Riverside County Health Department. 2008. 'The Work Summary of Building Advanced Traditional Chinese Medicine County in Rural Areas, Riverside, Sichuan' (Sichuan shen Riverside xian nongcun zhongyi gongzuo xianjin xian jianshe gongzuo zongjie) • Riverside County Health Department. 2008. 'The Arrangement Planning of Community Health Institution in the Riverside County' (Riverside xian shequ weisheng fuwu jigou shezhi guihua) • Municipal Health Department. 2013. 'Reform Plan for County-level Hospitals in the Next Five Years' (Xianji gongli yiyuan zonghe gaige shidian gongzuo shishi yijian)	These government reports supply important background information and useful data of local health sector, although their reliability may be questioned. Besides, they are useful to understand the government's rationales for particular health policies and reforms
	Other unpublished local documents I collected and used • Lists of patients who had received insurance reimbursements • Introductory materials about local hospitals and hospital regulations • Three autobiographies and two petition letters written by village doctors • Medical aid reports from the local Bureau of Civil Affair	These documents present original materials that not only serve as background information, but also provide useful cases and supporting data for this research
Media reports and on-line discussions	• Media reports about health reform and health care issues • Blogs and micro-blogs I followed including individual doctor's blog (e.g. 医哥子), several famous doctors' micro-blog, and some hospitals' blogs or micro-blogs • Health professionals' websites and medical forums I followed including Dingxiangyuan (丁香园), village doctors' forum and qq group (an on-line instant chatting group) • Three local forums where local residents discuss all kinds of issues on-line	Media reports provide compelling 'raw' accounts of traumas and tragedies of individuals, some of which may not be witnessed by researchers, such as the many cases I used to in this dissertation. The reason of choosing each individual media case is further explained in the middle of the dissertation The blogs and forums are filled with lively discussions about health care and reforms. Materials from internet and blogs are fragmented and personal; yet, they frequently express views that are different from the official ones, thus can supplement and contrast with the official discourses Besides, all these materials are used in relation to the local context and are carefully compared with the materials I collected in the local county